Health &
Social Care

Richard Smithson

Philip Allan Updates
Market Place
Deddington
Oxfordshire
OX15 0SE

tel: 01869 338652
fax: 01869 337590
e-mail: sales@philipallan.co.uk
www.philipallan.co.uk

ISBN-13: 978-1-84489-408-6
ISBN-10: 1-84489-408-8

Printed by Raithby, Lawrence & Co. Ltd, Leicester

Environmental information
The paper on which this title is printed is sourced from managed, sustainable
forests.

P00780

Contents

Contents

Chapter 9 Complementary therapies

Chapter 10 Psychological perspectives

Chapter 11 Study skills

Index

Introduction

This textbook is written specifically for students following the AQA AS specification in Health and Social Care.

How the book is organised

+ The chapter numbers correspond to the unit numbers — for example, Chapter 1 contains information relevant to Unit 1.
+ The first three chapters cover the three compulsory units; the following seven chapters cover the optional units.
+ In most of the chapters, the information is presented in the same order as it occurs in the AQA specification.
+ The final chapter gives guidance on study skills for examinations and for coursework.

How to use this book

Examined units

Chapters 1, 4, 5 and 6 cover the examined units. These chapters contain all the information expected to arise in questions in the unit tests. In some cases, additional detail is given. To prepare for a unit test, you should learn as much of the information as possible. There is no choice in the tests, so you should cover all the sections.

Each chapter includes some sections headed 'Try it out'. These comprise exercises and discussion points that should help increase understanding and facilitate learning. As many of the suggested activities as possible should be attempted.

Some chapters contain additional background information too. These sections are headed 'Did you know?' They contain material that might make the specification content a bit clearer. However, this background information does not have to be remembered.

Each chapter finishes with two specimen examination questions, followed by model answers.

Portfolio units

Chapters 2, 3, 7, 8, 9 and 10 cover the portfolio units, which are assessed by coursework. They include material to promote understanding of the basic ideas needed before tackling coursework. They also include practical guidance on planning, carrying out and reporting coursework tasks. You should read the relevant sections at each stage of your coursework.

These chapters also give guidance on how to score high marks in these units. However, they do not contain all the information you will need to complete portfolio reports. The main reason for this is that you will gain higher marks if you use a variety of sources (not just this textbook). Another reason is that some of the units contain so much choice that it would not be practical to include all the information you might want in this book. Suitable books and/or websites are suggested at the end of each chapter.

Chapter 2 is rather different from the others. It not only includes information and guidance relating to Unit 2, but also has a detailed section on designing and using questionnaires. This information will be needed when producing coursework for Units 2 and 3.

Additional exercises

Additional exercises for the compulsory units (1, 2 and 3) can be found in the workbook designed to accompany this text. This is available for purchase by teachers and includes a set of teacher notes with answers.

Effective caring

This chapter provides an introduction to health and social care services in the UK and contains the information you need to prepare for the examination of **Unit 1: Effective caring**. Key concepts and techniques, important to workers in those services and to informal carers, are explained. Examples from everyday care situations are also included, highlighted in green.

Life-quality factors

There are many factors that can affect quality of life. These are called **life-quality factors**.

Some of these factors, for example nutrition, are physical. This means that they affect the body directly. Other factors are more psychological — they affect beliefs, behaviour and emotions. An example of a psychological life-quality factor is the approval of other people.

If a life-quality factor is present in a person's everyday life, his or her quality of life is likely to be better than if that factor is absent. In reality, life-quality factors are usually present to some extent. In health and social care settings, care workers can help clients by increasing the extent to which various life-quality factors are present. However, these factors are important for everybody — not just for patients and clients in health and social care settings.

Psychological life-quality factors

There are many psychological factors that can affect the quality of a person's life. Some of these factors can be provided by care workers.

Psychological security

Psychological security means the absence of fear or distressing anxiety. Patients and clients might feel insecure if the people they meet are threatening or bullying. Insecurity can also result from having a serious disease, because a patient might worry about the treatment they will be given or the chances of dying soon.

Social contact

Social contact means having opportunities to be with other people. For many people, isolation from others reduces their quality of life. This is partly because social contact often provides other life-quality factors, such as stimulation and social support. In addition, a person's sense of self includes a feeling of belonging to a group.

For some elderly people, the husband, wife or partner is the major source of social contact. When the partner dies, the survivor might become socially isolated. Effective caring for elderly people can involve providing social contact, for example by arranging visits to a day centre.

Other people are much less dependent on social contact and are happy to be by themselves for long periods.

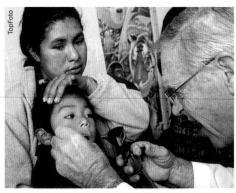
Family members provide social support

Social support

Social support means opportunities to be with familiar and trusted people who act in a person's own interest. Typically, family members and friends provide each other with social support but advocates, classroom assistants and other key workers allocated to individual clients might also provide this.

+ A daughter takes her mother for a hospital appointment and provides comfort and reassurance.
+ A parent takes a child to the dentist.

Approval

Approval means being shown positive regard, such as affection or praise. This can benefit a person by maintaining **self-esteem**. Most people like to be praised or complimented occasionally. The absence of this increases the risk that a person will develop negative feelings and **cognitions** about themselves (such as a feeling of not being liked). Clients in health and social care settings are particularly likely to have such negative feelings and cognitions. For example, if they are ill or disabled and unable to work or to care for themselves, then they might think of themselves as useless. Approval is particularly important in such cases.

In practice, positive regard is usually given conditionally. This means that it depends on what the person has done. For example, you might say, 'You're a clever lass' to a 4-year-old girl who has built a toy car out of plastic construction bricks, but you might avoid showing positive regard if she runs screaming through a supermarket.

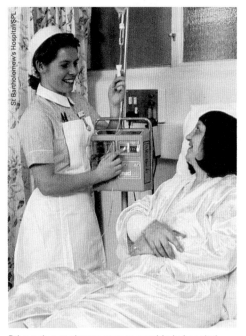
Privacy is not always easy to provide in hospital

Privacy

Privacy means opportunities to be undisturbed or unobserved by others in situations likely to cause embarrassment. Key situations where privacy is important include dressing and undressing, washing, bathing and going to the toilet. This privacy is not always easy to provide — for example, in the case of a person confined to bed in a hospital ward with other patients.

Privacy also refers to opportunities to spend time alone, perhaps to rest from the stimulation provided by contact with others. It also refers to having personal possessions that are not interfered with by other people.

Dignity

Dignity can be provided by showing a person respect and by the absence of demeaning treatment that could reduce a person's self-esteem. Examples of **demeaning treatment** include:

+ addressing people in overfamiliar ways (e.g. by using nicknames) rather than in the way they prefer
+ giving people orders instead of asking for their compliance

Confidentiality

Confidentiality means preventing sensitive information about a client from being made public unnecessarily. Confidentiality is maintained by staff not discussing clients or patients in public and by keeping information, such as medical records, filed in such a way that access is restricted to those who are authorised to see it. For example, a GP might refuse to give information about a patient's condition to a relative, unless it was clear that the patient wished the relative to have it.

Equitable treatment

To be treated equitably is to receive treatment that might not be the same as the treatment of others, but is seen as fair, appropriate and not significantly better or worse. **Equitable treatment** is fair if it takes account of the person's needs. Since people have varying needs, they could be treated differently without this being inequitable. Equitable treatment is the same as the absence of **unfair discrimination.**

People dislike inequitable treatment because it sends the message that they are less deserving, or less important, than others.

Some people think that treatment can be truly equitable only if everyone is treated the same. See what you think of the following examples.

Try it out

1 Kim is a patient in a hospital ward. At lunch time, she is offered the choice of three different main courses. She notices that the patient in the next bed has a different, special main course. This is because that patient is allergic to several types of food. Kim thinks that it is unfair that one patient should have a special meal, while others all have the same, limited choice.

2 Dave has had to wait 6 weeks for a knee operation with the NHS. He finds out that a private, fee-paying patient has had a similar operation, performed by the same surgeon after waiting only 1 week.

3 Johnny goes to the Accident and Emergency department of his local hospital to get a peanut removed from his ear. After waiting two hours for treatment, he sees another patient being brought in on a stretcher to be given treatment immediately. Johnny thinks the other patient has 'jumped the queue'.

In each case, is the difference in treatment inequitable?

Effective communication

Effective communication enables people to access information they need and to influence those around them. In care settings, this means:

+ enabling clients to find out, or be given information about, their treatment, future opportunities and prospects
+ giving clients coherent explanations of their condition and future treatment
+ enabling clients to ask questions and receive answers
+ listening to clients

During a consultation, a GP listens carefully to what a patient says about her symptoms, partly to help diagnose the disease, but also to find out how the patient feels about her condition.

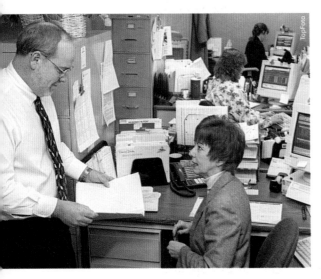

Having a job provides occupation; some jobs also provide social contact and stimulation

Occupation

Occupation means having something interesting or worthwhile to do, such as a job, hobby or sporting activity. It can give people the feeling that their lives are worthwhile. It can also motivate them to act in ways that are adaptive, i.e. that bring other benefits to them.

A client in a residential home takes part in an activities session involving making a greetings card. She later decides to start making some Christmas cards for all her friends and relatives. She paints each card and makes up a verse to write inside it. It takes her 3 months to make enough cards.

Stimulation

Stimulation means the presence of stimuli (events or activities) that increase a person's arousal to a comfortable level, making life interesting and challenging. Without stimulation, a person might feel bored. Most people actively seek stimulation, but there are situations in which a person is unable to do this, including some health and social care settings.

People with physical disabilities take part in an adventure sports holiday. They can choose activities such as sailing with an instructor in a specially adapted dinghy, and either abseiling or being lowered down a crag in a wheelchair. The people who take part can also benefit by becoming more independent and by making new friends.

It is easy to assume that occupation and stimulation are the same. However, an activity that provides stimulation does not always provide occupation (i.e. if it only takes up a small amount of time). An activity that provides occupation often also provides stimulation — but not always.

Try it out

1 Think of a situation in which you have been occupied — busy doing something — but not stimulated, because what you were doing was boring.

2 For 30 years, Viv worked at a machine, stamping out metal parts. During that time she often complained about how she hated work. Now she has retired, she is bored, and often talks about how much she used to enjoy working. Do you think Viv's work provided her with occupation, stimulation, or both?

3 A children's party should provide both occupation and stimulation. Think of one reason why children at a party should be provided with occupation.

Choice

Choice means having (or being given) the opportunity to make decisions about your situation. Choice gives people a sense of freedom. Examples of choice include:

+ deciding what to have to eat
+ deciding when to get up in the morning
+ making important decisions, such as what career to follow

Autonomy

Autonomy means having effective control over your actions and being free from coercion.

+ Klara decides not to start smoking, even though her friends try to persuade her. In this example, Klara has autonomy.
+ Mac would like to drink less alcohol, but is unable to cut down. In this example, Mac lacks autonomy.

Choice and autonomy are easily confused. One difference is that choice can often be about momentary events, such as where to sit when you enter a room. Autonomy is more about people's continuing or long-term ability to shape their lives. For example, a person who is confident and assertive often has more autonomy in life than a person who is easily persuaded or bullied into doing what other people want.

In care settings, a person can be given a choice, but cannot be given autonomy. People can only be encouraged to become more autonomous, perhaps by giving them opportunities to assert themselves and gain confidence.

People who have most choice and are most autonomous are usually powerful, wealthy adults. Most clients in care settings do not belong to this group. Effective caring requires careworkers to give choices to clients whenever possible.

Summary

Psychological life-quality factors are summarised in Table 1.1.

Table 1.1
Psychological life-quality factors

Factor	Simple definition
Psychological security	Feeling safe
Social contact	Being with other people
Social support	Having other people to share your problems
Approval	Being liked or praised
Privacy	Having your own space, or time alone
Dignity	Being treated with respect
Confidentiality	Personal information being kept secret
Equitable treatment	Being treated fairly
Effective communication	Being informed and listened to
Occupation	Having something to do
Stimulation	Having interests, fun, excitement
Choice	Having options
Autonomy	Having personal control and power

Physical life-quality factors

These include exercise, adequate nutrition, physical safety and hygiene, physical comfort and freedom from pain.

There are important long-term health benefits from exercise

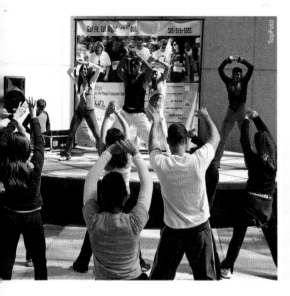

Exercise

Most people feel better after taking **exercise** and regular exercise has important long-term health benefits. Many clients or patients have only restricted opportunities for exercise, perhaps because of advanced age, disease or disability. In long-term situations, effective caring should involve opportunities for appropriate exercise.

A member of staff at a residential home encourages residents to take part in exercise sessions on two after-noons per week. All the exercises are done sitting down, so that residents who require wheelchairs can take part. Exercises include lifting the arms, waggling the feet and turning the head from side to side. Residents are also encouraged to do these exercises themselves every morning.

Nutrition

Nutrition contributes to the quality of life in a number of ways. People need a balanced diet in order to remain healthy, particularly if they have a condition such as pregnancy or diabetes, which might affect their health. Varied and appetising food can also contribute to a good quality of life. However, if energy intake exceeds energy use, this is harmful to the quality of life.

Physical safety and hygiene

+ Physical safety refers to the absence of serious risk of injury.
+ Hygiene means the absence of serious risk of infection.

Effective caring requires care staff to take precautions to reduce the risks of injury and infection to clients and patients.

+ Care homes are required to have covers on radiators to prevent residents accidentally burning themselves by contact with the hot metal.
+ Hospital staff are required to wash their hands when moving from patient to patient, to reduce the risk of spreading disease.

Physical comfort

Physical comfort means the absence of excessive cold, heat or unpleasant stimulation. Excessive stimulation might be a noisy environment or irritated skin. Physical comfort is particularly important in health and social care settings for clients who are unable to control their own environment.

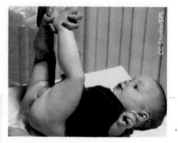

Infants depend on their carers for physical comfort

As a result of wearing a wet and dirty nappy for several hours, a young infant will experience discomfort. There is nothing the infant can do directly to reduce this — a carer (usually a parent) will have to change the nappy.

Freedom from pain

Clients and patients sometimes experience pain, usually as a result of their health condition. This could include people with heart disease, cancer or arthritis. Frequent or continuous pain can severely reduce the quality of a person's life. Effective care in these cases requires techniques of pain relief or pain management.

Look through the five physical life-quality factors and the 13 psychological life-quality factors described above. For each, decide whether or not it is present in your life. For those factors that are absent, think about the effect this absence has on your quality of life.

You might also try to think of occasions in the past when one or more of these factors has been absent from your life.

Try it out

Conflicting life-quality factors

Sometimes, a situation that provides one life-quality factor will tend to reduce another. For example, if clients have plenty of *choice* about what they eat, this might conflict with the quality of their *nutrition* – they might always choose to eat a lot of sugary foods. These conflicting factors might have to be balanced. In this example, choice could be restricted to those foods that are the best for health.

Another example is a possible conflict between privacy, social contact and stimulation. In a hospital ward, maximum *privacy* is available in a single room. However, a patient confined to bed in a single room has fewer opportunities for *social contact* than a patient in a room with several others. There is less activity to observe, so the situation is less stimulating.

Sometimes the balance between conflicting life-quality factors is a matter of comparing the benefits of an activity with the risks. For example, a young, disabled person might benefit from the stimulation provided by going on an adventure trip to Brazil, but might be exposed to increased risk of psychological insecurity and discomfort.

Individual differences in the impact of life-quality factors

People differ in the extent to which they value different life-quality factors. For example:

+ some people are quite happy when they lack occupation; others are never happy unless they are busy
+ some people are quite happy to spend most of their time alone; others are only happy when with other people
+ some people remain fairly content in conditions where some life-quality factors are minimal or absent; others soon suffer in such conditions

In the example of the hospital ward given above, some people would prefer privacy above social contact.

Try it out

1 Look at the list of 13 psychological life-quality factors in Table 1.1 and rank their importance to you. For example, if you think psychological security is the most important factor, give it a ranking of 1. Do not rank two or more factors equally. The factor you feel is least important should have a ranking of 13. The factors with the highest rankings (say, the top five) will be those which, if absent, would reduce the quality of your life most severely. Compare your rank order with those of other students.

2 You might have noticed that some factors that are important in your life are not included in the list of 13 factors. Try to think of at least one of these.

3 The following scenario illustrates several life-quality factors that are present, and some that are lacking:

Peter is in a hospital ward, waiting for a heart operation. He is woken at 7 a.m., which is earlier than he prefers. After lunch, a specialist surgical registrar visits him to explain about the operation and to answer any questions. Later, Peter's wife visits to cheer him up and pass on messages from friends. She has brought a book for Peter to read.

Peter finds it difficult to sleep that night, partly because he is anxious about the operation and also because the person in the next bed keeps talking to himself. However, there is nothing he can do about this. Next day, he is dressed in a surgical gown and put on a stretcher. He feels half-naked as he is wheeled along the corridors to the theatre.

Identify as many life-quality factors as you can, and link them with statements in the scenario. You might be asked to do this in an examination question.

Try it out

Treating people well

It is a belief of the health and care services that clients and patients should be treated well. There are ethical and practical reasons for this:
+ An ethical reason for treating people well is that being a care worker implies having a duty of care for clients.
+ A practical reason for treating people well is that clients who are well treated tend to behave agreeably and cooperatively. They also tend to recover more quickly and have fewer problems.

A simple way of thinking about how to treat clients well is to relate this to life-quality factors. To some extent, treating people well involves trying to provide such factors. For example, people can be treated well by ensuring that they have occupation, privacy, choice and so on.

In practice, treating people well is not always as easy as it sounds. This is because the most appropriate treatments are sometimes unpleasant. For example, to treat a client with dental caries well, it might be necessary to drill out the decayed tissue of a tooth. This is likely to be uncomfortable. Appropriate treatment for a client who is recovering from a stroke might be to get them to practise walking with support, which could be difficult and frustrating.

A more sophisticated view suggests that treating clients well involves taking actions that eventually — though not always immediately — help to provide life-quality factors. For example, drilling a person's tooth might cause immediate pain and psychological insecurity. However, it will help reduce or avoid more pain and insecurity in the future.

In any caring situation, the best way to treat a client might not be obvious. This is partly because it is not always possible to predict accurately how a client will respond to any particular treatment. The best a care worker can do is to think carefully about the client and his or her situation and to take whatever action seems to give the best prospect of improving the client's situation and well-being.

How clients are sometimes treated badly

In practice, there are a number of ways in which clients are sometimes treated badly.

Neglect

Neglect means ignoring or otherwise failing to attend to a person's needs. In other words, this means not considering, or not attempting to supply, important life-quality factors for the person. In terms of physical life-quality factors, neglect might involve not feeding clients or not washing them properly. In terms of psychological life-quality factors, clients can be neglected by, for example, not speaking or listening to them or by not providing social support.

Rejection

Rejection means showing the client in some way that the care worker does not accept the responsibility of caring for them.

Hostility

Hostility means expressing dislike or aggression towards a client, by verbal or non-verbal communication or by unsympathetic treatment.

Punishment

Punishment means responding to a client's unwanted actions with unpleasant consequences – for example, making residents go to their own rooms if they have disturbed or upset other residents. Punishment is intended to be unpleasant treatment, though it is rarely effective or appropriate in care situations.

Bullying

Bullying can take various forms, including physically abusing or intimidating a person, using demeaning language towards them or teasing them in a way designed to be unpleasant.

Violence

Violence means physically hurting a client, with or without producing detectable injury. An example is a parent smacking a child.

Unfair discrimination

Discrimination means acting differently towards certain people or groups of people. Discrimination is not necessarily a bad thing. For example, we expect a GP to discriminate between two people with different illnesses. People should be treated differently, according to their medical condition. Most care workers are able to discriminate between clients in terms of their personalities. They might speak in a light-hearted way to one client, who enjoys this, and in a more formal way to another client, who prefers this.

Unfair discrimination involves treating people differently not because of their different needs, but because of their membership of certain groups. There are several bases for this type of discrimination, including sex, sexuality, ethnicity, religion, social class, age and impairment:

+ **Sex discrimination** means treating people less well than others because of their sex. For example, a woman who is not offered a job purely because she is a woman — even though she is well qualified for the job concerned — has been discriminated against on the basis of her sex. Note that people of either sex can be discriminated against and that it is possible for people to discriminate against others of their own sex.
+ Discrimination on the basis of **sexuality** means treating people less well because they are gay, straight, bisexual or asexual.
+ **Ethnicity** is a difficult concept. It refers to the cultural origins of a person. Ethnicity can be defined by the nation (or region of a nation) that people feel they belong to — for example, being Australian. Alternatively, it can refer to race. The term 'Caucasian', for example, refers to white Europeans. Ethnicity may also be defined in terms of religion, when this is a major component of a particular culture. An example would be a person who thinks of himself or herself as a Muslim. For many people, ethnicity is a mixture of nationality, race and religion.

> **Did you know** ?
>
> Some white Anglo-Saxon people assume that ethnicity is something other people have, i.e. they think it refers to non-whites. However, everyone has ethnicity.
>
> As more people migrate from one country to make a life in another, ethnicity becomes complicated. This is especially true of Britain. People have emigrated from Britain in large numbers over the past 300 years. Their descendants live in North and South America, Africa, Australasia and, to a lesser extent, Asia. People from other countries have migrated to Britain for well over 2000 years.

Barriers to treating people well

Care workers sometimes fail to treat people well, even when they intend to do so. Barriers to treating people well can be internal to the carers, i.e. aspects of the care workers themselves. There are also client barriers that make poor treatment more likely.

Barriers internal to carers

Barriers internal to carers include attitudes and prejudices, stereotyping, lack of motivation, conformity with inappropriate workplace norms, preoccupation with their own needs and lack of skill.

Attitudes and prejudices

An **attitude** is a long-lasting set of beliefs, feelings and behaviour tendencies towards an individual, group or object. The attitudes held by people tend to shape the way they think about their world, including other people.

An attitude can act as a barrier to treating people well, for example by shaping the way a care worker thinks about clients. This can prevent the care worker from thinking about a client as an individual. One difficulty is that people are often unaware of being influenced by their attitudes. Instead, they tend to assume that the way they feel, think and act is somehow natural, reasonable and justifiable.

Dev works with adults who have physical disabilities. His attitude to disabled people includes strong feelings of pity, a belief that they are less fortunate than he is, and a tendency to try to compensate them for their disabilities.

As a result of this attitude, Dev tends to be overhelpful and overprotective of his clients. The clients do not like this, partly because Dev does not let them do things for themselves, which reduces their autonomy. They also dislike Dev's attitude, because it emphasises the difference between them and able-bodied people.

Dev's clients would prefer it if he treated them as equals who sometimes need his assistance, rather than as objects of pity. Dev has no idea that his attitude is a barrier preventing him from treating his clients well.

Prejudices are attitudes that are usually negative. Attitudes are called prejudices when they are generally disapproved of or seen to be socially unacceptable. For example, a negative attitude towards gay people is called a prejudice. Illogically, a similar negative attitude to politicians is not usually called a prejudice.

Behaviour tendencies that go together with negative attitudes include:

+ speaking critically about the object of the attitude – for example, saying 'I don't like French people'
+ showing hostility
+ unfairly discriminating

The definition of an attitude listed three features: beliefs, feelings and behaviour tendencies. Pick out the belief, feeling and behaviour tendency described in Dev's attitude to disabled people in the example above.

Try it out

Stereotyping

Stereotyping is an oversimplified belief that all members of a particular social group share some particular characteristic. For example, a person might believe that all women are interested in fashion – this is an example of a gender stereotype. Another example of a stereotype is the belief that elderly people are not interested in sex.

Stereotypes are culturally transmitted. This means that they are beliefs learned from other people, often parents or peers, but also from the mass media.

Stereotyping means noticing or assuming that a person belongs to a particular social group and applying a stereotype to them, i.e. assuming that the person has a characteristic believed to be shared by members of that group. It acts as a barrier because it leads care workers to make assumptions about clients, instead of really getting to know them.

A female nurse enters a four-bedded unit on a hospital ward, which is occupied by two men. The television is showing a documentary about the history of art. Without asking the men, the nurse changes to a television channel that shows football, on the assumption that they will prefer this.

In this example, the nurse has the stereotype that all men like to watch football. She first categorised the patients as men and then assumed that they would prefer to watch football.

You might think that the nurse was probably right. However, what is important is not whether a stereotype happens to be accurate in a particular case. The point is that stereotypes lead us to make assumptions, which will sometimes be right and sometimes wrong. The nurse could have avoided making the assumption that men prefer football by asking them whether or not they would like to watch it.

Think of four different groups in society to which you have either a strong positive or negative attitude. These groups might be based on occupation (e.g. police officers, teachers, sports players), ethnicity (e.g. white people, Scottish people), age (e.g. children, middle-aged people) or on another of the bases of discrimination listed above. For each of the four groups you choose, try to decide on:
+ a feeling you have about the group
+ a cognition (something you think you know, or believe about them)
+ the way you tend to act towards that group
Try to think of a stereotype for each of the four groups.

Lack of motivation

A person who lacks motivation might have few reasons for trying to treat clients well. **Lack of motivation** can occur when a person has a job that they do not enjoy or for which they have little aptitude. It can also occur when people perceive that they are not valued or well treated at work — for example, if they are low paid, frequently criticised and never praised.

Conformity with inappropriate workplace norms

A **norm** is a behaviour or belief shared by most members of a group. People who work together develop norms in the way they treat each other and do their jobs. For example, it might be the norm among a group of workers to 'cover up' for each other if something goes wrong — for example, by not saying anything that could get a fellow worker into trouble.

When a new member of staff starts work in an organisation, a process of socialisation begins by which that member of staff learns (usually by observation) what the workplace norms are.

In some cases, workplace norms might be inappropriate. For example, they could have potentially dangerous consequences. In care settings, norms such as these might lead to poor treatment of clients.

In a residential home, the residents are given a cup of tea just before one shift of staff goes off duty. Often there is not much time to do this and the staff members do not want to stay late. On some occasions, there is not enough time to wash the cups properly, so they are just rinsed under the hot water tap. A new member of staff points out that this is unhygienic. Staff tell him that he 'mustn't go shouting his mouth off about it'. He soon adopts the practice himself — in other words, he conforms to this norm.

Preoccupation with own needs and lack of skills

This is a barrier that mainly affects inexperienced care workers. If care workers find themselves in a new situation (e.g. treating a type of client they have not previously encountered), there is a tendency for them to focus on their own feelings rather than on the needs of the client.

> A newly qualified nursery-school teacher is told that one boy in her class is autistic. The teacher has not come across children with autism before and does not know how best to respond. As a result, the teacher tends to avoid contact with the autistic child. This means that the educational needs of the child are less likely to be met.

Client barriers

Client barriers include:

+ lack of status and power
+ a tendency to conceal real needs and concerns
+ a tendency to exaggerate needs and concerns
+ hostile or obstructive behaviour

Lack of status and power

In Britain, a person's **status** is influenced by occupation, abilities and wealth.

Many clients and patients have low status because of their age and condition. For example, young children and elderly people tend to have low status. People who are ill or have certain disabilities are less likely to be employed. Lack of status acts as a barrier to people being treated well because it commands less respect and gives these individuals less influence.

The **power** that people have is influenced partly by wealth, but also by their skill in asserting their wants. One reason why people with low status or little power are treated badly is because they cannot exert influence over others.

> A care worker who neglects a young child might escape criticism or punishment, because the child is unable to complain or even to recognise that neglect is occurring.
>
> Contrast this with an adult who receives poor service in a hotel. The adult is much more willing and able to make a complaint.

The fact that a client has low status or power does not result directly in poor treatment, but it makes it more likely.

Tendency to conceal real needs and concerns

Clients seeking treatment sometimes approach practitioners with a '**presenting problem**'. This is usually a minor condition that the client feels comfortable to speak about. Clients might conceal their real concerns until the practitioner has gained their confidence or invites more information.

There are several reasons why clients may conceal their real concerns. One is that they are embarrassed by a medical condition. Another is that they are afraid of appearing silly or irrational. Typically, a patient will visit a doctor complaining of an actual illness, such as a cold or a painful knee, when they really want help with a condition such as incontinence, impotence or the feeling that they are becoming mentally ill.

This could lead to poor treatment if the practitioner simply treats the presenting problem and fails to realise the existence of another ailment.

Tendency to exaggerate needs and concerns

The situation in which clients and patients seek attention and treatment is complicated. Clients sometimes feel that practitioners have to be manipulated in order to make them provide the treatment required. A common way to do this is to exaggerate or overstate symptoms.

A client in a residential home is worried about her health and believes that care workers should check her condition frequently. She often pulls the alarm cord during the night, complaining that her heart has stopped.

Exaggerating needs and concerns can lead to poor treatment because care workers may perceive this behaviour as time wasting and begin to expect that future complaints will be equally exaggerated.

Hostile or obstructive behaviour

Clients and patients sometimes behave in ways that make it more difficult for care-workers to treat them well. To be **hostile** means to show resentment and dislike in an over-assertive way. To be **obstructive** means to fail to cooperate or to deliberately make it difficult for care workers to do their jobs. For example, clients might be rude to, or harshly critical of, care workers or they might not cooperate during treatment procedures.

There are several possible reasons for this. Clients sometimes feel anxious or guilty, but misinterpret their own negative feelings and focus them on the care worker. Clients who have negative attitudes towards people in authority might mistrust, or show dislike to, NHS staff or social workers. In addition, drunkenness and some medical conditions can produce aggressive behaviour.

A patient with schizophrenia might react angrily to a psychiatrist for 'stealing his thoughts'. This is the result of disturbed and inaccurate cognitions that commonly occur as symptoms of this condition.

Caring skills and techniques

Practitioners and informal carers use a wide range of caring skills and techniques, often without being aware that they are doing so. For some care workers, these skills just seem to come naturally. For others, they are learned with practice.

This section introduces you to 15 such skills or techniques. Each is described separately, but in practice they overlap to varying degrees and are often used together.

Observation

Observation involves collecting information about clients by taking measurements such as temperature and blood pressure, or by weighing them. It also refers to noticing how a person is behaving — for example, whether they are eating or sleeping as usual or whether something has changed.

In everyday life, observation tends to be selective. We focus on the people we are most interested in and we notice aspects that interest us. For example, someone interested in hairdressing will notice other people's hair.

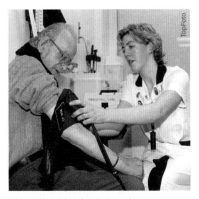

Measuring blood pressure is an important method of observation of clients with medical problems

Social perception

Social perception means being aware of a person's likely feelings, needs and intentions. These factors can be shown by facial expression, posture and tone of voice, as well as by what is said.

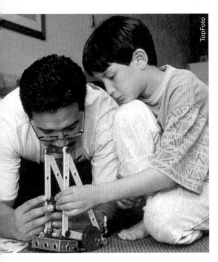

Working alongside clients is a good way of making contact with, and being accepted by, them

Working alongside

This means working in contact with a client either by doing what they are doing or by working on an activity in order to encourage them to join in. This is useful in situations in which clients might not like to be approached directly, and also when carers need to be seen more as equals and as less of a threat.

Imagine you are working in a special parent-and-toddler group that some of the parents are attending because they had previously neglected or ill-treated their children. These parents might be feeling guilty, defensive or resentful at having to be there. They might not like it if you start giving them advice. However, if you sit alongside them and play with the children who come and show an interest, the parents might begin to relax. By modelling their behaviour on yours, they might also learn effective ways of playing with their children.

Modelling

Modelling means observing and imitating the behaviour of another person. Practitioners can help clients to learn new, more effective ways of behaving by acting as models. Rather than telling someone how to behave, the practitioner demonstrates appropriate behaviour and encourages the client to copy this.

Unskilled parents, whose young children are believed to be at risk, can be invited to bring their children to play sessions. Expert play workers play with the children, and the parents can watch and join in. Observing and imitating the play workers is probably more effective for the parents than being told what they are doing wrong.

Setting challenges

This means suggesting tasks or activities to clients that will stimulate them, and perhaps help them to improve their abilities, skills or confidence. Some people lead lives that are restricted by their beliefs about what they can and cannot do. For example, a person might feel too afraid to go out of doors. Practitioners can help such people by suggesting challenges, such as walking a few metres to post a letter. People recovering from disabling illnesses and injuries can progress if they are set a sequence of achievable physical challenges that gradually become more demanding – for example, to walk across the room, to walk half a mile and then to walk 3 miles.

   Children can also benefit from challenges. For example, a child who can easily complete a familiar jigsaw could be asked to complete it with the pieces picture-side down, so that there is no colour to provide clues.

Communication

Communication does not just mean talking to someone. It also means listening, allowing people to ask questions and giving answers, using writing and reading, and non-verbal communication. As a skill used by a care worker, this is different from typical, everyday communication. You might chat to friends and ask them questions, but this is often for your own amusement. Communication in a care setting might often seem quite similar to this kind of chat, but the care worker will be communicating with the purpose of providing life-quality factors to the client.

An informal carer is chatting with her elderly husband who is beginning to develop dementia. She shows him an album of holiday photographs, so that he can try to recall some of the events that happened. The conversation helps to remind the man of who he is and to help him retain some of his more enjoyable memories.

Encouraging adaptive behaviours

Encouragement includes rewarding **adaptive behaviour**. Adaptive behaviour is behaviour that tends to increase the well-being of a client. In contrast, **maladaptive behaviour** tends to harm a client, either directly or by making other people become hostile to the client. Examples of maladaptive behaviour include aggression, dishonesty, self-harm and excessive use of drugs. People sometimes develop maladaptive behaviours because these bring short-term rewards. For example, a child who bullies other children has the reward of being obeyed by others and enjoying their fear. Care workers usually try to avoid rewarding or encouraging maladaptive behaviours; rather, they try to encourage more adaptive ones.

Showing approval

Showing approval means giving positive responses to the behaviour of a client – such as smiling and praise, or, if appropriate, a cuddle.

Physical contact

Physical contact can be used to comfort a client who is anxious or upset, as well as to show approval. Usually it takes the form of touching a person on the hand or arm, or a cuddle. However, physical contact can be misunderstood, for example, if it is seen as a threatening or sexual approach. It is most appropriate between carers and clients who know each other well, particularly between parents and their children.

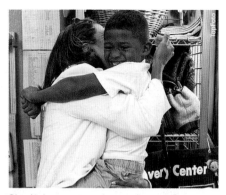

Physical contact can be used to comfort and to show approval

Creating trust

Creating trust means acting in such a way that a client is likely to judge the carer to be reliable, for example by behaving consistently — similarly in similar situations — and by following correct procedures and fulfilling promises.

A health visitor is due to pay a second visit to the parents of a young child. The health visitor reads her notes from the last visit carefully before arriving. When she arrives, it is clear to the parents that she remembers all the important details about their child. This helps to create trust. If the health visitor started by asking questions she had already asked on her previous visit or — worse still — confused the child with a child from another family, this would make the parents feel less confident in following the health visitor's advice.

Gaining compliance

Gaining compliance means getting the client to do what is required. The skill of gaining compliance is important in many caring situations. Examples include a GP trying to get a patient to stop smoking, a day-nursery worker trying to get children to wash their hands, and a radiographer trying to get an injured person to stay still for an X-ray.

Notice that a practitioner does not have the authority to order a client to do (or not do) anything. Nor should a practitioner coerce or threaten a client. The client has the choice of whether or not to comply. In most situations, clients do comply, partly because they trust practitioners but also because they perceive that what the practitioner wants them to do is in their own interests — that is, it will benefit them.

One effective way of gaining compliance is for practitioners to explain the reason for their request, for example by saying: 'Could you roll up your sleeve, please. I want to take a small drop of blood to have it tested for any sign of diabetes.'

Another way is to offer a limited range of choices, so that the client can comply, but still feel empowered. For example, a physiotherapist wants to provide passive exercise to the legs of a client. The client is unwilling to cooperate at first, so the physiotherapist asks: 'Shall we do the left leg first or the right leg first?'

Distraction

This technique is most often applied to help the management of temporary pain and anxiety. Normally, if people feel pain or anxiety, they tend to concentrate on it – in other words, they give it a lot of attention. However, the pain a person experiences is *greater* if they focus attention on it. Distraction is a way of making people focus their attention on something other than their pain. This can lessen the pain and reduce the distress felt. An example is waving a cuddly toy at an infant just as they are receiving an injection. This distracts the infant from feeling anxious about the strange situation.

Women who attend antenatal classes are sometimes taught a self-distraction technique to help them cope with the pain they will experience before giving birth, when the uterus is contracting. Some women are told to say a nursery rhyme to themselves when the pains begin. Having to concentrate on the words means that their attention is divided between the pain and the nursery rhyme, thus lessening the pain.

Try this exercise. Prepare a list that you can memorise, such as an A–Z list of singers or bands. Next time you stub your toe, or have a tooth cavity drilled, repeat the list to yourself.

Try it out

Reducing negative feelings and behaviours

Clients often experience **negative feelings**, such as anxiety, sadness or anger. Sometimes, they behave in **negative ways**, such as being apathetic, self-harming, destructive or hostile.

These feelings and behaviours might result from ill health, difficult circumstances or the personality of the client. Care workers can sometimes help to reduce negative feelings and behaviours by the way they respond to the client. One way to do this is to try to avoid responding negatively. For example, if a client has become hostile, responding aggressively by shouting back is unlikely to defuse the situation. In conflict situations, it is sometimes best to disengage from the client temporarily (see below).

If a care worker remains calm, a panicking client is more likely to calm down. A care worker who shows positive feelings, such as approval and respect for a client, can help the client to feel better about himself or herself.

One useful way to think about this technique is that the aim is to reduce the 'emotional temperature' of the situation – to cool the client down emotionally.

Disengagement

Disengagement means temporarily withdrawing from contact with a client. This can be useful when the client has become hostile. To be effective, this disengagement should not itself be a hostile act. It would not be a good idea to storm out of the room and slam the door. Rather, it is much better to behave neutrally, perhaps giving a reason for withdrawing.

Using eye contact and facial expression

Eye contact is important in effective communication with clients. Making occasional eye contact during conversation can help to signal to clients that they are being listened to and taken seriously. Eye contact is also useful to support speech. People with partial hearing might need to see facial (especially lip) movements if they are to understand what the care workers are saying. By making eye contact, care workers can see whether clients are looking at them, and if not, can attract their attention before speaking.

Eye contact can also help to establish trust between care workers and clients. If practitioners do not establish eye contact with clients, the clients might assume the practitioners are concealing something from them.

Facial expressions are important as well in communicating intentions. In particular, smiling tends to produce a positive response from clients.

However, frequent eye contact is not always helpful in encounters with clients. The effect that eye contact has on a client depends partly on the client's interpretation of the situation. A client who feels neglected is likely to respond positively to eye contact, whereas a client who is angry and feeling guilty is more likely to interpret eye contact as being accusatory and hostile.

Summary

Caring skills and techniques are summarised in Table 1.2.

Table 1.2
Caring skills and techniques

Skill or technique	Example
Observation	Measuring blood pressure
Social perception	Noticing that a client is annoyed, but is trying to hide it
Working alongside	Going on a joint shopping trip with a client
Modelling	Putting a hearing aid in one's own ear to show how it is done
Setting challenges	'Now see if you can send an e-mail all by yourself'
Communication	Asking if the client has any questions
Encouraging adaptive behaviours	Rewarding a child for apologising
Showing approval	Looking pleased with a client's response
Physical contact	Shaking a client by the hand
Creating trust	Keeping a promise to a client
Gaining compliance	Explaining to a patient why an enema is necessary
Distraction	Reading a story to a child who is in pain
Reducing negative feelings and behaviours	Using a calm voice with an angry client
Disengagement	Switching attention to another task or client
Using eye contact and facial expression	Smiling at a child who is anxious

Services and how they are accessed

NHS services

The **National Health Service** (NHS) is a public-sector organisation directly funded by central government and paid for largely by taxation. It is one of the largest employers in the world, with nearly 1 million employees.

The NHS provides many services including general practitioners (GPs), hospital services, community nursing, health visitors and advice from NHS Direct.

GP services

General practitioners work in local GP practices and health centres. Local people usually have to book an appointment before they visit the GP, although in an emergency the GP will visit a patient at home.

The local GP practice usually keeps the medical records of its patients and each patient is allocated a named GP. Patients can change their GP if they wish. GP services are for dealing with illnesses that do not require emergency treatment — for example, where patients notice symptoms, but can wait perhaps a few days to see a doctor.

A visit to the GP is called a **consultation**. During a consultation, the GP will try to diagnose any illness the patient is suffering from. Sometimes, the GP will delay diagnosis until a blood test has been carried out. Following the diagnosis, the GP might prescribe treatment, most commonly by issuing a written prescription for the patient to take to a pharmacist, who provides the medication.

However, the GP does not always provide treatment. He or she might decide that no treatment is needed or might recommend that the patient self-treats, for example with painkillers.

If the GP diagnoses a serious illness, or is uncertain of the diagnosis, the patient might be referred to a medical specialist, such as a hospital consultant. Access to a hospital consultant is through the GP. If the GP believes that the patient does not need to see a consultant and can be treated better by the GP, referral to a consultant will not be made. GPs therefore act as gatekeepers, controlling access to hospital consultants.

+ Access to GP services can be obtained by people who have registered with a GP.
+ Access is most commonly by self-referral. This means that the patient makes the decision to visit the GP.

Hospital services

Most general hospitals provide a range of services.

Accident and Emergency department

An **Accident and Emergency department** is staffed day and night to provide emergency medical care for people who have been involved in accidents or who have been taken ill suddenly.

Access to this service is gained by:

+ being taken by an ambulance crew, following a 999 call. This is usually for people with life-threatening conditions or severe injuries.
+ self-referral. This is for people who can travel independently and who need medical attention for a non-life threatening injury such as a broken limb.

Soon after arrival at Accident and Emergency, patients are assessed briefly to decide on the seriousness of their condition. Assessment is carried out by a triage nurse or a senior house officer. Those patients with the most serious conditions get priority treatment. People with less serious conditions might wait for a long time, and find that people who came in after them receive treatment before them.

As a result, patients can wait up to four hours to receive treatment. The waiting time depends on how busy the department is — Friday and Saturday nights are usually the busiest times.

The services provided in the department include diagnosis (often with the use of, for example, X-rays and blood tests) and treatment (such as stitching and dressing wounds, and setting broken bones).

Patients are then either discharged if they are well enough, or admitted to a hospital ward for further treatment.

Day surgery

During the last 20 years, surgical techniques have been developed that enable some operations to be performed in a way that does not require a stay in hospital. This is called **day surgery**. Day surgery leads to a much faster recovery and reduces the risk to patients of contracting infections in hospital. It is also much less expensive to perform.

One technique that has made this possible is called **endoscopy**. An endoscope is a tube carrying a tiny camera and light that can be inserted into the patient's body to examine tissues, without the need for surgically opening the abdomen or thorax. Some operations can be performed using tiny instruments attached to the endoscope. This is sometimes called '**keyhole surgery**', because only a small incision (a cut in the skin) is needed. An example of an operation that can be carried out using this technique is the removal of a diseased gall bladder.

Cataract operations can be performed using local anaesthetics. This enables the patient to be treated and discharged within two hours of arriving at hospital.

+ Access to day surgery is through the hospital consultant, who is usually the surgeon who will perform the operation.

Community nursing

Community nursing is nursing care provided by qualified nurses who are typically based in local health centres or GP practices. In some areas, community nurses are called district nurses.

Community nurses visit patients in their own homes and provide services such as changing wound dressings, giving injections and monitoring health.

This service is provided for people who are ill or disabled (especially elderly people) but who do not require hospital treatment. The clients are often people who have recently been discharged from hospital following treatment.

+ Access to community nursing is by professional referral — for example, by a GP or a social worker who has assessed the needs of the client.

Health visitor developmental assessment

A health visitor is a trained nurse whose main role is health education.

The health visitor visits people in their own homes and specialises in the prevention of illness rather than in treatment. An important part of the job of a health visitor is to visit families with very young children and perform screening tests to check that the child is developing normally. These tests include checking hearing, vision, gross and fine motor skills and general health. Health visitors also provide parents with information about the development of their child and give guidance on how they can help with this.

+ Access to health visitors is by professional referral, usually following the birth of a child.

Advice from NHS Direct and NHS Direct Online

People sometimes experience fairly minor symptoms. As a result, they might be unsure whether or not to visit their GP. It is possible that if they decide to visit the GP, the visit might turn out to be unnecessary. However, if they decide not to visit, it is possible that early symptoms of a serious disorder might not be picked up. NHS Direct was set up to help people in this situation — and also to reduce the number of unnecessary demands on GPs' time.

NHS Direct is a low-cost telephone helpline that people can call to obtain information or advice on health matters. The calls are answered by nurses, who try to find out what is wrong and then give advice for people to treat themselves, to seek a GP appointment or to make an emergency 999 call. The service is available 24 hours a day in most areas of the UK.

+ Access to NHS Direct is by self-referral, i.e. by calling the number.

NHS Direct Online is a website that provides information and advice on health matters. It also provides access to information on a wide range of diseases.

+ Access to NHS Direct Online is by self-referral.

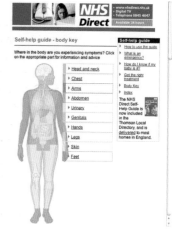

NHS Direct Online gives advice and information on a wide range of diseases

Informal care

Informal care is provided by people who are unpaid. Informal carers are not usually trained practitioners. They are often family members; occasionally they might be friends or neighbours.

Informal care can range from simply providing social contact and stimulation (e.g. by visiting an elderly neighbour who is unable to go out), to feeding, bathing and toileting.

The most common type of informal care is that provided by parents for their children, especially when young. Informal care is also provided for some elderly relatives who might have become disabled and for disabled people of any age.

Informal care is work, but it is unpaid and largely unrewarded. People provide informal care partly because they want to maintain the well-being of family members, partly because of a feeling that they ought to do this and partly because this is encouraged by the culture in which they grew up.

✦ Access to informal care depends on the availability and willingness of family members or friends.

Early-years care

Apart from the informal care provided in the home, **early-years care** is usually provided by day nurseries, crèches, playgroups and nursery schools. It is provided for infants and children up to the age of 5 years.

A **day nursery** is usually equipped to cope with children aged from a few months to 5 years. Children attend during the hours in which their parents are at work. Some day nurseries are provided by local authorities; others are run by private providers. Play activities, sleeping areas and meals are provided.

A **crèche** is a day nursery supplied by a workplace and is usually at or near that workplace. It enables employees with pre-school children to continue working, yet be in easy reach of their children should it be necessary.

Playgroups provide activity sessions for children aged 3 and 4 years. Children can attend one or more times a week, typically for around two hours at a time. Playgroups provide social contact and stimulation for children and can help to prepare children for school.

A **nursery school** provides more structured activities than a playgroup and is staffed by qualified nursery teachers and nurses. Children aged 3 and 4 years usually attend part time (for example, on weekday mornings). This provides a preparation for school. Nursery schools are provided free of charge by local education authorities.

✦ Access to nursery schools is restricted to children living within the local area.

Care of elderly people

As people get older, some begin to develop ailments that affect their ability to look after themselves. They might become unable to provide themselves with nourishing meals, keep themselves and their homes clean or keep in contact with other people. This can lead to illness and to a reduced quality of life.

Needs assessment

Elderly people at risk have a right to an assessment of their needs. This is likely to be carried out by social workers, during a home visit. Social workers assess both the living conditions and independent-living skills, such as the ability of the clients to cook and to wash themselves.

As a result of a needs assessment, a social worker can recommend a range of services that might help the elderly person, including those described below.

+ Access to a needs assessment is by:
    + self-referral — although usually a relative or informal carer will contact the social services department
    + professional referral — for example, by a social worker based in hospital when a patient is about to be discharged

Home (or domiciliary) care

Home care means care provided for clients in their own homes. The aim of providing **domiciliary care** is to enable people to be independent for as long as possible.

Home care usually involves home-care workers visiting their clients at home to perform services such as helping them get up and dressed in the morning, cleaning their homes and cooking meals. Home-care workers also provide a useful opportunity for social contact and stimulation.

Day centres

A **day centre** is a place that people can visit once or twice a week to spend the day. Sometimes, transport is provided to and from the centre, usually by a community transport organisation. At the centre, activities such as crafts, singing and reminiscence sessions are provided, as well as a meal. At least one member of staff is likely to be nurse-trained and is therefore able to monitor informally the health of the clients. The social contact and stimulation provided are important aspects of this service.

Day centres are provided by local authorities and voluntary organisations such as Age Concern. They are sometimes sited on the premises of residential homes.

+ Access to a day centre is by:
    + a request from the clients or their relatives
    + a recommendation from a practitioner, such as a social worker

Nursing and residential home care

A **residential home** provides long-term accommodation and social care for elderly people who are unable to live in their own homes, even with support. Usually, residents have their own bedrooms, which often have a small bathroom and toilet attached. Residents are provided with meals, a laundry service and day rooms in which they can be with other residents, watch television or take part in activities. Help is given as required with bathing, toileting, getting dressed and going to bed. Hairdressers, chiropodists, GPs and opticians sometimes visit the home to provide their services.

Care workers in a residential home include care assistants and, usually, some staff with nursing qualifications. The staff administer any medication that has been prescribed for the residents.

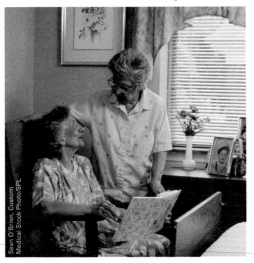

Each room is provided with an alarm system, enabling staff to know which resident is calling for attention. Residents and their relatives are usually encouraged to personalise the bedrooms with favourite items of furniture, pictures and so on. Most homes try to encourage a family-type atmosphere, for example, by celebrating each resident's birthday with a party.

Some residential homes are owned and run by local authorities; others are run by voluntary, not-for-profit organisations such as housing associations; some are run for profit by individuals or organisations in the private sector. In all three types of home, some residents are supported by funds from the local authority social-services budget, while those who have more money pay fees.

Residents are encouraged to personalise their bedrooms

Nursing homes are similar, although they specialise in caring for people with greater health problems, for example those who are severely disabled or with terminal illnesses. Nursing homes have a higher proportion of qualified nursing staff and charge higher fees to reflect the cost of caring for high-dependency clients.

+ Access to residential and nursing homes depends on who will pay for the care:
    + For fee-paying clients, access is by applying directly to the home.
    + For clients who will be funded by social services, access is by a needs assessment (usually carried out by a social worker).

Special educational needs

Services are available for children who have **special educational needs**, usually because they have some sort of disability that makes it harder for them to take part in education (e.g. deafness or a physical disability) or that means that they have an impaired ability to learn (a learning disability).

Children who cannot be adequately educated by mainstream school provision are assessed by practitioners (usually including an educational psychologist) and provided with a statement of special educational needs. This process is called 'statementing' and provides the child with access to special education. Special education may take place either in special schools or through special provision made in mainstream schools.

Special schools

Special schools educate pupils with significant disabilities. They are designed and equipped to be accessible to children with a variety of disabilities and some or all of the teachers are specially trained. The proportion of children who need to attend special schools is quite small, so there are far fewer of them than there are mainstream schools. This often means that the nearest special school is too far for daily travel, so some are residential – pupils board at the school during term time.

Support within mainstream schools

Children with disabilities can also be educated in special units in mainstream schools. In addition, mainstream schools provide extra support within lessons for children with special educational needs. This support is usually a classroom assistant who works with the child in some lessons on the school timetable.

+ Access to special units and extra support is by the recommendation of a member of school staff called the Special Educational Needs Coordinator (or SENCO) and sometimes, after an assessment, by an educational psychologist.

Access to services

The method of access to each service is described above.

Barriers to access

Access to services is not always instant or easy. Barriers include inadequate resources, ignorance, physical difficulties and communication problems.

Inadequate resources

The term '**resources**' refers to funding, staff and equipment. A lack of these creates barriers to accessing services in a number of ways, including long delays before receiving treatment.

1 Elderly people assessed as needing residential care might have to wait several weeks, or even months, because the local authority social-services budget for that year has already been spent.

2 A patient requires a brain scan. However, the local general hospital does not have the right sort of scanner, so the patient has to travel a long distance to another hospital.

The problem of inadequate resources can be overcome by increasing funding. One way of doing this is by raising local or national taxation. To increase the social-services budget, a local authority could increase council tax. To increase funding for the NHS, the government could increase taxation, for example, on alcoholic drinks, cigarettes and petrol.

However, increased funding does not always overcome the problem of inadequate resources. It will allow an NHS trust hospital to employ more nurses and consultants, but if there are not enough suitably trained people, the problem of inadequate resources remains. This can be overcome by increasing the number of training places and by improving conditions of employment (such as salaries) to encourage more people to enter the health and caring professions.

Ignorance

Another barrier to accessing services is the ignorance of clients. Some people are not aware that particular services exist, so they do not access them. For example, elderly people might not know that they can receive a flu jab each autumn from their local health centre. This barrier can be overcome by education, including publicity campaigns such as public service advertisements on television.

Physical difficulties

Sometimes people are aware of services, but find it difficult to reach them. For example, people whose work often takes them away from home might not be able to attend a GP appointment. People living in rural areas who do not have their own car might find that a lack of public transport makes it difficult to visit the nearest optician or dentist. Elderly and disabled people might have difficulty in using any form of transport.

These barriers can be overcome in various ways:

+ NHS walk-in health centres can be used without making an appointment. They operate for longer hours than most health centres or GP surgeries.
+ Local voluntary organisations sometimes provide 'community transport' to take people to appointments and day centres.
+ Some services (e.g. community nurses) provide home visits for clients with mobility problems.

Communication

Another barrier to access is caused by communication problems. These can occur when care workers and clients do not speak the same language, or if clients are deaf. Access to written information is a problem for clients who are blind or illiterate.

These barriers can be overcome in various ways, including giving out information on services in multi-language and Braille versions, employing translators, sign-language users or advocates who can speak on behalf of clients.

Rights and responsibilities of service users

Rights

Clients and patients in the health and social care services have certain rights. Some of these are included in the document *Your Guide to the NHS* under the heading, 'The NHS core principles'. Each principle is shown in a separate box.

The NHS will provide a universal service for all, based on clinical need, not ability to pay.

This means that every person who has a need for the services provided by the NHS will receive them. It also means that access to NHS services should not be influenced by how much money people have.

This means that there will be no gaps in service provision, i.e. that people throughout the country should have access to the same range of services. It is questionable whether this actually happens at present. For example, in several areas it is very difficult to get access to an NHS dentist. Therefore, many adults have to pay the full cost of their treatment, so access to dentistry depends on the ability to pay.

This means that services will be more patient-centred and responsive to the particular situations of patients, rather than providing standardised services that might be more convenient for practitioners.

This statement recognises that the same practices and procedures might not be appropriate in different parts of the country. In particular, it recognises that members of different ethnic groups might have different needs and preferences.

NHS hospital trusts collect data to find out how well they have performed. They use a range of performance indicators, such as waiting times and patient satisfaction. This information provides a guide that indicates which aspects of services need to be improved.

Mistakes occur in all organisations. In healthcare, the consequences of mistakes can be extremely serious. One example is that of a patient who had a diseased kidney. An operation to remove the kidney was performed, but the surgeon removed the healthy kidney by mistake and the patient died. The response to such mistakes is to design procedures that make similar mistakes less likely in future.

This refers to good employment practice, including the absence of unfair discrimination in promotion, and the provision of appropriate in-service training.

Some NHS resources are shared by the private healthcare sector. For example, some NHS hospital consultants also take private (i.e. paying) patients. This principle is designed to reassure people that NHS funding — which comes from taxpayers — will not be used to subsidise the treatment of private patients.

This means that NHS staff will communicate with staff from other organisations (such as local authority social-services departments), so that when a patient is transferred from the care of one organisation to another, the necessary information about them is handed over. This avoids delay, confusion and discomfort. For example, when a patient is ready to be discharged from hospital, any domiciliary care will already be in place.

The NHS will help keep people healthy and work to reduce health inequalities.

This statement implies a commitment to the prevention of illness, rather than just providing treatment for those who are already ill. Reducing health inequalities is partly about ensuring that effective health services exist in all parts of the country. However, health inequalities also exist because of lifestyle differences between communities — for example, in smoking behaviour and taking exercise.

The NHS will respect the confidentiality of individual patients and provide open access to information about services, treatment and performance.

This is really two items combined. The first is about keeping information secret; the second is about giving information.

Maintaining confidentiality about the health of a patient is regarded as very important in the NHS. For example, an adult whose mother is ill might ask the mother's GP about her illness. Unless it is clear that the patient wishes relatives to be told, the GP is likely to refuse to give this information.

Open access to information does not include information about particular patients. Better access to information about services, treatment and performance can help to build confidence among members of the community. In the past few years, NHS trusts have been much more active in providing this information, both in leaflets and on websites.

Responsibilities

Your Guide to the NHS also lists the following responsibilities of service users under the heading, 'Your commitment to the NHS'. These responsibilities are more specific than the statements of principles listed above.

Look after your own health and follow advice on a healthy lifestyle.

This is designed to reduce the number of people who become ill because they smoke, abuse drugs (e.g. by drinking alcohol excessively), avoid exercise or eat too much.

Care for yourself when appropriate. (For example, you can treat yourself at home for common ailments such as coughs, colds and sore throats.)

This is designed to reduce the number of people seeking medical help for trivial illnesses, which usually get better without treatment.

Give blood if you are able, and carry an organ donor card or special needs card or bracelet.

If most people carried an organ donor card, there would be enough organs for transplants. At present, people are dying unnecessarily while waiting for donor organs.

People who have special needs, or specific medical conditions, can carry a card or Medic Alert bracelet so that if they are involved in an accident, practitioners will know that they require special treatment.

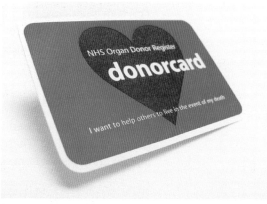

Carry an organ donor card

Listen carefully to advice on your treatment and medication. Tell the doctor about any treatments you are already taking.

This is designed to avoid misuse of medicines and possible adverse reactions when two or more medicines are taken. Some patients misuse prescription medicines by keeping drugs they were prescribed for a previous illness and taking them again when they become ill. Some people give prescribed drugs to friends or relatives.

Another potentially risky situation occurs when a patient who has to take medication to control high blood pressure (hypertension) visits a GP about a different condition. It is important for the GP to know about the existing medication, in case drugs prescribed for the second condition would cause an adverse reaction.

Treat NHS staff, fellow patients, carers and visitors politely, and with respect. We will not accept violence or racial, sexual or verbal harassment.

The section on page 33 about 'Violence from clients' explains why this item is included in the list of responsibilities.

Keep your hospital appointment or let the GP, dentist, clinic or hospital know as soon as possible if you cannot make it. Book routine appointments in plenty of time.

This is intended to prevent staff-time being wasted. A surprising number of people fail to attend appointments. Staff would be able to fit in another patient if they knew that someone would not be attending.

Return any equipment that is no longer needed.

This applies to equipment, such as crutches, that can be used by other patients.

Pay NHS prescription charges and any other charges promptly when they are due and claim financial benefits or exemptions from these charges correctly.

Some people, including pensioners and those receiving some benefits (e.g. Income Support and Child Benefit), are exempt from prescription charges.

This item is designed to remind people that they should not mistakenly or fraudulently claim exemption, for example, by indicating on the prescription that they are receiving benefits which they are not.

Risks and safe working

Although work in health and social care usually takes place in a safe environment, there are some risks. These include HIV and hepatitis infection, MRSA, lifting injuries and violence from clients.

HIV and hepatitis infection

HIV (human immunodeficiency virus) is the virus that can lead to AIDS (acquired immune deficiency syndrome). Although HIV is normally transmitted through sexual intercourse, it is also spread when blood and other bodily fluids from an infected person come into contact with mucous membranes or exposed tissue.

Hepatitis is a viral disease causing inflammation of the liver. It is spread in a similar way to HIV.

Precautions that care workers should take include:

+ covering any cuts, sores or open wounds with a dressing or plaster
+ avoiding being pricked or cut by used needles or scalpels by immediately disposing of them in a 'sharps' container
+ cleaning up spills of bodily fluid using sterile latex gloves and disinfectant

MRSA

Washing hands before contact with each patient helps to reduce the risk of MRSA

MRSA (methicillin-resistant *Staphylococcus aureus*) is a strain of the bacterium *Staphylococcus aureus* that has evolved during recent years to be resistant to the antibiotic methicillin. MRSA is often found in hospitals. It is extremely dangerous to young children, elderly people and those whose immune systems are weakened — for example, by an immune system disorder such as AIDS, or by chemotherapy to treat cancer.

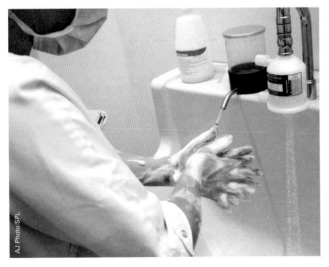

Although newspaper stories give the impression that the spread of MRSA is caused by 'dirty hospitals' or poor cleaning routines, the main problem is that some people (staff, patients and visitors) carry the bacterium into hospital, where it is spread by physical contact. The large increase in this kind of infection has been caused by the rapid evolution of the bacterium.

Precautions that practitioners can take to reduce this spread include:

+ washing their hands with an antibacterial soap or alcohol gel before touching any patient
+ keeping wounds covered by dressings
+ isolating infected patients in single rooms
+ keeping wards free from dust, which can harbour the bacterium

Lifting injuries

Patients in hospital and clients with physical disabilities (including many elderly people in nursing and residential homes) sometimes have to be handled or lifted. This usually happens when they are being washed, bathed, taken to the toilet or put to bed. Clients with physical disabilities are sometimes overweight because of a lack of exercise, so lifting and handling often impose stresses on the bodies of care workers.

Precautions against these injuries include receiving training on techniques of lifting and handling to minimise the risk of harm. These techniques include keeping the backbone vertical, using the strength of the legs to lift and using hoists.

Violence from clients

Clients can sometimes be violent to care workers. There are several reasons for this:

+ People often have accidents or are injured in fights when they are drunk. They then require treatment — often in a hospital Accident and Emergency department. Drunkenness increases the likelihood of violence.
+ Clients might be violent as a result of the disorder from which they are suffering. For example, people with some types of brain damage can become very impulsive, while mental disorders, such as schizophrenia, occasionally lead to outbursts of aggression.
+ Some people have a culturally acquired dislike of authority figures, such as police officers, and see hospital staff in the same way.
+ Patients and their relatives are often extremely anxious or guilty, but interpret the strong emotion they feel as anger.

Precautions that care workers can take to reduce the risk from violent clients include:

+ staying within the range of CCTV cameras. Provided there are notices in the building warning clients that cameras are in operation, this can inhibit violent behaviour.
+ making sure they are never alone with potentially violent clients
+ carrying personal alarms that either produce a piercing noise when activated or automatically send a message to get help
+ using calming techniques such as avoiding eye contact with the potential aggressor, avoiding shouting or becoming angry and apologising calmly for problems the client is facing (such as a long wait for treatment)

Risks and safe-working precautions for care workers are summarised in Table 1.3.

Table 1.3
Risks and safe-working
precautions

Risk	Precautions
HIV and hepatitis infection	Cover open wounds
	Take care with sharp medical equipment
	Clean body fluid spills with disinfectant
	Wear sterile latex gloves (discard after one use)
MRSA (methicillin-resistant Staphylococcus aureus)	Wash hands between patients
	Protect wounds with dressings
	Isolate infected patients
	Keep rooms free from dust
Lifting injuries	Lift with an upright, straight back
	Receive training in handling clients
	Use hoists when available
Violence from clients	Stay within range of CCTV cameras
	Carry a personal alarm
	Stay within range of other staff
	Use calming techniques

Sample examination questions with model answers

The model answers given would score full marks. In some cases, alternative answers would be acceptable.

1 Joanna is nearly 5 years old. She has a severe learning disability.

(a) Suggest one type of provision that is likely to be suitable for Joanna and justify your suggestion. (3 marks)

A special school would be suitable, because Joanna's disability is probably too great for her to manage in a mainstream school. Staff in special schools are trained to help disabled children learn. The school is also likely to have equipment such as specially adapted computers.

(b) Outline how the service you suggested in your answer to part (a) is accessed. (2 marks)

Joanna will be assessed, probably by an educational psychologist, and a statement of educational needs will be made.

(c) Suggest and describe two barriers to access that might make it difficult for Joanna to use the service you suggested in your answer to part (a). (4 marks)

One barrier to access might be a lack of resources. There might not be a suitable special school near where she lives, or the school might be full.

Another barrier could be the physical difficulty of getting to school. The school might be a long way away and travel might be difficult for her.

(d) Suggest two caring skills or techniques that might be appropriate for teachers and care workers to use to help Joanna as she starts her education. Justify your answers. (6 marks)

Physical contact might be useful, because Joanna will probably be feeling anxious at first. Giving her a cuddle might help to comfort her.

Working alongside could also be useful, as Joanna would probably not know anyone at the school. This would be a way of showing her what to do, as well as providing her with social support.

Total: 15 marks

2 Isobel is 90 years old and lives alone. She receives neither formal nor informal care. She has osteoarthritis, which makes it difficult for her to move about and handle objects. She recently scalded herself when she spilt a pan of boiling water.

(a) Suggest three different physical life-quality factors that Isobel is likely to lack. Illustrate each with reference to the description of Isobel. (6 marks)

Isobel might lack physical safety because her arthritis increases the risk of accidents. She probably dropped the pan because she could not grip it properly.

She will not have freedom from pain if she has to do everything for herself. For example, she does not have anyone to do her shopping.

Isobel might not have adequate nutrition because her condition will make it more difficult for her to cook. Sometimes she might not bother.

(b) A relative has recently suggested that Isobel should move into a residential home.

(i) Suggest two psychological life-quality factors that would probably be improved for Isobel by moving into a residential home. Explain your answers. (4 marks)

Isobel would have more social contact in the residential home. She would be able to talk to the staff and other residents.

Isobel would probably have more psychological security because she would not be so worried about having an accident. There would be an alarm call system in case she needed help.

(ii) Suggest one life-quality factor that would probably be decreased
if Isobel moved into a home.   (2 marks)

Isobel might experience a loss of autonomy, because she will have to fit in
with other people. For example, she might not be able to get up when she
wants to. This might depend on the availability of staff.

(c) Briefly describe one alternative type of social care (apart from
residential care) that could benefit Isobel, and state how this
could be accessed.   (3 marks)

Isobel could receive domiciliary care. This would mean that a care worker
would visit her several times a week to help her with daily living tasks, such
as getting up in the morning. This would probably be accessed as a result of
an assessment by a social worker.

Total: 15 marks

Further reading

Komaroff, A. L. (ed.) (2003) *The Harvard Medical School Family Health Guide*
(UK edn), Cassell.
Moore, S. (2002) *Social Welfare Alive!*, Nelson Thornes.
Your Guide to the NHS (2002), Department of Health.

Websites
The Department of Health:
www.dh.gov.uk
The King's Fund (a charitable foundation researching health care):
www.kingsfund.org.uk
NHS Direct:
www.nhsdirect.nhs.uk
The National Health Service:
www.nhs.uk

Effective communication

This chapter introduces you to the skills and techniques needed for **Unit 2: Effective communication**.

The first section is about factors that influence the effectiveness of communication. These factors have to be understood in order to prepare and deliver the talk that forms the basis of the unit assessment.

The second section gives detailed guidance on preparing the talk that forms the basis of the Unit 2 assessment, collecting feedback and writing the report.

The third section contains information on using questionnaires, which is needed for the assessment of Units 2 and 3.

Factors influencing the effectiveness of communication

Language and non-verbal communication

Language is a form of communication that uses words. A spoken word is a set of speech sounds (called phonemes), a written word is a set of visual symbols (called letters) and a word in sign language is a gesture with an agreed meaning. Therefore, language may be oral (i.e. spoken), visual (i.e. written or printed) or gestural.

Language can be defined as verbal communication. 'Verbal' means 'using words'. Some people mistakenly use the word 'verbal' to mean just 'oral' — for example, people talk about a 'verbal warning' when they mean a spoken (but not written) warning.

Another common mistake is the assumption that all communication is through language. However, people are able to communicate some things without using words at all, for example by frowning when they disapprove of something. Non-human animals, such as ants, fish, dogs and birds, do not use language yet communicate effectively.

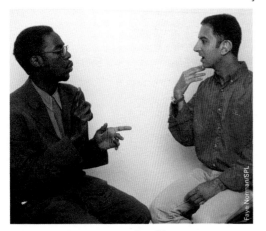

Each gesture in sign language has a specific meaning

This non-language type of communication is called **non-verbal communication**. In human beings, it involves visual signals — especially from the face — and auditory signals, such as laughter. Some people call non-verbal communication 'body language'. This creates confusion because, by definition, non-verbal communication cannot be language.

Some people think that sign languages (such as British Sign Language and Makaton) are not languages because they use gestures. This is a mistake. It is true that the gestures most people use in everyday conversation are not language, because they do not have specific meanings. For example, shrugging your shoulders can express a variety of feelings, but not a single, specific meaning. In contrast, the gestures that are words in sign language do have specific meanings and can be translated directly into other forms of language such as speech.

Effective communication requires competent performance of both verbal and non-verbal skills. For example, when explaining a treatment to a client, good verbal skills are needed to give clear information and good non-verbal skills are required to manage the emotional aspects of the communication, such as appearing reassuring and supportive.

This does not mean that there is only one correct way of using language and non-verbal skills. There are noticeable differences between individuals. What is effective for one person might not work so well for another. This is partly because people have different personalities.

While it is useful for students to model their communication skills on those of experts — such as some teachers — it is also good to have personal styles.

Factors in verbal communication

The first five factors are concerned with matching the language and style of the communication to the audience.

Use of technical terminology

As in other fields of study, health and social care has its own **technical terminology.** Practitioners use terms such as 'hypertension', 'empowerment', 'reinforcement' and 'separation anxiety', which are unlikely to be understood by all clients. For this reason, practitioners use technical terminology with their colleagues, but tend to avoid it when talking to clients. When talking to clients, practitioners should try to paraphrase technical terms. This means they should use more familiar words to say what they mean. For example, on speaking to patients it would be better to use the phrase 'high blood pressure' rather than 'hypertension', and 'stroke' rather than 'cerebrovascular accident'.

Sentence length and complexity

The ability to understand a sentence depends partly on the capacity and duration of the working memory. (This used to be called the short-term memory.) Typically, working memory can hold information for anything between 5 and 30 seconds. Long sentences are a problem, because to understand the sentence, the start has to be remembered while listening to the rest of it. People with a low working-memory capacity, such as infants and some elderly people, might not understand a long sentence.

Sentence complexity refers to the number of clauses the sentence contains. An example of a simple sentence is: 'For my breakfast I usually like to have fresh orange juice, porridge, fried egg, sausage, bacon, tomato, baked beans, white toast, marmalade and black filter coffee.'

An example of a more complex sentence of similar length is: 'I asked the lady, who had fallen and now seemed confused, whether she felt able to go home on her own or whether she needed a lift.'

The second example sentence requires more cognitive effort to understand.

Use of humour

Humour can be useful in care situations. A practitioner can use it to help a client relax. In meetings or training sessions humour can help to keep people alert and interested. In these situations it is being used with the aim of assisting communication.

However, humour is sometimes used in a way that does not help. For example, when a serious situation is being discussed, humour can make a person seem uncaring and flippant.

Formality of style

A **formal communication style** usually means a conventional, respectful way of communicating, without any kind of joking familiarity. This is often appropriate in written communication, for example in an examination or when writing a report. In caring situations it is also sometimes appropriate. For example, clients who do not think of care workers as their friends might prefer to be addressed formally as 'Mrs Williams', rather than 'Helen' or 'love'. However, other clients are not comfortable with this kind of formality and prefer a warmer, friendlier style. The skill of matching style to audience often depends on judging, or asking, what level of formality a client would prefer.

Use of colloquialisms

Colloquialisms are a feature of an informal language style. They are not always widely understood, because they are often used only by subsections of the population, such as young people or people from a particular area. Sometimes, they are restricted to one family. The result is that people from different groups might fail to understand, or might misunderstand, what is being said.

+ An elderly man says that his heart is 'on the blink', meaning that he has a heart disorder.
+ A woman tells her GP that she often unexpectedly has 'waterworks', meaning that she often becomes tearful. The GP might think she is referring to incontinence.
+ A care worker responds to a rude joke made by a client by saying, 'What are you like?'

You can see the problem — colloquialisms often do not mean what they say. The care worker in the example above is not actually asking a question. The meaning is really something like, 'I'm amused by your naughty sense of humour'.

Colloquialisms are appropriate for use with an audience from the same cultural background and in a situation that calls for an informal style. They are not appropriate with an audience drawn from a wider age or cultural range. Think of the difficulty that might be experienced by a person who is learning to speak English and is told, 'Any worries, give me a bell, OK?'

Try it out

1 Make a list of colloquialisms you hear among friends or on television during a single day. Find out whether your teacher knows what they all mean.
2 Rewrite the following paragraph in an informal style for an audience that does not understand the technical terminology. It is not necessary to replace all the technical terms. However, the language and style of your version should be much more informal.

> Parental neglect can lead to the development of maladaptive behaviours in infants. The child seeks stimulation from his or her caregivers and when this is not forthcoming is likely to engage in disruptive behaviours that are more successful in securing attention. For example, the child might engage in destructive behaviour or periods of intense vocalisation. This is likely to elicit a hostile or punitive response from the caregiver. Even this attention might be preferable to the child than its absence. Consequently, the caregiver is actually reinforcing the behaviour that they are seeking to discourage.

The following four factors apply equally to written or oral communication.

Logical progression

An extended communication — such as a talk or report — is easier to understand if it follows a logical order. For example, to explain what happened in an accident in which you were involved, the logical order would be to describe events in the order in which they occurred.

For a talk or essay about a sexually transmitted disease, a logical progression might be as follows:

+ an introduction, outlining what is to be included in the talk/essay
+ a description of the signs, symptoms and outcome of the disease

+ an explanation of how the symptoms are caused
+ an explanation of how the disease is transmitted
+ an explanation of how it can be prevented
+ a description of how it can be treated

The particular order shown here is not the only one that is logical. For example, treatment could be discussed before transmission and prevention.

A more interesting way of introducing this talk would be to start with an example, such as: 'Martina was infected with chlamydia at the age of 18. She had no idea of this until 10 years later when a gynaecologist told her that she might not be able to have children.'

This acts as a kind of trailer for the talk, which should then follow logically as in the list given above.

Avoiding ambiguity

An **ambiguous statement** is a statement that can be interpreted in more than one way. The result is that the person receiving the information might understand it to mean something different from what the person giving the information intended.

The most striking examples come from newspaper headlines, such as 'INJURED BABY NAMED AFTER SMASH', which could lead some readers to think that parents have decided to name their child after a brand of instant potato.

'A large garden is needed for growing children' could also be interpreted in two ways.

Sometimes, ambiguity occurs because the correct technical terminology is not used. For example, the statement 'Bernard has a problem with his nerves' could be interpreted to mean that Bernard has an anxiety disorder — a type of extreme nervousness, unconnected with nerve tissue. Alternatively, it could be interpreted as Bernard having a condition that affects his nerves and nerve cells, such as multiple sclerosis.

Appropriate use of words

Inappropriate use of words can arise when the meaning of a word is unclear. For example, the word 'ignorant' means 'lacking knowledge', but people sometimes use it to mean 'bad-mannered'.

Lack of precision is another problem, i.e. a word is used with a related, but not quite correct, meaning. For example, the word 'privacy' is sometimes misused to mean the same as 'confidentiality'. It is wrong to assume that because a friend, parent or teacher uses a word in a particular way, this meaning is correct. If in doubt, check using a dictionary.

The words 'access' and 'assess' are easily confused.

Fluency

Fluency refers to how well words flow in speech or writing. Fluency in speech comes with much practice.

Read the two alternative versions below:

Version 1: The NHS has converted most mixed-sex wards (which is what they mostly used to be) to single-sex wards because one of the things patients said they didn't like, when they were asked in quality-assurance surveys, was whether there was enough privacy in hospital and this is one of the things they said.

Version 2: Quality-assurance surveys showed that hospital patients were concerned about a lack of privacy on mixed hospital wards. As a result, the NHS has converted most such wards to single-sex wards.

Version 2 flows better and is easier to understand. It uses two relatively simple sentences, whereas version 1 is one complex sentence.

Paralanguage factors

The effectiveness of spoken communication is also affected by factors that are not themselves aspects of language, but which are features associated with speech.

Speed, clarity and loudness

Clarity of speech refers to how precisely speech sounds are made. Some people have slurred speech in which different speech sounds run together or are not fully sounded. This makes it difficult for a listener to pick out the words. Clarity can be improved by speaking more slowly. Conversely, very precise speakers can speak quickly and still be understood.

Volume or loudness is also important. A quiet voice is much harder to follow, while a very loud voice can be tiresome and irritating to listen to for long.

Clarity and volume are very important in talking to clients, particularly those who have impaired hearing or for whom English is not their first language.

Pitch and tone

Pitch refers to how high or low the voice is on a musical scale. Deep, bass voices are low pitched. Young children hear high-pitched sounds better than low-pitched sounds. Parents and care workers recognise this and often use high-pitched voices. In contrast, some older people with progressive hearing loss have difficulty in hearing high-pitched sounds and find it easier to hear mid-range voices.

Tone can vary from a mellow voice to a hard-edged, quite piercing voice. A mellow tone is more restful and soothing; a piercing voice is easier to hear.

Speech sounds more interesting if pitch and tone are varied. Speech in which the voice is all on one note (a monotone) sounds dull (monotonous).

Hesitations and filled pauses

Hesitations are silent pauses in speech, during which the speaker is thinking how to continue. They tend to give the impression that the speaker is unsure of the facts or lacks confidence. Sometimes this impression is correct. Being unprepared or lacking in confidence leads to anxiety, which occupies the attention of the speaker, making it more difficult for the speaker to concentrate on the content of the talk.

However, in some situations, speakers hesitate intentionally. For example, when counselling or interviewing clients, hesitations provide opportunities for clients to intervene.

Filled pauses are words or sounds that do not contribute to the meaning of what is being said, but serve to conceal hesitation. They prevent another person from interrupting, while giving the speaker time to think of what to say next. Typical pause-fillers are 'erm', 'you know', 'and so on' and — a recent favourite — 'to be honest'. Frequent repetition of such sounds or phrases can become noticeable to an audience and distract attention from what the speaker is actually saying.

Filled pauses such as 'uh-huh' and 'mm' can also be used to indicate to another person that we are listening and want him or her to continue.

Improving verbal communication and paralanguage skills

An awareness of the factors that influence effective communication makes it easier to avoid mistakes. One common mistake in written communication is a tendency to show off by using unnecessarily complex sentences or impressive-sounding words.

A useful way to improve your writing skills is to read out loud what you have written. Places where the writing is too complex or lacks fluency will be easily noticed. The sentences that do not 'sound right', or that are difficult to say, can then be rewritten.

Speech can also be recorded and played back later. You can listen for paralanguage factors such as loudness, pitch and filled pauses. You might find that you are trying to read too quickly, in which case you should practise speaking more slowly.

Factors in non-verbal communication

Non-verbal communication is mainly used to support language. It is particularly effective at communicating emotions and intentions.

Eye contact

Eye contact is important in everyday conversations. A quick glance at the other person's eyes signals interest and attentiveness. It can also be used to keep another person's attention and to signal the end of a statement. Eye contact is hardly ever noticed unless it is too prolonged or absent. Prolonged eye contact can make a person feel uncomfortable — it might seem like an aggressive stare.

Absence of eye contact can make communication more difficult. A person who does not make eye contact can appear untrustworthy or acutely self-conscious.

In a conversation with another person, eye contact comes automatically to most people. With a larger audience, it might require a conscious effort to occasionally glance at different audience members.

Facial expressions

Facial expressions are effective in communicating emotions. In communicating, it is sometimes necessary to conceal our emotions. One way to do this is by controlling facial expressions.

+ You are listening to a teacher whom you respect. You feel a bit tired and bored. Just as you begin to yawn, the teacher looks at you. You quickly convert the yawn into an interested expression.

+ You are caring for a child who for some reason is trying to make you angry. You will not allow yourself to be manipulated by the child, so you keep a calm expression on your face, even though you feel angry.

Body orientation and proximity

Body orientation refers to your position in relation to people with whom you are communicating. A face-to-face orientation is often useful for communication because it allows eye contact and facial expression to be easily visible. It is particularly important for people with a hearing impairment because it allows them to lip-read.

However, in some situations a face-to-face orientation might seem threatening, particularly if there is much disagreement or criticism in the content of the communication. In these circumstances, a side-by-side orientation can be useful.

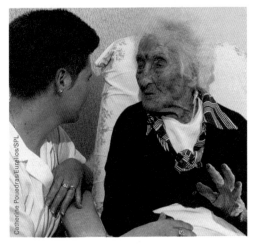

A face-to-face orientation helps a deaf person to lip-read

Turning your back on an audience is very rarely a useful orientation!

Proximity refers to how close a speaker is to the audience. In one-to-one conversations, proximity depends on how well the people involved know each other. A stranger is likely to feel uncomfortable if someone stands or sits very close during conversation.

When talking to an audience, a speaker often feels more comfortable with a separation of at least 2 metres. However, members of a distant audience might feel that the speaker cannot see them very well, so they can reduce their attention without it being noticed. Closer proximity prevents this and makes it easier to involve the audience.

Gestures and body posture

Arm gestures are sometimes used to emphasise speech, but mostly serve to indicate how relaxed and involved a speaker is. Frequent gesturing can be distracting, while an absence of movement can also seem strange. Anxious and inexperienced speakers often produce unnecessary movements (such as face touching and head scratching), which tend to communicate their anxiety.

An upright posture is usually the most effective for face-to-face communication. Inexperienced speakers sometimes adopt a sagging, head-down posture.

In some situations, upright posture is not appropriate. For example, when communicating with a child or a seated person it is often useful to squat down. This means that your face is at the same level as that of the other person and also prevents the other person from feeling dominated.

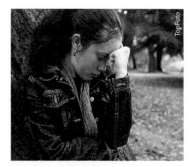

Gestures and posture can communicate anxiety

1 Try this exercise with a friend you know well. Do not tell them what you are doing. In an ordinary conversation make eye contact for longer than usual. What is the effect on communication? Now try having a conversation without looking at the other person at all. Afterwards, explain what you were doing and why. Apologise if necessary.

2 Watch a person who is having a telephone conversation, but not using a video-phone. Are they using non-verbal communication? See if you can spot changes in expression, gestures and so on.

Try it out

Improving non-verbal communication skills

Most people automatically use appropriate non-verbal communication skills in everyday conversation. However, in situations such as communicating in care settings or giving a talk to an audience, non-verbal communication skills might need to be developed.

The best way of doing this is to videotape yourself talking and watch the recording carefully. Notice how often you establish eye contact (in this case how often you look at the camera), your posture, orientation and gestures. At first, this can be quite embarrassing. However, the benefits of seeing yourself as others see you should outweigh the disadvantages.

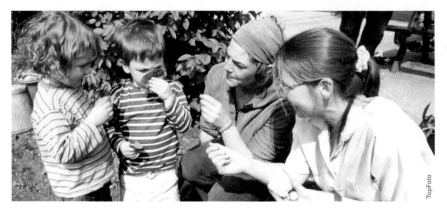

Getting down to the same level — a useful posture for working with infants

Communications in care settings

Most of the factors described above relate to speaking and writing. However, in care settings, one of the most important skills is **listening**.

Listening

People often think of listening as a rather passive activity. In conversation with friends, listening is sometimes the boring bit, while waiting in turn to speak. For care workers, listening is an active skill, which improves with practice. A useful rule of thumb in care situations is to spend more time listening than talking.

Listening can serve several functions, including receiving information, providing support and maintaining dignity.

Receiving information

It is often important to find out how a client is feeling. For example, a GP will listen carefully to a patient's description of symptoms. Care workers learn that clients do not always tell them the whole story and that careful listening, combined with other observations, can reveal this. For example, a GP might become aware that a patient is describing a 'presenting problem' rather than talking about a condition that embarrasses them (such as incontinence).

Providing support

People who are upset often benefit from being able to talk to someone. This is only really effective if the other person actually listens to them. Experienced care workers are able to encourage this kind of talk, while less experienced care workers often interrupt and give advice, or talk about their own similar experiences.

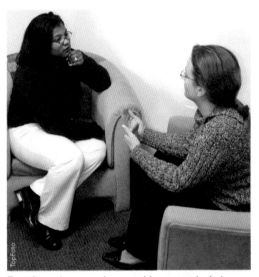

Experienced care workers provide support by being good listeners

Maintaining dignity

If people are not listened to, they can get the impression that they are regarded as unimportant. Not being listened to is associated with low social status. Some people habitually show a lack of respect to others of lower status. This is most commonly experienced by children and elderly people, who, in comparison with younger adults, lack power.

Some clients, especially those in an unfamiliar setting, are very sensitive to this perceived loss of status. For example, consider a female patient in hospital being visited by a consultant and a group of medical students. A discussion might take place about the patient in which she is not included. The patient might get the impression that she is not regarded as a person. Including her in the discussion, and taking what she has to say seriously, would help to preserve her dignity.

Communication difficulties

Clients in health and social care are more likely than other people to have **communication difficulties**. For example, elderly people are likely to have impaired hearing because of the progressive hearing loss that occurs with age. Partial sight in this group also leads to difficulties in reading written communications, such as letters.

Strokes are fairly common in this age group. If a stroke occurs in the hemisphere of the brain that controls speech, there are likely to be difficulties in speaking. For most people, this is the left hemisphere. A typical pattern is for a person to have paralysis and loss of muscle tone in the right-hand side of the body, as well as speech impairment. This is because the motor area in the left-hand side of the brain controls muscle movements in the right-hand side of the body. In contrast, stroke patients who show paralysis in the left-hand side of the body are less likely to have a speech impairment.

Speech impairments resulting from strokes are called **aphasias**. Damage to Broca's area results in loss of the ability to produce speech (Broca's aphasia); damage to Wernicke's area results in loss of the ability to understand speech (Wernicke's aphasia).

Dementias, such as Alzheimer's disease, can also result in speech difficulties — in particular, the inability to remember words while speaking.

People with severe learning disabilities have much less ability than others to perceive, understand and respond to their environment. They are unlikely to be able to read, and might also have difficulty in producing and understanding speech.

Some young children experience difficulties in language development, particularly in producing some speech sounds. These can often be overcome with the help of a speech and language therapist. Some children suffer from a condition known as 'glue ear', which impairs hearing.

Unit 2 assessment

Preparing the talk

Before starting on any of the activities needed for the assessment of this unit, read the section of the specification that describes the assessment tasks.

Choosing your topic

Your talk should be about communication skills for a particular type of client. You might choose a type of client with whom you are already familiar. For example, if you have an elderly relative with partial hearing, or an infant brother or sister, you might choose one of those types of client. Whatever your choice, try to get some first-hand experience of the type of client that you are going to talk about.

You might decide to focus on a client with a specific communication problem. This would enable you to talk about techniques and aids available to clients and care workers in this situation. For example, your talk could include a demonstration of voice-operated software, such as *ViaVoice*.

Alternatively, you might focus on a broader range of communication skills used in working with clients who do not have specific communication problems. There is a wide range of topics to choose from, including communication skills:

+ for working with people who have dementia
+ for working with victims of accidents
+ for working with stroke patients in hospital
+ for helping infants to acquire language

If you choose the last topic, your audience would have to imagine they were the parents of young children.

You will also benefit if your topic is different from those chosen by your classmates.

Finding relevant sources

Assembling your talk will be easier if you find some good sources of information.

While it is appropriate to refer to textbooks, you should also try to find sources specifically related to the type of client you have chosen. For example, textbooks on developmental psychology often include sections on the role of parents in the development of language. Books and websites for people with partial hearing or partial sight are likely to contain useful information — for example, on communication aids.

You should also try to make personal contact with relevant clients and/or practitioners — for example, speech and language therapists.

These sources should be listed in the appendix to your report. It is a good idea to list published sources separately from website addresses and from personal contacts. For more guidance on writing references, see Chapter 11, pp. 298–299.

What to include in your talk

You might be anxious that you will not have enough material for a talk lasting from five to ten minutes. In fact, it would probably be a mistake to include a great deal of information. Instead, you should think about how to illustrate your talk with examples.

Suppose that your talk is to be about effective communication with hospital in-patients. You might ask someone who has recently spent time on a hospital ward how staff communicated with him/her about his/her condition and treatment. For example, how were the results of tests communicated to the patient? How long after the results were known were they given to the patient? Did the patient have opportunities to ask questions? Did the patient understand the information?

You might also ask a practitioner his or her opinion about effective communication with the type of client you are interested in.

You would then be able to use these examples, and quotations from the people you spoke to, to illustrate your talk.

Rehearsal

Your talk is not likely to be very effective if you simply read out what you have written. This approach would restrict your ability to make good use of non-verbal communication skills. At the opposite extreme, you might not feel confident to give your talk without using notes. You could learn your talk by heart or you could use some form of written prompt. One way of doing this is to print the main points of your talk in a large point size on two or three sheets of paper or card. During your talk, you can glance at the next heading and then talk from memory about that, before going to the next heading.

An alternative is to display your main headings using overhead transparencies or PowerPoint slides, and use these as cues to remind you what to say.

In any case, you should practise giving your talk (perhaps using a friend or family member as an audience). As a result of this practice, and the feedback you get, you should be able to make improvements.

Design decisions

These are decisions you will have to make during the planning and preparation of your talk.

Order of presentation

You should think carefully about this. The topics you cover should follow a logical progression.

Whether or not to use visual aids

Visual aids can add interest and clarity to a talk. For example, a short video clip showing a nursery nurse working with an infant could be used to illustrate what you are saying. A possible drawback is that the equipment you are using does not work properly, so a rehearsal, using the same equipment, is vital.

Whether or not to encourage audience participation

Audience participation can make a talk more enjoyable for audience members because they become more involved. It can also make the situation less threatening for the speaker because the audience is helping you – not just listening. Encouraging participation could involve:

+ asking if there are any questions
+ using a volunteer to demonstrate a particular technique
+ teaching a few signs in sign language

A disadvantage of audience participation is that the situation might become more difficult to control. For example, someone could ask you a question to which you do not know the answer, or the audience contributions might deflect you from the main topic.

Collecting feedback

An important part of the assessment for this unit is collecting and analysing feedback about your talk.

There are several ways of collecting feedback. One is to ask for comments at the end of your talk and to note down what people say. Comments from your teacher will probably be particularly useful.

To meet the assessment requirements of this unit, you should design, print and copy a questionnaire for members of your audience to fill in immediately after your talk. You should collect the completed questionnaires. Your ability to design a questionnaire is assessed too, so you should follow the guidance given in the section on questionnaires later in this chapter.

The questionnaire should include items on all the important aspects of communication covered by your talk, including content, language, paralanguage and non-verbal skills. For example, if you decided to use visual aids, you should include an item or items about these.

In order to meet the requirements of the assessment, some of your questionnaire items should be 'scorable'. For example, you might include the item:

How interesting was the talk? Please underline one of the following:
Very interesting/Quite interesting/Undecided/Not very interesting/ Not at all interesting

You could analyse this item by counting how many respondents said the talk was 'very interesting', how many said it was 'quite interesting' and so on. Alternatively, you could give a score to each response (e.g. 5 to 'very interesting' down to 1 for 'not at all interesting').

Your questionnaire should include both open and closed items.

Feedback analysis

Having collected the feedback, you need to analyse the questionnaire data. Guidance for doing this is included in the section on questionnaires later in this chapter.

Writing the report

Before writing your report, you should be aware of the assessment criteria given in the specification for this unit. The marks given are for:
+ knowledge of communication skills (AO1)
+ application of communication skills (AO2)
+ research and analysis (AO3)
+ evaluation (AO4)

AO1 marks: knowledge of communication skills

In your talk, you should show your knowledge of communication skills by identifying and explaining the skills that are relevant to the particular type of client you have chosen. Accuracy and completeness are important, so you should avoid making mistakes such as ignoring listening skills or assuming that 3-year-olds can read.

Your knowledge of communication skills should also be shown in the way your talk is structured (is it in a logical order?) and in the range of items included in the questionnaire. Your questionnaire should ask about all the skills important to your talk. For example, it would be a mistake to leave out items on non-verbal communication.

AO2 marks: application of communication skills

These marks are for competent use of communication skills. Your talk should be well planned and well written; items in your feedback questionnaire should be clear, unambiguous and relevant. Your knowledge of communication skills should be specifically applied to the type of client you have chosen, rather than being a general description of good communication skills that could apply in almost any situation.

AO3 marks: research and analysis

Marks are gained here by the correct use of data processing and presentation methods when analysing the feedback. For example, you might show median scores on each scored questionnaire item and illustrate these with a bar chart. Effective analysis enables the reader to see at a glance which aspects of your talk went well and which went less well.

In the appendix to the report you should list the sources of information you used during the preparation of the talk.

AO4 marks: evaluation

In the evaluation section of the report you should make judgements (based on the feedback you obtained) about the effectiveness of your communication in the talk. You will not lose marks in this section if you performed a skill poorly – for example, if your speech was not very audible. The key point is that your evaluation should be a true reflection of the quality of your talk and should be consistent with the results of your feedback.

You might find it useful to divide this section of the report into subsections, such as the following:

+ **Design decisions** – in this subsection, you could explain why you decided to structure the talk the way you did and comment on whether the decisions you made turned out to be good ones.
+ **Communication skills** – in this subsection, you could comment on your performance of the range of communication skills, illustrating your comments with reference to the information in the research and analysis section.
+ **Possible improvements** – in this section, you could suggest ways in which the content and performance of your talk could be improved. Again, these suggestions should be linked to the feedback obtained.

Questionnaires

What is a questionnaire?

A questionnaire is a printed or electronic document featuring questions or items that the respondent has to read, understand and record responses to. One advantage of a questionnaire survey is that large amounts of data can be collected quickly and easily, compared with the interview-survey method.

What are questionnaires used for?

One important use of questionnaires is for research – to find out information about a group of respondents. If that group of respondents is typical (or representative) of their population, the data collected are likely to be valid for that population. This kind of data gathering is important for research in health and social care – for example, in assessing treatments, evaluating patient care and patient satisfaction, and in measuring public attitudes to health risks and treatments.

Questionnaires are also important in other areas of research – for example, in carrying out a national census.

Some psychometric tests are in the form of questionnaires – for example, careers-interest inventories. Application forms for social-care benefits also include questionnaire items.

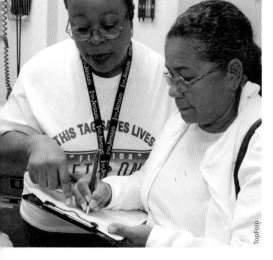

Customer-satisfaction questionnaires are often used to obtain feedback about a service

TopFoto

However, questionnaires are often used for other purposes. One is as a marketing tool; consumers are asked to fill in questionnaires about their interests (often with the reward of discount vouchers or the chance to win a prize). The data collected are then used to target advertising material at those consumers. Advertisers sometimes use questionnaires that repeatedly feature the product they are marketing, to increase the probability that the respondent will buy it.

Customer-satisfaction questionnaires are often used to obtain feedback about a service provided, such as a holiday or a meal in a restaurant. In some cases, the feedback is used to improve the service. However, such questionnaires are sometimes used simply to give the customers the impression that the service provider cares about them.

Writing questionnaire items

A questionnaire is made up of a list of items. Not all items on a questionnaire are questions, which is why the word 'item' is preferred. It is useful to number the items in a questionnaire. The people who fill in a questionnaire are called respondents or participants.

There are several types of item that can be used. These can be divided into open questions and closed questions (including forced-choice items).

Open questions

Open-question items are those in which there is no restriction on the response. For example, 'Please suggest one way in which the service could be improved'.

Free-response items are open questions that request information and provide a large space or box for the respondents to write their answers in. For example, 'Please use the box below to say what was good about your stay in hospital'.

Advantages of open-question items

+ Respondents are free to write what they want, instead of being restricted to choosing from a narrow range of responses.
+ They can produce unexpected responses that you might not have obtained in any other way.

Disadvantages of open-question items

+ They are time-consuming to record and to process.
+ It is difficult to compare different groups of respondents.

Closed questions

Closed-question items are those for which there is a limited range of possible answers. For example:

Please write your age in years in the box provided. ⬚

Most closed questions are of the **forced-choice type**, in which the respondent is restricted to a range of possible responses that are printed on the questionnaire. For example:

What sex are you?   Female ☐   Male ☐   Please tick one box.

Forced-choice items often include more than two alternatives. For example:

On how many days per week, on average, do you drink alcohol?
0 ☐   1 ☐   2 ☐   3 ☐   4 ☐   5 ☐   6 ☐   7 ☐   Please tick one box.

Some forced-choice items allow respondents to give alternative answers outside the specified range, by stating: 'Other – please specify'. For example:

Which of the following physical or sporting activities do you do 3 or more times a year?
Please tick any boxes that apply.
Swimming ☐   Gym training ☐   Organised group exercise/yoga ☐
Indoor ball games ☐   Outdoor ball games ☐   Dancing ☐
Running ☐   Cycling ☐
Others (please specify) _____

Forced-choice items can ask respondents to give a rating on a 5-point scale (or sometimes a 3- or 7-point scale). For example:

Please show how important you think regular exercise is for you by ticking one box.
Not at all important ☐ Not very important ☐ Undecided ☐
Quite important ☐ Very important ☐

Sometimes rating scales are used with statements to which respondents are asked to agree or disagree. These are called **Likert-type items**. For example:

'Exercise makes very little difference to a person's general health.'
Agree strongly ☐ Agree ☐ Undecided ☐ Disagree ☐ Disagree strongly ☐

The advantages of closed-question items are that they are very easy for the respondent to use and the data collected are easy to process. For example, the number of respondents who reported taking part in swimming can be counted. This makes it easier to draw general conclusions from the data.

The disadvantage is that respondents might not have the opportunity to say what they really feel about the topic.

Collecting different types of data

A questionnaire is usually designed to collect several different kinds of data. These include what groups or categories respondents belong to, and information about their behaviour, cognitions, feelings, preferences and wishes.

Items to categorise respondents

Categorising means finding out, for example, the sex, age, family status (e.g. whether living alone, or with a spouse, partner or children) and occupation of the respondents.

The main reason for collecting data categorising respondents is to make comparisons between groups – for example, to compare the attitude of people of different ages to diet.

A typical item for categorising respondents is shown below.

What sex are you? Female ☐ Male ☐ Please tick one box.

Items to find out about behaviour

Researchers often want to know how their respondents act. For example, someone researching eating habits might want to know what a sample of respondents eats for breakfast. This information could be collected using either a closed or an open item. An example of a typical closed item for collecting such data is:

Which of the following foods do you usually eat for breakfast? Tick any items that apply.
Cereal ☐ Porridge ☐ Toast ☐ Egg ☐ Bacon ☐ Sausage ☐ Fried bread ☐
Baked beans ☐ Fruit ☐ Jam/marmalade/honey ☐
Others (please list) _____
_____
_____

An example of a typical open item collecting similar data is:

Please list the foods you usually eat for breakfast.

_____

_____

Usually closed items are better for finding out about commonly occurring behaviours. In the breakfast items above, the closed item lists foods, so the respondent is unlikely to miss one out – which might happen with the open item.

Sometimes data are collected about the frequency of specific behaviours – for example, asking respondents to estimate how many cigarettes they smoke in a typical day or how often they weigh themselves. Frequency items often give a range of frequency categories, as in the following example:

How many cigarettes do you smoke in a typical day? Please tick one box.
1–10 ☐   11–20 ☐   21–30 ☐   31–40 ☐   41–50 ☐   More than 50 ☐

Items to find out about cognitions

Cognitions are beliefs and perceptions. They influence behaviour, so it is often useful to know about them. For example, if a health-promotion researcher is interested in studying condom use, it could also be important to find out what beliefs people have about condoms. The researcher might find that some people who do not use condoms believe them to be ineffective in protecting against disease.

Likert-type closed items are often used to find out about beliefs. They do this by stating a belief and asking the respondent to what extent they agree with it. For example:

'Exercise makes very little difference to a person's general health.'
Agree strongly ☐   Agree ☐   Undecided ☐   Disagree ☐   Disagree strongly ☐

The problem with this type of item is that the questionnaire might not include those beliefs that are most important to the respondent. An open question might be more successful at finding these out, as in the example below:

Please outline your main reasons for taking part in sport or exercise.

_____

_____

_____

Items to find out about feelings, preferences and wishes

Data about feelings can be collected in a similar way, using Likert-type items such as:

'My mood usually improves soon after smoking a cigarette.'
Agree strongly ☐   Agree ☐   Undecided ☐   Disagree ☐   Disagree strongly ☐

However, open questions allow respondents to report those feelings that are most important to them.

Preferences and wishes can be studied using forced-choice items, as in the following example from a careers inventory:

Would you prefer to work alone ☐ or as part of a team ☐ ?   Please tick one box.

An open-item alternative might ask respondents to describe their preferred working environments.

Ranking preferences

Another technique for assessing preferences is to ask a respondent to rank alternatives in order of preference.

The following item is designed to find out what hospital patients think is most important to them:

Please rank the following items in order of importance for you. Write the number 1 next to the most important item and 7 next to the least important item. Please do not give any items an equal ranking.

☐ Quiet
☐ Privacy
☐ Access to television
☐ Contact with other patients
☐ Good lighting
☐ Appetising food
☐ Flexible visiting times

In practice, this is not a good way to collect data, partly because respondents might not understand the instructions. Processing the data poses more of a problem. You could count how many respondents gave 'Quiet' a rank of 1 and treat all the other items similarly. However, counting how many second, third, fourth, fifth, sixth and seventh rankings each item was given is complicated and time-consuming. For this reason a rating scale is much preferred. For example:

How important is privacy for you in the hospital ward? (Please circle one number.)
Very important   7   6   5   4   3   2   1   Not at all important

Attitude questionnaires

Attitude questionnaires usually include items about behaviour, cognitions and feelings. For example, a questionnaire about parents' attitudes to immunisations for their children would probably find out whether or not the children had been immunised, what parents believed about the advantages and disadvantages of immunisation and what anxieties they felt. Attitude questionnaires are often designed so that data from several items can be combined to give one attitude score for each respondent.

Questionnaire design

In order for a respondent to be able to read, understand and respond to a questionnaire, it must:

+ be written using simple, non-technical language
+ be well laid out with a clear route through the items
+ include clear instructions on how to record responses

Some questionnaires have a branching structure in which, depending on the answer given in one item, the respondent is guided to a later item. For example:

If you answered 'No' to this item, please go to item 15.

Deciding on aims

To be effective, a questionnaire should be designed to meet a clearly stated aim. For example, a researcher might have the aim: 'To find out how patients use prescribed medicines'.

A statement of aim is useful in two ways:

+ First, it guides you in thinking of questionnaire items. For example, the researcher above might think of items such as:

 + 'Do you stop taking a prescription medicine as soon as you start to feel better?'
 + 'Do you keep leftover prescription medicine to use next time you get ill?'

+ Second, a statement of aim helps you to edit your questionnaire by removing irrelevant items. For example, an item based on the question 'Are you disappointed if the GP does not prescribe any medicine for you?' is really about the attitude of the patient to the consultation with the GP and not about how prescribed medicine is used. Therefore, this item should be cut out of the questionnaire.

When using a questionnaire to obtain feedback on your performance when giving a talk, your aim should be something like: 'To find out what was good and what was bad about my talk, and how I could have improved it'.

Order of presentation

The order in which items are presented in a questionnaire can make a difference to the quality of data collected.

Suppose you were designing a questionnaire investigating the attitudes and behaviour of adults to their elderly, infirm relatives. You might want to know how much informal care the respondents provide to their elderly relatives. This could range from respondents who live with elderly people and provide many care needs to those with elderly relatives in residential homes who receive very little informal care from the respondents. You might also want to measure how positive or negative the attitudes of the respondents are to elderly people.

In the above example, it would be much better to include the attitude items first in the questionnaire, followed by the items on the level of informal care provided.

The reason is that respondents who do not provide much care might feel guilty about this. If they are asked about the level of informal care first and then asked to indicate their attitude to elderly people, they might be tempted to exaggerate how positive their attitudes are. In this case, asking about attitudes first would probably produce more accurate data.

Ethical treatment

As with all social research methods it is important to follow ethical guidelines:

+ Informed consent – potential respondents should be informed of the purpose of the questionnaire and given anonymity. Respondents should understand that they do not have to take part and that, if they do, they have a right to leave answers blank if they wish. This information should be stated to respondents and also included on the questionnaire.

+ Items should be chosen and worded so as to avoid offending respondents, either because of the subject matter or because of the wording. For example, 'Would you describe yourself as fat?' is likely to be considered offensive by some.

+ Items that seriously invade a person's privacy should be avoided – for example, 'How many times per week do you take illegal drugs?'

Methodological issues

Social desirability bias

It is easy to give clues to respondents about what the most 'socially desirable' responses are. For example, in a questionnaire on smoking and health, most respondents will be aware that our society disapproves of smoking. This could result in some participants being biased into giving inaccurate answers, for example by understating how frequently they smoke.

The problem of social desirability is that it tempts respondents to give the responses they feel they ought to give, or think you want, rather than saying what they really feel, think or do.

Suppose that a questionnaire on smoking and health starts with a section on smoking behaviour and then goes on to ask about health status. The risk is that non-smokers could be tempted to understate any health problems they have, because not smoking tends to be associated with good health. Similarly, smokers might be tempted to overstate their health problems. This could lead to poor-quality data, giving an exaggerated impression of the link between smoking and health status.

One way of reducing this kind of social desirability effect is by careful choice of the order in which the items are arranged. Using the example given above, it would be better to ask about health status before asking about smoking.

Another way to reduce the influence of social desirability is to try to make the questionnaire neutral overall – for example, by including some statements that are positive about the topic and some that are negative. In the example below, item 6 is positive and item 7 is negative.

(6). 'Smoking is a good way of reducing stress.'

Agree strongly ☐   Agree ☐   Undecided ☐   Disagree ☐   Disagree strongly ☐

(7). 'Smoking increases the speed of ageing.'

Agree strongly ☐   Agree ☐   Undecided ☐   Disagree ☐   Disagree strongly ☐

Response bias

Response bias is a slightly different problem. It sometimes happens that a series of items in a questionnaire follows a similar pattern. For example, a feedback questionnaire following a residential course might include the following items:

Please rate the following aspects of your course by circling one number for each item.

Quality of accommodation

Very poor 1 2 3 4 5 6 7 8 9 Excellent

Quality of the first presentation (Mrs Obaid)

Very poor 1 2 3 4 5 6 7 8 9 Excellent

Quality of the second presentation (Mr Atkinson)

Very poor 1 2 3 4 5 6 7 8 9 Excellent

Quality of the third presentation (Ms O'Leary)

Very poor 1 2 3 4 5 6 7 8 9 Excellent

Helpfulness of centre staff

Very poor 1 2 3 4 5 6 7 8 9 Excellent

What can happen is that, for example, a respondent starts by circling '6' for the first item, then '6' for the second item, '6 'for the third item and then stops giving proper attention to the remaining items, assuming that the other responses will be the same.

The way to get around response bias is to prevent the items from following the same pattern, so that the respondents have to keep thinking about what they are doing.

When Likert items are included, response bias can be avoided by including some positively and some negatively worded items. It is usually possible to rewrite a positive item so it becomes a negative one and vice versa. If positive and negative items alternate, the respondent is less likely to answer in a careless, repetitive way.

Trialling

It is very difficult to write questionnaire items that are clear and that succeed in finding the information you want. For this reason, it is important to try out a questionnaire on a few people who will tell you how easy or difficult it was to follow. Items that did not work well can be changed or deleted.

You should also try processing the data collected in the trial, so that you can iron out any other problems that might arise.

Producing the questionnaire

The final questionnaire should be word-processed and printed, so that copies can be made.

Depending on your intended sample, you might have to decide whether to produce copies in languages other than English, or in bilingual (e.g. English/Welsh) versions.

Carrying out a questionnaire survey

Sampling

Sampling is the process by which a researcher finds people to be participants in a research study. Ideally, the sample studied should be large and selected to be representative of the population from which it is drawn.

Questionnaires are sometimes distributed by post to hundreds or thousands of people, with the expectation that only a fairly small proportion will be completed and returned. This can still result in a large sample. However, the sample might not be representative of the population, because the people who take time to fill in the questionnaire might be those who have more leisure time than most — perhaps retired people. The result is a self-selected sample.

Fewer sampling problems occur when the population to be studied is small and easy for the researcher to access. For example, a hospital trust might want to measure satisfaction among patients who have received hospital treatment. A representative sample could be obtained by asking patients to fill in the questionnaire before they are discharged from hospital, or possibly at a follow-up appointment.

For your student research, the recommended approach is to make personal contact with the people you wish to have as participants. You might leave the questionnaire with them and return to collect it. In some cases, it might be possible to wait while the questionnaire is filled in. It will rarely be practical to study a large sample.

Initial request

Ideally, you should recruit participants by asking them to take part in your questionnaire study, outlining what it is about and why you are doing it. You should ensure that each potential participant has a real opportunity to refuse to take part. It is not a good idea to persuade people to take part. If they are not keen, the quality of data you will collect is likely to be poor.

You should also make clear whether or not the questionnaire is genuinely anonymous. If it is, then no one, not even you, will know who has filled in which copy of the questionnaire.

One way of showing this is by having a large envelope with 'Completed questionnaires' written on it. When a respondent hands you the questionnaire, do not read it, but immediately put it into the envelope.

Conditions statement

Your questionnaire should also have a statement at the start indicating whether or not it is anonymous and restating the right of the respondent to withdraw or not to fill in all items.

At the end of the questionnaire, you should include a statement thanking the respondent.

If you are not intending to collect the questionnaire yourself, you should include instructions for returning it.

Data processing

The data recorded on a questionnaire (ticks in boxes, lists and written answers) are called 'raw data'. Raw data do not provide immediate answers. If you look through a pile of completed questionnaires to obtain an impression of what they show, you are likely to end up quite confused. There are simply too many data. The purpose of data processing is to summarise the raw data so as to be able to pick out any patterns that are present.

Measures of central tendency

This section introduces you to the use of calculations to find the **mean**, **median** and **mode** of sets of scores.

The mean, median and mode are sometimes called '**measures of central tendency**' because each is used to summarise a set of scores with a single number that is usually at or near the middle of a set of scores. Being able to summarise a set of scores with one number is very useful when making comparisons.

For example, if you studied how much exercise a sample of male and female students took, it would be useful to end up with one number representing male exercise and one number representing female exercise. You could then draw conclusions about whether there was a difference between the sexes in the amount of exercise undertaken.

You might ask: 'Why have three measures of central tendency instead of just one?' If you had to choose just one measure of central tendency, the mean would be the best because it makes use of all the data available. One reason for having other measures is that in some situations the mean cannot be used – the next best measure is usually the median.

The mean

The mean can be used with data that are on a scale with a zero point and equal intervals. Statisticians sometimes call this a ratio scale.

Examples of ratio scales include measurements of length, time and frequency of behaviour reported by individual respondents. For example, you could use the mean with pedometer readings from people who recorded how far they walked in a day at work. You could also use it with respondents' reports of the number of visitors they met in a week.

The mean of a set of scores is easy to calculate. You just add up the scores of all the respondents and divide the total by the number of respondents.

Respondent number	Number of minutes spent reading to child
1	10
2	55
3	0
4	15
5	25
6	0
7	20
8	10

Table 2.1

Table 2.1 shows the number of minutes that eight parents of 3-year-old children said they spent reading to the child on a single day. Each respondent (parent) is given a respondent number.

To work out the mean reading time:
+ add up the eight reading times — the total is 135 minutes
+ then, divide this by the number of respondents, which is 8 — this gives a mean time of 16.875 minutes

It is fairly clear that the reading times are estimates to the nearest 5 minutes, so we should not state the result to one thousandth of a minute. This would give the impression that the data were measured much more accurately than was the case. In this case, the total would be rounded to the nearest minute. Therefore, the mean reading time is 17 minutes.

In the above example there is quite a degree of variation in the data, with one parent reading for nearly an hour and two parents not reading at all. This shows a drawback of summarising data. While it is useful to give a mean score, it is also important to comment on the pattern or range of scores.

The median

In cases where numerical scores have been collected that are not on a ratio scale, the median can be used. In questionnaires, this most often happens when rating scales are used. For example, if a person is asked to rate how interesting a talk was on a scale of 1 to 5, the ratings would be on what statisticians call an 'ordinal scale'. Data on an ordinal scale should not be divided or multiplied, so the mean cannot be used.

The median is the middle score of a set of scores, once those scores have been put in rank order.

Table 2.2

Respondent number	Rating of interest (5 is high)
1	3
2	4
3	2
4	3
5	3
6	5
7	4
8	5
9	4

Table 2.2 shows ratings given by a group of nine students asked to judge how interesting a talk was.

The scores are ranked as follows:

2, 3, 3, 3, 4, 4, 4, 5, 5

The middle value of these nine scores is 4. This is the median.

Finding the median is easy when there is an odd number of scores, as in the example above. However, when there is an even number of scores, there is no middle value. The usual way to deal with this is to split the difference between the middle two scores.

For example, consider the following ranked set of eight scores:

1, 3, 3, 3, 4, 5, 5, 5

The two scores nearest the middle are 3 and 4, so the median is 3.5.

The mode

The mode is the least useful of the measures of central tendency. It is the most frequently occurring score in a set of scores. This is no use when all the scores are different and not much use when two scores occur an equal number of times. For example, in the ranked scores:

1, 3, 3, 3, 4, 5, 5, 5

there are two modes, 3 and 5 — both numbers occur three times.

The only advantage of the mode is that it can be used where responses are not numerical. For example, if you asked a sample of people what their favourite sport was, you would collect data in the form of names of sports, such as cycling, football, swimming and so on. The mode would be the sport that was mentioned most often (if there was one).

Example questionnaire

Below is a questionnaire investigating pet ownership and life satisfaction among retired people who live alone. The main aim of the questionnaire is to find out whether there are differences in life satisfaction between people who own pets and people who do not. A researcher might use this questionnaire as a first step in finding out whether the quality of life of single retired people could be improved by owning a pet.

This questionnaire is referred to in the following section on scoring and analysis of questionnaire items.

This questionnaire is about everyday experience of life, including keeping a pet. If there are any items you would prefer not to fill in, please leave them blank.

Section A

In the items below, please show to what extent each statement is true for you, by ticking the appropriate box.

(1) I feel contented most of the time.

Agree strongly ☐   Agree ☐   Undecided ☐   Disagree ☐   Disagree strongly ☐

(2) I often feel lonely.

Agree strongly ☐   Agree ☐   Undecided ☐   Disagree ☐   Disagree strongly ☐

(3) I sometimes wonder whether my daily routine is worth the effort.

Agree strongly ☐   Agree ☐   Undecided ☐   Disagree ☐   Disagree strongly ☐

(4) I hardly ever worry about myself.

Agree strongly ☐   Agree ☐   Undecided ☐   Disagree ☐   Disagree strongly ☐

(5) My life at the moment is quite rewarding.

Agree strongly ☐   Agree ☐   Undecided ☐   Disagree ☐   Disagree strongly ☐

(6) I sometimes get anxious about unimportant matters.

Agree strongly ☐   Agree ☐   Undecided ☐   Disagree ☐   Disagree strongly ☐

Section B

(7) Do you own a pet or pets at present? Yes ☐ No ☐

If you answered 'No' to the last question, please go to the end of this questionnaire.

(8) In the space below, please list the type and number of pets you own (e.g. 1 dog, 4 goldfish etc.).

_____

_____

_____

Section C

In the items below, please show to what extent each statement about your pet or pets is true for you, by ticking the appropriate box.

(9) Having a pet provides me with companionship.

Agree strongly ☐ Agree ☐ Undecided ☐ Disagree ☐ Disagree strongly ☐

(10) I enjoy having a pet to look after.

Agree strongly ☐ Agree ☐ Undecided ☐ Disagree ☐ Disagree strongly ☐

(11) Having a pet makes me take exercise.

Agree strongly ☐ Agree ☐ Undecided ☐ Disagree ☐ Disagree strongly ☐

(12) Using the space below, please write down any other reasons why you have a pet or pets._____

_____

_____

Thank you for taking time to fill in this questionnaire.

Read the questionnaire carefully.

+ Pick out one open question and one closed question.
+ From section A, pick out one positive item and one negative item.
+ Why does section A contain both positive and negative items?
+ Which section of the questionnaire is aimed at studying behaviour?
+ Which section of the questionnaire is most likely to raise ethical issues?

Scoring and analysis of questionnaire items

Questionnaires produce a lot of data. These data are of value if they can be summarised to produce a conclusion or a set of conclusions, i.e. to answer the research question asked. The purpose of data analysis is to process the data so that valid conclusions can be drawn.

Should poor-quality data be analysed?

A questionnaire might produce poor-quality data because:

+ some or all of the items are poorly written
+ the respondents have not taken it seriously

Some people think that all questionnaires are a waste of time. This could be because they have been asked to fill in many badly designed questionnaires in the past.

Some people seem to resent being restricted to closed and forced-choice items and respond by trying to express themselves by giving silly answers.

The result in both these cases is that the data collected will be of poor quality – they will not reflect what the respondent actually feels, thinks or does. Therefore, it is best to be cautious when using these data, and it may even be justifiable to ignore them.

In reporting a questionnaire study, it is important to state if data have been ignored and to explain why.

Methods of analysis

There are various ways of analysing questionnaire data, depending on the type of item. These analytical methods are illustrated with reference to the example questionnaire on pages 63–64.

Collating results

Some closed items can be processed by counting the number of each type of response. In the example above, item 7 can be processed by counting the number of respondents who said 'Yes', and the number who said 'No'. Item 7 is likely to be used to sort the questionnaires into two categories – those completed by pet owners and those completed by non-owners. This will enable differences between these two groups to be found.

Working out the number of respondents who gave one particular answer is called 'collating' the results.

It would also be possible to use the data from item 8 to separate cat owners from dog owners, in order to look at differences between these two groups.

When an item is used to collect data about the frequency of behaviour, the data can be summarised by calculating the mean. The data are on ratio scales. Item 8 produces such data. By reading the responses, the number of pets owned by each respondent can be found.

Table 2.3 shows the number of pets owned by a sample of ten respondents. The respondents are given numbers from 1 to 10.

If required, the mean number of pets owned can be calculated by finding the total number of pets listed and dividing by the number of pet owners:

total number of pets = 19
number of pet owners = 10
mean number of pets = 1.9 per owner

Scoring rating-scale items

Rating-scale items can be scored by collating, i.e. counting the number of times each rating is given.

For example, in item 9, the number of respondents who 'agree strongly' that a pet provides them with

Respondent number	Number of pets owned
1	3
2	1
3	1
4	1
5	5
6	2
7	1
8	2
9	1
10	2

Table 2.3

companionship would be counted, then the number who 'agree', were 'undecided', who 'disagree' and who 'disagree strongly'.

Table 2.4 shows responses to the statement that 'a pet provides companionship'.

Table 2.4

Respondent number	Agree strongly	Agree	Undecided	Disagree	Disagree strongly
1		✔			
2	✔				
3	✔				
4			✔		
5		✔			
6		✔			
7				✔	
8		✔			
9		✔			
10	✔				
Total	**3**	**5**	**1**	**1**	**0**

These data can be summarised by reporting that:

Item 9 – 'Having a pet provides me with companionship' – produced the following responses:

+ 3 respondents agreed strongly
+ 5 agreed
+ 1 was undecided
+ 1 disagreed
+ No respondents disagreed strongly

There are several ways of processing these data further, if required. One way is to calculate the percentage of respondents who showed agreement. This includes those who ticked the 'agree strongly' box and those who ticked the 'agree' box. The total is eight participants out of ten, or 80%.

Another way is to assign numerical values to the ratings. With a 5-point rating scale (as used in item 9), the values given are normally 1 to 5. With item 9, it seems best to give 'agree strongly' a rating of 5 and 'disagree strongly' a rating of 1.

The rating scale with numerical ratings is shown below.

Agree strongly ⑤ Agree ④ Undecided ③ Disagree ② Disagree strongly ①

The table showing responses to item 9 is reproduced again on the next page, but this time with numerical ratings instead of ticks (Table 2.5). The data are the same, but in numerical form.

To summarise these data, you might be tempted to add up all the ratings and divide by the number of respondents to get a mean rating. This is not a bad idea.

Respondent number	Agree strongly	Agree	Undecided	Disagree	Disagree strongly
1		4			
2	5				
3	5				
4			3		
5		4			
6		4			
7				2	
8		4			
9		4			
10	5				

Table 2.5

However, rating-scale data (which are on an ordinal scale, i.e. just show an order of preference) should not be divided or multiplied (unlike data that count, for example, frequencies of events or time taken). In this case, the median should be used.

In rank order, the ratings from the table above are:

2, 3, 4, 4, 4, 4, 4, 5, 5, 5

There is an even number of scores, so there is no middle score. Therefore, we take the two scores that are closest to the middle and split the difference. The data from item 9 have a fifth place score of 4 and a sixth place score of 4. The median is therefore 4.

Processing attitude scores

The methods of data processing described so far are adequate to deal with most of the items in sections B and C of the example questionnaire. Section A requires a different approach. Section A is designed to find out about the general satisfaction with life of each respondent. The expectation is that if respondents are satisfied with their lives, they will agree with such statements as, 'I feel contented most of the time', and disagree with such statements as, 'I sometimes wonder whether my daily routine is worth the effort'.

These items are designed to be taken together, as a measure of life satisfaction. Therefore, a way of combining the data from all six items is needed, in order to obtain one score for each respondent. This is achieved by converting the verbal ratings to numerical ones (as described above) and then adding up the ratings for all six items for each respondent.

Some of the statements are positive (statements 1, 4 and 5); some are negative (statements 2, 3 and 6). Therefore, the rating for 'agree strongly' will not always be 5.

The decision is made that a person who feels satisfied with life should be given a high score and a dissatisfied person should be given a low score. This means that the 'agree strongly' rating should be 5 for the positive items and 1 for the negative items.

Section A is reproduced below with these ratings included.

(1) I feel contented most of the time.
Agree strongly ⑤ Agree ④ Undecided ③ Disagree ② Disagree strongly ①

(2) I often feel lonely.
Agree strongly ① Agree ② Undecided ③ Disagree ④ Disagree strongly ⑤

(3) I sometimes wonder whether my daily routine is worth the effort.
Agree strongly ① Agree ② Undecided ③ Disagree ④ Disagree strongly ⑤

(4) I hardly ever worry about myself.
Agree strongly ⑤ Agree ④ Undecided ③ Disagree ② Disagree strongly ①

(5) My life at the moment is quite rewarding.
Agree strongly ⑤ Agree ④ Undecided ③ Disagree ② Disagree strongly ①

(6) I sometimes get anxious about unimportant matters.
Agree strongly ① Agree ② Undecided ③ Disagree ④ Disagree strongly ⑤

The highest score a person could obtain on this life-satisfaction scale is $6 \times 5 = 30$. The lowest score is $6 \times 1 = 6$.

Work out the life-satisfaction score for a person who ticked the boxes as follows:

Try it out

(1) I feel contented most of the time.
Agree strongly ☐ Agree ☐ Undecided ☐ Disagree ☑ Disagree strongly ☐

(2) I often feel lonely.
Agree strongly ☐ Agree ☐ Undecided ☑ Disagree ☐ Disagree strongly ☐

(3) I sometimes wonder whether my daily routine is worth the effort.
Agree strongly ☐ Agree ☐ Undecided ☑ Disagree ☐ Disagree strongly ☐

(4) I hardly ever worry about myself.
Agree strongly ☐ Agree ☐ Undecided ☐ Disagree ☑ Disagree strongly ☐

(5) My life at the moment is quite rewarding.
Agree strongly ☐ Agree ☐ Undecided ☑ Disagree ☐ Disagree strongly ☐

(6) I sometimes get anxious about unimportant matters.
Agree strongly ☑ Agree ☐ Undecided ☐ Disagree ☐ Disagree strongly ☐

You could also fill in section A yourself and work out your own life-satisfaction score.

Once scores have been found for each participant, a comparison can be made between pet owners and non-owners, to find out whether or not people who own pets are more satisfied with life than those who do not.

Table 2.6 shows life-satisfaction scores from ten pet owners and nine non-owners.

Table 2.6

Respondent	Pet owners' score	Respondent	Non-owners' score
1	17	1	16
2	21	2	12
3	14	3	14
4	18	4	10
5	12	5	11
6	15	6	11
7	23	7	13
8	18	8	15
9	14	9	16
10	16		

To find out whether there is a difference between the two groups, the median score for each group is calculated:
+ For pet owners, the rank order of the scores is: 12, 14, 14, 15, 16, 17, 18, 18, 21, 23
+ The median (because there is an even number of scores) is 16.5.
+ For non-owners, the rank order of the scores is: 10, 11, 11, 12, 13, 14, 15, 16, 16
+ The median (and middle score) is 13.

From these data, the non-owners seem to be slightly less satisfied with their lives than the pet owners. This might be because owning a pet really does make you feel more satisfied.

You have probably noticed that there are different numbers of pet owners and non-owners. This is not a problem, as long as the median scores of the two groups are compared, rather than the overall total scores.

Processing data from open questions

Some open questions are quite easy to process. Item 8 on the example questionnaire asks respondents to list the number and type of pets they own. As we have already seen, numerical data can be extracted simply by counting the number of pets listed. The data can also be sorted into categories, according to type of pet (e.g. dogs, cats, birds, fish). Information can then be extracted about the commonest types of pet for the group of respondents. Comparisons could also be made between, say, cat owners and dog owners. It would not be surprising to find differences between these in responses to item 11: 'Having a pet makes me take exercise'.

Item 12 on the example questionnaire invites respondents to list reasons for owning a pet. Responses to this could be processed by finding the number of times the same (or similar) reason is given. For example, several participants might say that having a pet dog makes them feel safe at night because it could deter burglars. The most commonly occurring reasons could then be reported.

Data from open questions can also be processed by selecting quotations that can be used to make a point in the report. For example, it might be worth quoting a respondent who wrote, 'My dog seems to know how I'm feeling. If I'm a bit down, he tries to cheer me up. It usually works, too'.

Drawing conclusions

After analysing and processing summarised data, it is important to draw correct conclusions from these data. It is best to restrict those conclusions to the sample of respondents studied. Referring to the example questionnaire, you might conclude that 'pet owners in the sample reported slightly higher levels of life satisfaction than non-owners'.

Generalising to the target population

It is tempting to draw conclusions about the population from which the respondents were drawn. A conclusion such as this might say, 'Single, retired pet owners are more satisfied with their lives than single, retired non-owners'. This conclusion would be justified only if you could be sure that the sample of respondents studied was truly typical or 'representative' of all single, retired people. With a sample smaller than several hundred randomly selected respondents it would be difficult to justify drawing such a conclusion.

Drawing conclusions about cause and effect

In the example questionnaire, we found that pet owners were slightly more satisfied with life than non-owners. You might be tempted to conclude that owning a pet was the reason for this difference in satisfaction. It might be, but the data do not justify such a conclusion. The data show that, in this sample, there is a link between pet ownership and life satisfaction, but not how it is caused. It is quite possible that people who are more satisfied with their lives are more likely to buy pets. Some non-owners might be discontented people who hate animals and perhaps hate other things too. For such a person, buying a pet might lead to a decrease in life satisfaction, rather than an increase.

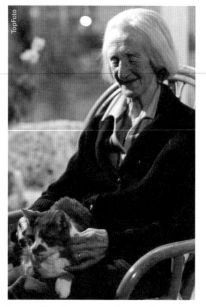

It could be that pets make people more contented; alternatively, discontented people could be more likely to hate animals

Try it out

One reason why it is so easy to fall into this trap is that lots of other people do. A study once revealed that people who prayed tended to live longer than people who did not. A newspaper reported this with the claim that 'prayer can prolong your life'. Try to think of differences in the way people who pray and people who do not pray might behave. Could some of these differences be more likely explanations of the difference in lifespan?

Just because two things go together, we should not assume that one must cause the other. This assumption is a kind of trap.

Data presentation

Once the raw data have been processed, the findings should be displayed so that they are clear to someone reading the research report. This can often be achieved by the use of tables, bar charts and pie charts.

All tables and charts must be clearly introduced and preferably titled, so that the content can be understood. If the data have units of measurement (e.g. kilograms, seconds or metres), these should be stated. It is sometimes useful to give maximum and minimum possible scores, so that a reader can judge whether the respondents' scores were high, low or in-between.

Tables

Tables are sometimes used as a convenient way of presenting raw data that have been extracted from a set of completed questionnaires, but not processed. Table 2.4, showing responses to item 9 in the pet questionnaire, is an example of this.

This table is reproduced below (Table 2.7), with an extra row in which the raw data have been processed.

Respondent number	Agree strongly	Agree	Undecided	Disagree	Disagree strongly
1		4			
2	5				
3	5				
4			3		
5		4			
6		4			
7				2	
8		4			
9		4			
10	5				
Total	**3**	**5**	**1**	**1**	**0**

Table 2.7
Responses to the statement that 'having a pet provides companionship'

A table could be used to present the processed data:

Level of agreement	Agree strongly	Agree	Undecided	Disagree	Disagree strongly
Total responses	3	5	1	1	0
Percentage of all responses	30	50	10	10	0

Table 2.8
Total responses and percentage of all responses to the statement 'having a pet provides companionship'

Bar charts

A bar chart is a simple method of presenting data graphically. A bar chart could be used to display the data from the table above (see Figure 2.1).

Figure 2.1
Percentage levels of agreement with the statement that 'a pet provides companionship'

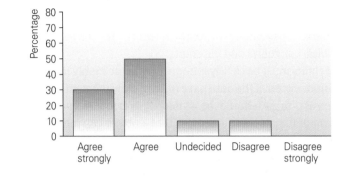

Bar charts can be presented with either horizontal or vertical bars. Key features of simple bar charts are that:
+ there is a space separating each bar from the next
+ if the bars are vertical, there is a scale on the vertical axis
+ if the bars are horizontal, there is a scale on the horizontal axis

A second example illustrates the use of a table and a bar chart to present a difference between two groups.

Table 2.9
Median life-satisfaction scores of pet owners and non-owners

Category of respondent	Median score (minimum = 6; maximum = 30)
Pet owners	16.5
Non-owners	13

The best way to present these data graphically is with a bar chart, showing two bars (Figure 2.2).

Figure 2.2
Median life-satisfaction scores of pet owners and non-owners

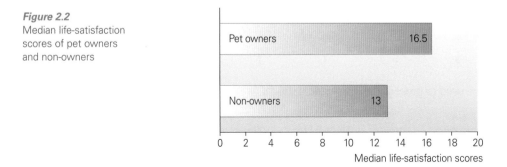

Compound bar charts can be used, for example to make comparisons between males and female on a range of different issues (Figure 2.3).

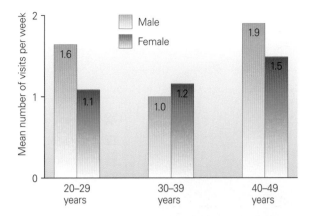

Figure 2.3
Mean frequency of visits to a sports centre by males and females in three age groups

Graphs and tables should express data clearly. The best way to do this is to keep them as simple and uncluttered as possible. A complicated bar chart with many bars might seem impressive, but it is unlikely to show findings clearly.

Pie charts

A pie chart is a simple method of presenting data graphically. Pie charts are best used for data that show how a fixed total is divided up.

For example, a fixed total might be the 24 hours in a day. Suppose a researcher carried out a survey into how hospital patients spent their time each day. Patients could be asked to estimate how long they spent asleep, how long they spent in conversation with others (e.g. visitors), how long they spent receiving care or treatment (including bathing and eating) and so on. The mean times for each category for a sample of respondents could be found, and then expressed as proportionate slices of a pie (Figure 2.4). The whole pie represents 24 hours.

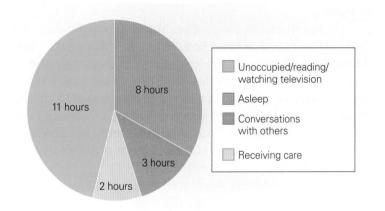

Figure 2.4
Mean time taken up by different activities for hospital patients in a 24-hour period

Pie charts can also be used to show the proportion of respondents in each of several categories. For example, the number of patients whose condition after treatment is categorised as fully recovered, significantly improved, marginally improved, unchanged or worsened (Figure 2.5). The fixed total in this case is the number of patients in the sample.

Figure 2.5
Outcomes of treatment for 36 patients

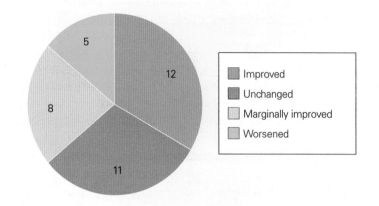

Data expressed as percentages can also be displayed using a pie chart. In this case the fixed total is 100.

A common error

It is a common error to use both a bar chart and a pie chart to present the same data. Only one method of graphical presentation should be used for any one data set. The more appropriate method should be chosen.

Common errors in questionnaire design

Writing questionnaire items is more difficult than people think. It requires a very clear, careful and precise use of language. One problem is that the person writing the item knows what they mean but a respondent might interpret the item differently.

For example, you might write the question, 'Would you say you drink too much?' The intention of your question might be to find out how many respondents drink alcohol excessively. However, respondents who drink excessively might answer 'No', meaning that however much they drink they do not think it is too much. Other respondents, taking the question literally, might answer 'No' meaning that even if they did drink too much they would not admit it. Others might not realise that the question is about alcohol. Such respondents might not drink alcohol but could be aware of the health benefits of drinking plenty of water every day. These respondents might answer 'Probably not enough'.

The problem with the question 'Would you say you drink too much?' is that the writer has not thought carefully enough about the intention behind the item. It could be an item intended to collect data about drinking behaviour or it could be about the attitudes of the respondents to their own drinking.

If the intention were to collect information about drinking behaviour, it would be better to use an item asking participants to report their actual intake.

Respondents could be asked how often they drink alcohol or to estimate the number of pints (or other measure) they drink each week.

If the intention were to measure attitudes to drinking alcohol, this would be better done using a Likert-type item such as: 'I am worried that I drink more alcohol than is good for me'.

Another problem is caused by writing items that respondents cannot be expected to answer accurately. For example, the question 'How many times have you been to a pub or licensed club this year?' is unlikely to produce accurate answers unless respondents have been previously asked to keep a diary. The question 'How many times have you been to a pub or licensed club in the past week?' is much better.

An effective questionnaire item is likely to be the result of much editing and rewriting, as well as trialling with respondents, including some from the population to be studied. This means that trying out a questionnaire with fellow students might not be enough. They might think in the same way as you and therefore not spot problems that, say, an older person might experience.

Specific errors in writing questionnaire items

Below is a list of some of the more common problems that occur in writing questionnaire items. You should familiarise yourself with these, and use them to evaluate questionnaires written by yourself and by others.

+ **Inadequate indication of how to respond** – this means that respondents are not told clearly how they should show their answer. It is important to give guidance such as 'Tick one box', 'Tick any boxes that apply' or 'Please write your answer in the box provided'.
+ **Inadequate category ranges** – items asking people to categorise themselves according to age or behaviour should have categories to fit all respondents. For example, in a questionnaire about smoking, if people were asked to indicate whether they were either a 'cigarette smoker' or a 'non-smoker', someone who was a pipe-smoker would not be able to respond.
+ **Overlapping categories** – another common mistake is to use categories that overlap, so some respondents might fit into two categories. This would be a problem if they had been asked to tick one box. For example, if you asked cigarette smokers how many they smoked on a typical day and gave them categories such as '10 to 20', '20 to 30' and so on, people who smoked 20 a day could fit into two categories and would be unsure how to respond.
+ **Non-discriminating items** – items that most respondents are likely to answer in the same way are unlikely to yield useful information and should be deleted. An example of a non-discriminating item is, 'Would you agree that growing children need a good diet?'
+ **Lack of precision** – items written imprecisely often appear clear and unambiguous to the writer, but not to the respondent. An example of an

imprecise question is, 'When they talk about healthy eating, do you think "Why bother?"?'

+ **Technical language** — unless respondents are known to have particular technical knowledge (e.g. nurses), the wording of items should avoid technical terms. For example, a questionnaire item asking people to estimate the number of units of alcohol they drink in a typical week would create problems for those respondents who are not aware how much a unit of alcohol is.

+ **Leading questions** — a leading question is one that hints that the researcher wants the respondent to answer in a particular way. This is a problem because the data collected might not reflect the actual views of the respondents. An example of a leading question is, 'Most people think smoking in public is anti-social. Do you agree?'

+ **Presuming questions** — these are items that appear to make assumptions about the respondent. For example, the item 'Do you drink more alcohol at weekends than you do on weekdays?' presumes that the respondent does actually drink alcohol. However, this would not be a presuming question if you had already asked respondents to categorise themselves as drinkers or non-drinkers and you had diverted the non-drinkers away from this item.

+ **Double questions** — items that contain two linked questions. It will not be clear what the respondents intend by their answers. An example of a double question is, 'Do you think that smoking makes people less healthy and less attractive? *Yes/No*'. If the respondent answers '*Yes*' or '*No*', we cannot be sure whether the answer relates to the 'healthy' part of the question or the 'attractive' part of the question, or both. This item should be divided into two.

Sometimes, a single, badly written item might feature several of these errors. For example, an item that is a leading question is also likely to be non-discriminating, because most respondents will answer it in the same way.

General errors in the questionnaire

Below is a list of some of the more common problems that occur in writing questionnaires. You should familiarise yourself with these, and use them to evaluate questionnaires written by you and others.

Inadequate guidance through the items

This is mainly a problem in branching questionnaires. If there is a point requiring a choice, the respondent should be told which item to go to next. For example, 'If you answered "Yes" to the last item, please go to item 15'.

Risk of bias

Bias can occur for several reasons:

+ The researcher has strong opinions about the topic, which are obvious to the respondents. Researchers should try to avoid revealing their own opinions or biases.

+ The topic gives rise to social-desirability effects, as mentioned on page 58.

+ Response bias can occur if there is a series of positive (or a series of negative) items. A good questionnaire should appear to be neutral towards the topic. Neutrality can be achieved by writing neutral items or by writing a mixture of positive and negative items.

Over-restricted response opportunities

Respondents might feel frustrated when completing a questionnaire on a topic about which they feel strongly but in which there are no opportunities to say how they feel. For this reason, occasional free-response items are useful.

Unnecessary or irrelevant items

A common fault in questionnaires produced by inexperienced writers is to include items to 'pad out' a questionnaire. A good questionnaire is the shortest one that achieves the aim of the researcher. Respondents often dislike filling in long questionnaires and the dislike is even stronger if they feel that some of the items are pointless. For example, in a questionnaire on cigarette smoking and health, an item asking which brands of cigarette are smoked is not really relevant. More relevant would be to ask whether respondents mainly smoke filter or non-filter cigarettes, low-tar cigarettes and so on.

Unethical practices

These include failure to:

+ indicate the purpose of the questionnaire
+ inform respondents of their freedom to take part or not
+ ensure anonymity (if this is required)

They also refer to questionnaires that are discourteous in tone or contain items that are potentially upsetting or insulting to some respondents.

Example of a poor questionnaire

The following example questionnaire about pet ownership illustrates the specific errors listed above. First, read it from the point of view of a person who does not have a pet. Then read it from the point of view of a person aged 70, who is very fond of her pet cat. Try to identify as many errors as you can in this questionnaire, before reading the comment section that follows it.

The aim of this anonymous questionnaire is to find out about pet ownership among adults.

(1) Please print your name here: _____

(2) Please tick the box which shows your age.
    20–30 ☐   30–40 ☐   40–50 ☐   50–60 ☐

(3) Do you own a pet? Yes ☐   No ☐

(4) What sort of pet is it?
    Cat ☐   Dog ☐   Guinea pig ☐   Mouse ☐   Hamster ☐   Fish ☐

(5) How did you get it?

_____

(6) What was your reason for getting a pet? Tick one box.
Felt lonely ☐   Like animals ☐   Children wanted one ☐

(7) Do you agree that pets are expensive to keep and a lot of trouble to look after?
Yes ☐   No ☐

(8) Do you agree that cruelty to animals is a bad thing?
Yes ☐   No ☐

(9) There is a high risk of children contracting toxocariasis from cat faeces. Tick one box.
Agree strongly ☐   Agree ☐   Undecided ☐   Disagree ☐   Disagree strongly ☐

(10) It is wrong to own a pet that eats meat when there are starving people in the world.
Agree strongly ☐   Agree ☐   Undecided ☐   Disagree ☐   Disagree strongly ☐

(11) Animals should not be kept in captivity.
Agree strongly ☐   Agree ☐   Undecided ☐   Disagree ☐   Disagree strongly ☐

(12) Most people who own pets do not have enough time to care for them properly.
Agree strongly ☐   Agree ☐   Undecided ☐   Disagree ☐   Disagree strongly ☐

Thank you for completing this questionnaire.

Comments on the poor questionnaire

Generally, the questionnaire reveals the attitude of the writer — someone who is opposed to pet ownership. It is not effective at finding out what respondents think. Specific errors include:

+ **Unethical practice**:
    + The questionnaire claims to be anonymous, but item 1 asks for the name of the respondent.
    + Items 10, 11 and 12 are potentially insulting to some pet-owning respondents.
+ **Overlapping categories**: in item 2, the ages 30, 40 and 50 each appear in two boxes.
+ **Inadequate category range**:
    + Item 2 — adults over 60 cannot respond
    + Item 4 — rules out other pets; should ask, 'Other, please specify'
    + Item 6 — probably better as a free-response item
+ **Inadequate guidance through the items**: if a respondent answers 'No' to item 3, items 4, 5 and 6 are not relevant to them. Appropriate guidance might be, 'If you answer "No" to item 3, please go to item 7'.
+ **Inadequate indication of how to respond**: in item 5, perhaps some response-choice boxes have been omitted, or perhaps this is supposed to be a free-response item. Either way, the respondent should be given guidance on how to respond.
+ **Double question**: item 7
+ **Leading question**: item 7
+ **Risk of bias**: items 7 and 9 to 12 are all negative

+ **Undiscriminating item**: item 8
+ **Technical language**: in item 9, terms such as 'toxocariasis' and 'faeces' might be a barrier to some respondents.
+ **Lack of precision**:
  + Item 5 — it is not clear whether this is asking about the source of the pet (e.g. pet shop, Cats Protection League) or whether it is asking how it was transported home.
  + Item 10 — it is not clear what the link is between starving people and, say, tinned catfood.
+ **Over-restricted response opportunities**: there are no free-response items that pet owners in particular might wish to respond to.
+ **Unnecessary or irrelevant questions**: it is difficult to see the focus of the questionnaire. Items such as 5, 8 and 10 seem irrelevant.

Checklist for evaluating questionnaires

In questionnaires you design, use this list to check for errors.
+ Is the questionnaire so long that respondents will lose interest?
+ Are any items unnecessary?
+ Do all the items include response boxes (or similar)?
+ Are category ranges complete but not overlapping?
+ Are all items precise and discriminating?
+ Is the language appropriate (e.g. not too technical)?
+ Are any items leading, presuming or double questions?
+ Is there a risk of bias (e.g. response bias) in individual items or the questionnaire as a whole?
+ Is there a combination of open and closed items?
+ Is the questionnaire ethical?

Useful website

There are several websites giving useful advice on questionnaire design — for example, www.statpac.com/surveys/.

3

Health, illness and disease

This chapter provides information and guidance to help you prepare for the portfolio assessment of **Unit 3: Health, illness and disease**.

Concepts of health and ill health

The terms 'health' and 'ill health' do not mean the same to everybody. This section is designed to develop an understanding of what people mean when they talk about health and ill health.

When people become ill they usually develop **symptoms**. A symptom is something that is noticeable to the affected person (e.g. itching or pain). It might be noticeable to other people too (e.g. a rash or a lump).

Soon after developing symptoms, people begin to think of themselves as ill and decide to take some action. This might be to buy some medication or to visit their GP. The GP might then confirm that the person is ill and diagnose the disease.

However, there are sometimes situations in which this pattern is not followed. For example, people might think of themselves as ill but a GP or a hospital consultant might be unable to detect any disorder. Sometimes, people might have a disease but not notice any symptoms, or might notice symptoms but not think of themselves as ill. For example, a person might catch a cold, but ignore it and carry on as normal.

It might surprise you that there are several different opinions about what is meant by being healthy and also a range of views about what is meant by being ill. These differences are illustrated by the examples below.

Claire says, 'My GP tells me that I'm healthy. She says that all signs of my infection have gone. But I know she's wrong, because I don't feel right in myself. I've lost all my confidence.'.

In this example, Claire and her GP disagree about whether she is ill or healthy. The disagreement is really about what each person means by the terms 'health' and 'illness'.

During a routine health check, a practice nurse discovers that Younis has high blood pressure. Younis is surprised. He does not feel ill and he does not think that he needs any treatment. The practice nurse thinks that there is something wrong with Younis's circulatory system. In this example, the practitioner and the patient again disagree because they are using different concepts of what being ill means.

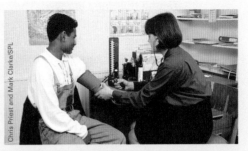

Younis does not feel ill, but the practice nurse knows something is wrong with his circulatory system

Concepts of health

You need to understand the differences between holistic, positive and negative concepts of health.

A holistic concept of health

A **holistic concept** of health is the belief that being healthy means being without any physical disorders or diseases and being emotionally comfortable. For example, a person who feels anxious or who has low self-esteem would, according to this concept, not be well. People with this view are likely to label themselves as ill when they experience a wide range of unpleasant feelings, not just physical discomfort or pain. They are likely to interpret minor discomforts, such as tiredness, as symptoms of illness.

A person with a positive concept of health believes that being healthy means taking active steps to stay well

A positive concept of health

A positive concept of health is the belief that being healthy is a state achieved only by continuous effort. People with this belief take active steps to maintain their health — for example, through their choice of food, by taking exercise and other activities they believe will keep them well. Such people are likely to feel responsible for their own health. They will take credit for the continued absence of disease and blame themselves if they develop symptoms. According to this view, people who do not take action to maintain their own health (for example, by 'healthy eating') cannot be healthy — even if, at any one time, there is nothing wrong with them.

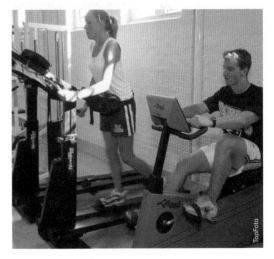

A negative concept of health

A **negative concept** of health is the view that being healthy is the absence of illness — for example, not having any symptoms of disease, pain or distress. People with this view are likely to believe that good health is normal and to take it for granted that they are well. They assume they do not need to take any special actions to keep healthy. They are unlikely to think of themselves as ill when they have minor discomfort caused by colds or headaches, or when they feel tired or depressed.

Try it out

A researcher asked a sample of people, 'Is your health good, average or poor?' When a respondent gave the answer 'good', the researcher asked, 'When you say your health is good, what do you mean?'

Read the following replies from different people and decide which concept of health best fits each answer. The three concepts of health you should use are:

+ a holistic concept
+ a positive concept
+ a negative concept

Answer A: 'I mean that there's nothing wrong with me, as far as I know.'

Answer B: 'I mean that I look after myself, stay fit and that sort of thing.'

Answer C: 'I mean that I feel well balanced. My body and my mind are working well together.'

When you have decided on your answers, check them against those given at the end of this chapter (see p. 101).

Now try to decide which concept of health is closest to the way you think about your health.

Did you know

When thinking about your own health, you might have realised that you use more than one of the three concepts of health, or perhaps you use all three. Do not be surprised by this. The fact that there are different concepts of health does not mean that your attitude to health necessarily belongs to just one of them. You will probably find that you apply one concept in some situations and others on different occasions.

You might also be wondering whether there is any advantage or disadvantage in holding one or other of these views.

Holistic concept

One result of having the holistic concept is that it tends to make people sensitive about their health. This can be an advantage because it can help them to notice symptoms more quickly than other people. They notice when something does not feel right and pay more attention to their bodies.

However, this can also be a disadvantage. Over-sensitivity can lead people to believe that they are ill when they are not. It can lead to unnecessary worry and result in people wasting their GPs' time.

It can also result in people not leading a lifestyle that is good for their health, such as going to work, taking strenuous exercise and going on holiday.

Positive concept

One result of having a positive concept of health is that people tend to take plenty of exercise, avoid smoking and excessive intake of alcohol, and eat a balanced diet. This is likely to be advantageous to them. Another advantage is that if such people become ill, they are likely to adopt attitudes and behaviour that contribute to getting better. There is some evidence that the chances of surviving cancer are influenced by the attitude of the patient. People who believe they can recover and avoid feeling defeated by their illness tend to do better than those who believe that they are doomed to die. People with a positive concept tend to be active rather than passive in relation to their own health.

One disadvantage of this concept is that, by taking responsibility for their own health, people might blame themselves for their illnesses and feel guilty when they become ill.

Negative concept

One result of having a negative concept of health is that people are unlikely to spend much time thinking about their health. One advantage of this is that it can save a lot of unnecessary worry. For example, a person with this concept is likely to ignore the symptoms of minor illnesses that usually get better without any treatment.

A disadvantage is that such people are less likely than others to take health advice seriously. For example, they might have a fatalistic attitude that allows them to continue smoking. This attitude is expressed in statements such as 'We've all got to die sometime. I could be killed tomorrow crossing the road'. This is an irrational attitude, because the more risks people take with their health, the more likely they are to die prematurely. The lung-cancer sufferer who has had both legs amputated because of circulatory problems linked to smoking is very likely to die prematurely from the condition and very unlikely to be killed crossing the road.

Another disadvantage of the negative concept of health is that, once they become ill, people are more likely to see themselves as victims and to respond passively, making it less likely that they will recover from a serious illness.

Acquisition of concepts of health

Concepts of health are acquired socially and culturally, as are other attitudes. This means that our views of health tend to be influenced by the people around us. Children of parents with a negative concept of health will tend to adopt the same concept themselves. People with friends who regularly go to a gym are more likely to have a positive concept of health. Students who study health and social care are likely to develop a sophisticated view of health, including all three concepts.

Concepts of ill health

Among the different views or concepts of ill health are 'ill health as illness' (a subjective sensation), 'ill health as disease' (a set of symptoms) and 'ill health as a disorder' (a malfunction of a body tissue, organ or system).

Ill health as the subjective sensation of illness

A subjective sensation of illness means feeling ill. People might feel ill when they have some disease symptoms; they might also feel ill when no symptoms are present. By this definition, ill health exists when people decide that they feel ill or describe themselves as being ill. People who are very anxious about, or sensitive towards, their health are likely to think of themselves as ill even when symptoms are very mild or absent. Other people refuse to think of themselves as ill even when there are obvious signs that something is wrong.

Ill health as having observable symptoms of disease

Disease refers to a diagnosable problem, which might be physiological (a physical disorder) or psychiatric (a mental disorder). This view of ill health is objective, i.e. ill health is something for which there is likely to be publicly available evidence — for example, two people with medical knowledge agreeing that a patient has a disease.

Ill health as a disorder

The term '**disorder**' refers to some malfunction of a body tissue, organ or system. This concept is based on the idea that body systems can go wrong. This definition is the one that the writer of a medical textbook is likely to have in mind.

A researcher asked a sample of people the question, 'What does "ill health" mean to you?' Read the following replies from different people and decide which concept of ill health best fits each answer. The three concepts of ill health you should use are:

+ ill health as a subjective sensation of illness
+ ill health as disease symptoms
+ ill health as disorder or malfunction

Answer A: 'It means having things like heart disease or something blocking your intestines.'

Try it out

Answer B: 'All sorts of things. You know, sickness and diarrhoea, unbearable pain, lumps growing on your skin.'

Answer C: 'It's when you don't feel well.'

When you have decided on your answers, check them against those given at the end of this chapter (see p. 101).

(see p. 101).

How concepts of ill health overlap

Students can have difficulty in telling the difference between the three concepts of ill health. This is partly because they sometimes overlap. For example, 'ill health as a subjective sensation' can overlap with 'ill health as having symptoms of disease'. This is because some of the symptoms of ill health (e.g. pain and tiredness) are themselves subjective sensations.

This overlap is most noticeable with mental disorders. Unlike physical illnesses, mental disorders often have no symptoms that are detectable through observation, blood tests, scans and so on. For example, a person suffering from depression is likely to have no observable symptoms apart from complaining of overwhelming feelings of misery and helplessness. In this case, 'ill health as a subjective sensation' is the same as 'ill health as disease symptoms'.

In other situations it is easier to tell the difference. For example, a person with a skin rash (observable disease symptom) might not think of himself or herself as ill (subjective sensation), particularly if the rash is not accompanied by pain.

The concept of 'ill health as disease symptoms' can also overlap with 'ill health as a disorder or malfunction'. This is usually the case when the symptoms correspond very closely to the malfunction. For example, a person with a lung disorder such as pneumonia will experience difficulty in breathing.

However, in other situations these two concepts of ill health can be distinct. For example, a person could experience symptoms, such as sneezing and a runny nose, that are not caused by malfunction of any body tissue, organ or system. Rather, those symptoms are the result of effective functioning of the immune system to overcome a cold virus. In this case, 'ill health as disease symptoms' is distinct from 'ill health as disorder or malfunction'.

A contrasting example is that a person can have a serious malfunction of body tissue (such as a tumour growing on the spleen) but not feel ill or report any symptoms. Tumours in some parts of the body, including the abdomen and brain, can grow for many months before they are noticed. This is because there are few sense organs in these parts of the body. Symptoms are unlikely to be felt until the tumour is pressing on surrounding tissue that has more sense organs.

Another situation in which 'ill health as symptoms of disease' and 'ill health as malfunction' do not overlap is when the symptoms could be the result of a range of malfunctions. For example, a person feels constantly tired and out of breath. A blood test reveals that the person is anaemic (has too few red blood cells). The symptoms of tiredness, shortness of breath and anaemia do not arise from any one particular disorder or malfunction. The anaemia could be caused in several ways – for example, by a disorder of the bone marrow, by internal bleeding or by a dietary deficiency. Only by further tests and investigations could a specific disorder or malfunction be detected.

However, in most people who are seriously ill, these three aspects of ill health occur together. People will think of themselves as ill, they will notice symptoms (e.g. partial paralysis) and they will have an organ malfunction (e.g. a stroke or bleed into the brain).

Table 3.1 gives several examples in which two or more of these views of ill health sometimes overlap and sometimes do not.

Table 3.1
Concepts of ill health

Patient's name	Illness as a subjective sensation	Disease as symptoms	Disorder as malfunctions of tissue, organ or system	Conclusion
Bob	Yes — Bob thinks he is ill	No — there are no obvious signs or symptoms	No — there is nothing physically wrong	Illness as a subjective sensation; no overlap with the other concepts
Shabeena	No — Shabeena does not think she is ill	Yes — she has a runny nose and keeps on sneezing	No — no system is malfunctioning	Disease as symptoms; no overlap with other concepts
Simon	No — Simon does not think he is ill	No — he has no symptoms	Yes — he has a brain tumour that has not yet been detected	Disorder as a malfunction of brain tissue; no overlap with other concepts
Polly	Yes — Polly thinks she is ill	Yes — she has noticed a lump in her breast	Yes — she has breast cancer	All three concepts of ill health occur
Finbarr	No — Finbarr does not think he is ill; he just feels thirsty and tired	Yes — he often feels tired and thirsty, and often needs to urinate	Yes — he has a malfunction of the pancreas, causing diabetes	Disease as symptoms and disorder as malfunction overlap

Example 1

Claire says, 'My GP tells me that I'm healthy. She says that all signs of my infection have gone. But I know she's wrong, because I don't feel right in myself. I've lost all my confidence.'

(a) Which concept of health is Claire using?
(b) Which concept of ill health is implied by what she says?
(c) Which concept of health is the GP using?
(d) Which concept of ill health is the GP using?

When you have decided on your answers, check them against those given at the end of this chapter (see p. 101).

Try it out

Example 2

During a routine health check, a practice nurse discovers that Younis has high blood pressure. Younis is surprised. He does not feel ill and he does not think that he needs any treatment. The practice nurse thinks that there is something wrong with Younis's circulatory system.

(a) Which concept of ill health is Younis using?
(b) Which concept of ill health is the practice nurse using?

When you have decided on your answers, check them against those given at the end of this chapter (see p. 102).

Factors affecting health and well-being (lifestyle factors)

The specification requires a basic level of understanding of the following six factors:

+ eating sensibly, in order to maintain a balanced diet
+ taking regular exercise, in order to maintain physical and mental fitness
+ monitoring weight, in order to avoid weight-related illness or premature death
+ limiting alcohol consumption, in order to avoid alcohol-related disorders
+ not smoking, in order to avoid tobacco-related diseases
+ visiting the GP, to obtain medical advice and appropriately prompt treatment

For each factor, you need to understand the underlying principles and the reasons why the factor is important. You also need to understand how the different factors interrelate.

Note that these factors provide a useful list of precautions for maintaining health.

Eating sensibly

Principle 1: allowing for growth, **energy intake** should balance **energy output**. This is sometimes called the **energy equation**.

Daily activities, such as walking, talking and thinking, are powered by chemical energy obtained from food, which is released in body cells. Most foods contain chemical energy (fats and sugars contain the most, by weight).

People who eat too little use more energy than they take in. The result is that they convert body tissue, such as muscle, into energy. This is bad for health, unless they have a lot of spare body tissue in the form of fat.

People who eat too much will store some of the excess energy as fat. This is also harmful to health.

People differ in their need for energy. For example, a person who regularly plays a strenuous sport, such as rugby, will need much more energy than a person who sits around all day.

Principle 2: a person's diet should include all the **macro-nutrients** and **micronutrients** he or she needs.

Macronutrients are needed in relatively large amounts. They include fats, proteins and carbohydrates. Micronutrients are needed in relatively small amounts. They include minerals, such as iron, and vitamins. Water and dietary fibre are also necessary.

Fats and carbohydrates are important sources of energy; proteins help to build tissues. Micronutrients are essential for biochemical processes in the body, such as the growth and repair of tissues.

Eating a varied diet, with many different kinds of food, helps to get the right balance of these nutrients. Some unbalanced diets, such as those containing high levels of fat and carbohydrate, are harmful to health. This is partly because they contain more energy than necessary and partly because they lack important nutrients.

People who take part in strenuous sports will need much more energy than people who sit around all day

Taking regular exercise

Principle 1: the human body has been adapted by evolution for frequent and prolonged activity, so exercise is needed to keep it in good working order.

Until the last few thousand years, most humans obtained food by hunting and gathering. Typically, this involved a lot of walking and running, for which the human body is very well adapted. A reasonably fit adult can cover at least 20 miles in a day on foot and some can manage two or three times this distance. Because of this adaptation, some people suffer reduced health and well-being when they do not take exercise.

In most people, exercise helps to maintain physical fitness. Exercise helps to keep the body supple and strong, maintains stamina and helps to limit body weight. In contrast, a lack of exercise often leads to a gradual loss of muscular strength, speed and lung capacity.

Principle 2: exercise can also contribute to psychological well-being.

This is partly because it can give a sense of achievement (particularly in sport) and boost self-esteem and confidence and partly because it leads to the secretion of body chemicals called endorphins, which produce feelings of pleasure and contentment.

Today, regular exercise is important for people because the circumstances of life are different from those during most of human evolution. Very few jobs now require the use of physical strength, and people travel without exertion and many have far more leisure than ever before. Entertainment opportunities, such as television and electronic games, often result in people sitting still for hours at a time.

Exercise maintains physical fitness and helps people to feel good about themselves

Monitoring weight

Principle 1: weight changes often indicate changes in health and fitness.

An increase in weight may be a sign of disease. For example, fluid retention (oedema) in body tissues, which could result from heart failure, leads to a weight increase. However, more often weight gain is not a sign of illness, but indicates that a person is eating too much, taking too little exercise, or both. Gain in weight can indirectly lead to illnesses, such as heart disease, and can also reduce the likelihood of a person taking exercise because this becomes more difficult.

A decrease in weight can also be a sign of disease. For example, intestinal disorders can result in poor absorption of nutrients from the intestine into the bloodstream.

Principle 2: increases or decreases in weight are usually gradual and are likely to be unnoticed unless people check their weight regularly (e.g. once a month).

A judgement about whether weight is normal for height is made using height and weight charts and a body mass index table.

Limiting alcohol consumption

Principle 1: habitual heavy consumption of alcohol has harmful short-term and long-term effects on health.

The short-term effects include an increased risk of accidental injury. This can occur after drinking three or four units of alcohol. (A unit is half a pint of beer, a small glass of wine or a single shot of spirits.)

The long-term effects include alcohol dependence, damage to the stomach, liver and kidneys, coronary heart disease, hypertension, strokes and impairment of brain function. These long-term effects can take many years to become apparent, so some people convince themselves that their excessive drinking is not doing them any harm. Unfortunately, when the effects do occur, they are usually irreversible.

The Department of Health recommends a maximum daily consumption of alcohol of up to three or four units for men and up to two or three units for women. In addition, it is recommended that people have alcohol-free days and avoid binge drinking.

Excessive consumption of alcohol seems to be increasing in the population. This is partly because of the huge increase in wealth, compared with 100 or even 50 years ago. It might also be caused by cultural beliefs, particularly among young people, that being very drunk is a desirable state. Young people tend to have more difficulty than older people in resisting the social pressure to get drunk.

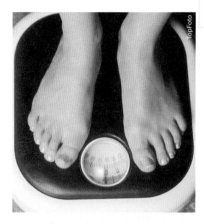

Principle 2: small amounts of alcohol are beneficial for health and well-being. Alcohol has been a popular drug for thousands of years. In small quantities (one or two units per day) it produces feelings of contentment and is associated with reduced risk of stroke and coronary artery disease.

Regular monitoring of weight can give warning of ill health

Not smoking tobacco

There is only one principle related to smoking, and that is that it should be avoided by people who wish to maintain good health.

Unlike alcohol consumption, smoking tobacco confers no health benefits. Smoking can produce pleasant sensations and people often use tobacco to manage their mood, for example to reduce anxiety. However, there are other equally effective ways of managing mood, such as taking exercise. In addition, smoking can suppress appetite, which is one reason why smokers are sometimes reluctant to give up — they think they will gain weight.

Smoking increases the risk of:

+ heart and circulatory diseases
+ respiratory diseases, including bronchitis, emphysema and lung cancer
+ many other cancers

Towards the end of their lives, smokers sometimes have circulatory problems that are so severe that they develop gangrenous infections in their legs, which then have to be amputated. This helps to extend life because without the legs, the heart and lungs are better able to maintain an adequate oxygen supply to the tissues.

Breathing in smoke from other people (passive smoking) causes significant health risks, particularly to members of a smoker's family.

Smoking is harmful because of three components of tobacco smoke:

+ nicotine, which tends to produce addiction
+ carbon monoxide, which reduces the oxygen-carrying capacity of the blood and can contribute to hardening of the arteries
+ tar, which irritates the respiratory system and causes cancer

The more serious ill-health effects of smoking can take many years to develop. This is partly because the lungs have a much greater capacity for gas exchange than is usually needed. Only when about half of the effective lung capacity has been lost do people become aware of shortness of breath. However, stopping smoking, even late in life, can help to prevent further damage.

Visiting the GP

Visiting a general practitioner is important to obtain prompt treatment and/or access to hospital services. It also allows people to be given health checks and useful advice. Practice nurses can carry out blood tests and check blood pressure. Regular visits (at least once every 5 years) are recommended for older people, even if they have no obvious symptoms.

How these factors interact

There are obvious links (interrelationships) between these factors:

+ Monitoring weight provides useful information about whether or not food intake and exercise patterns are correct. Eating and exercise are interlinked. Exercise helps to use up food energy and avoid accumulating too much fat in the body. It can also help to suppress appetite. A rapid loss in weight should prompt a visit to a GP to find out the cause.
+ Alcohol consumption is also linked with nutrition and weight. Alcohol contains a lot of chemical energy and excessive consumption can lead to weight gain. In addition, a significant proportion of the energy needs of an alcohol-dependent person might come from alcohol. Therefore, the person might not eat other foods that would contribute to a balanced diet. A person who is dependent on alcohol can obtain advice and treatment by visiting a GP.
+ Smoking can affect appetite, so is also linked with nutrition and weight.

A combination of adverse lifestyle factors makes a much greater contribution to ill health than one factor alone

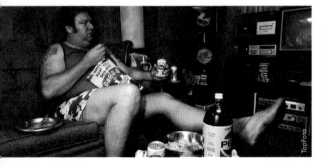

The combination of these factors makes a much greater contribution to health or ill health than any one factor alone. Therefore, people who hardly ever take any exercise, smoke, drink heavily, eat a diet high in fat and sugar and low in minerals and vitamins, do not monitor their weight and never bother to visit their GP are taking much greater risks with their health than people who take all but one of the precautions listed.

Individual, group and cultural differences

Individual differences

Individuals differ in how important they think these health factors are. Carrying out the questionnaire study that is part of the assessment for this unit might indicate some of these differences. For example, some people are significantly overweight but quite unconcerned about it, whereas others, who are in the normal weight range, believe that they need to lose weight.

Group differences

There are also group differences. For example, two families might have different views about health and nutrition. In one family there might be a tradition of eating a wide range of foods, including plenty of fresh fruit and vegetables; in another family, there might be no tradition of thinking about nutrition.

Group differences also occur between males and females. For example, men and women might have different attitudes and behaviour towards drinking alcohol, taking exercise and monitoring weight. Men are also believed to be less willing than women to visit a GP for advice and health checks.

Cultural differences

Cultural differences might reflect beliefs. For example, an individual might be a vegetarian or have religious beliefs that make taking exercise less likely.

People might also be influenced by subcultures. For example, they might drink excessively or take up smoking because their friends or workmates do.

Questionnaire on concepts and health factors

One part of the assessment for this unit is to design and use a questionnaire. Chapter 2 contains detailed guidance on designing and using questionnaires and on processing and presenting the data collected.

Overall design of the questionnaire

The questionnaire is likely to contain two parts — one about the respondents' concepts of health and ill health and the other about their behaviour and attitudes in relation to the six factors affecting health and well-being that are identified in the specification. You have to decide whether to start the questionnaire with items about concepts of health or to start with items about the six factors affecting health and well-being.

Choosing the respondents

You will have to decide which group or groups to study.

+ You could use the questionnaire to find out the attitudes and behaviours of one particular group of people, for example middle-aged men. Alternatively, you could use it to compare the attitudes and behaviours of two groups, for example young men with middle-aged men.
+ Probably the simplest option is to use the questionnaire with people you happen to know, such as adult family members and friends of different ages. You do not

have to have a large number of respondents: six should give a varied range of responses; three is probably an acceptable minimum.

+ You should consider trying to get respondents from more than one cultural or religious background. This is likely to produce more differences between responses and will help you meet the assessment criteria for this unit.

+ You could choose two respondents (one male, one female) who are from the same ethnic group as yourself and two (one male, one female) from a different ethnic group. These could be students from your school or college who are not studying health and social care. The advantage of this approach is that it would enable you to compare the responses of males and females and also of two ethnic groups.

+ It is not a good idea to use people younger than 16 as respondents, partly for ethical reasons but also because adults have more experience of life and are more likely to have formed opinions on the topics.

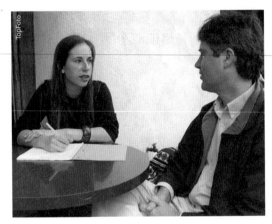

Your questionnaire will probably work better if you use it as an interview schedule

Methods of obtaining the data

Another decision you will have to make is whether to give a copy of the questionnaire to each respondent to fill in or whether to use it as an interview schedule.

With the sort of questions you are likely to ask, it will probably work better as an interview. This means that you would read out each item to a respondent and write down the responses. However, this is rather time-consuming, so if your sample is going to be larger than ten people, you should probably use the normal questionnaire procedure.

If you intend using your questionnaire as an interview schedule, you should phrase your items informally, to avoid sounding like an interrogator.

One advantage of using your questionnaire as an interview schedule is that you can ask further questions if necessary. For example, if a respondent gives a very brief or puzzling answer, you could say, 'Could you explain that a bit more please?'

Ethical issues

In designing your questionnaire, you should decide how you are going to handle ethical issues such as informed consent, confidentiality and the right to withdraw.

Probably the best way to do this is to use a prepared statement when you ask a person to take part. This statement should:

+ outline the aim of the questionnaire and what it is about
+ indicate how long it is likely to take
+ give the opportunity to refuse to take part or to withdraw after having started to answer
+ give the opportunity to refuse to answer some questions

You should be aware that the topics included in the section of your question-naire dealing with lifestyle factors raise ethical issues that might offend or upset some respondents. For example, suppose one of your respondents is noticeably overweight. If you ask about weight monitoring, he or she might think that you are indirectly commenting on — and possibly disapproving of — his or her weight. Unless respondents know that they are all being asked the same questions, they might be offended.

Respondents who have lifestyle-related illnesses might be upset if you ask about topics such as drinking alcohol and smoking. You could avoid this by checking whether or not this sort of question would be acceptable before you start.

It is always important to avoid seeming to be judging your respondents in any way.

As well as avoiding asking potentially embarrassing questions, you should allow respondents to opt out of the research if they wish or to avoid answering partic-ular questions. You should also ensure that they remain anonymous. For example, in your report you should refer to them just as Respondent 1, Respondent 2 and so on.

Items to investigate respondents' concepts of health and ill health

Designing the questionnaire items

Items to investigate the concepts of health and ill health held by the respondents should be designed to generate the sort of responses given to the questions on pages 82 and 84. Think about whether an open item or a closed item would be more likely to obtain this kind of answer.

It is important to phrase questions in a way that will generate the type of answer you want. For example, it would not be effective to ask, 'What is your concept of ill health?' You will only obtain the data you need if you use clear, non-technical language.

Analysing the responses

The aim of this analysis is to decide what views of health and ill health each respondent holds.

Suppose you asked the question, 'Some people have different ideas about health. What does "good health" mean to you?'

You might get an answer along the lines of 'Good health? That's what you say when you have a drink, isn't it? Seriously though…well, it's obvious isn't it? Good health is not being ill. It's when you are feeling OK.'

You then have the task of trying to decide what concept or concepts of health are held by this person. The key sentences in the example above are: 'Good health is not being ill' and 'It's when you are feeling OK'. These sentences illustrate a negative concept of health. The second sentence also illustrates the view of ill health as a subjective sensation, because it refers to 'feeling OK'.

From the replies to your questionnaire items, you should try to identify the concepts of good health and ill health shown by your respondents. However, you should not be surprised if you find that:

+ all your respondents share the same concepts of health and ill health
+ some of your respondents show evidence of more than one concept of health
+ some of your respondents produce statements that do not give clear evidence of any of the concepts described

If you claim that a respondent holds a particular view, you must be able to provide evidence for this by reference to one or more statements made by the respondent.

Your analysis might also include comparisons between individual respondents, which you might be able to relate to their gender, age, culture, ethnicity or occupation. For example, respondents who work in healthcare might have different views from those who do not.

Items to investigate respondents' behaviour and attitudes relating to factors that affect health and well-being

The assessment criteria for this unit state that you should use a 'wide range of relevant information from a good variety of different sources'. This means that you should not just rely on the description of the factors affecting health and well-being given earlier in this chapter. You should use additional sources to do some of the following:

+ Find out what is meant by a balanced diet and how people can check whether what they eat amounts to a balanced diet.
+ Find information on recommended types and frequencies of exercise.
+ Find out what the normal weight range is for people of different heights. Height–weight charts and body mass index charts will tell you this.

Designing the questionnaire items

Your questionnaire should include items on all six factors that affect health and well-being.

A typical item should find out whether or not the respondents take action on a particular factor — for example:

+ whether or not they smoke
+ whether or not they do anything to ensure their diet is balanced

A follow-up item should find out to what extent the respondents take the relevant action — for example:

+ how often the respondent smokes
+ what they do to manage their diet

You might also want the respondents to rate how important they think each of the six factors is to their health.

Analysing the responses

If you have used a small sample of people of different ages, you should summarise the responses each person has made and try to relate them to what you know about that respondent. For example, you might find that a young person visits a GP much less often than an older person. This might be explained by the young person feeling ill less often.

As a further example, you might find that female respondents show more concern about their food intake than male respondents. If so, you could try to explain this in terms of social and cultural pressures.

You should also analyse your data in terms of interrelationships between factors. For example, do people who smoke or drink excessively avoid visiting their GP?

Suggestions for presenting the questionnaire and results

In order to meet the assessment criteria relating to the questionnaire, you have to:
+ show sound understanding of the concepts of health and ill health and of the importance of the six lifestyle factors to different individuals and groups of different cultures, beliefs and/or contexts with a minimum of three respondents
+ show that you have collected relevant information from a wide range of sources
+ show that you can collate and analyse the data collected, judge their validity and accuracy and use logical, reasoned judgements to draw conclusions

There are several alternative ways of presenting your questionnaire material so as to meet these criteria. One of these is described below.

Aims

Start by stating the aims of the questionnaire.

Section on factors affecting health and well-being

The section covering the factors affecting health and well-being should be divided into six subsections — one for each factor.

In each subsection, you should make clear the importance of that factor for health and well-being and illustrate this with references to sources you have used. For example, when writing about limiting alcohol consumption, you might write, 'According to the British Nutrition Foundation website (www.nutrition.org.uk), men should consume no more than four units of alcohol per day'.

You should also refer to some of the responses to your questionnaire. For example, you might say, 'Respondent 4 pointed out that this factor did not apply to him because his religion does not allow him to drink alcohol'.

Illustrating the importance of each factor with reference to data collected using the questionnaire will enable you to show understanding. For example, if you asked a question about visiting a GP and a respondent answered, 'I've been healthy all my life, so I don't need to start visiting the GP at my age', you might write that this respondent was elderly and therefore more likely to need regular monitoring than younger people.

Illustrating this section with quotations like these will help to show that you have applied the lifestyle factors to different individuals, perhaps from more than one culture. Quotations can also be used to provide evidence for judgements you have made.

In this section you could also point out any links (interrelationships) you find between factors.

Concepts of health and ill health

In the section on the concepts of health and ill health, you should describe the three concepts of health and the three concepts of ill health and explain how some of these can overlap. Again, you should illustrate this section with selected responses from your questionnaire. For example, the statement quoted above — 'I've been healthy all my life, so I don't need to start visiting the GP at my age' — could be used as an illustration of the negative concept of health.

Analysis of data

Start the section on data analysis with an uncompleted copy of the questionnaire. (The completed copies should be included in an appendix at the end of the report.) You should outline how you intend to analyse the data.

This section could include a subsection collating the data from all respondents. For example, you could report the number of respondents who smoke, the number who show a positive concept of health and so on. Guidance on processing data is given in Chapter 2. It is not necessary in this assessment to present data graphically, although you might wish to do so. At the end of this subsection, you should make some conclusions, such as 'Overall, the respondents were much more likely to try to control their weight by dieting than by exercise'.

It is also advisable to include a subsection commenting on each respondent (provided the number is not too large). This will enable you to demonstrate that you can judge the validity and accuracy of the data. For example, you might comment that '...this respondent did not take the questionnaire very seriously, so the data collected probably do not reflect how they actually think or behave'. Of course, you might find the opposite — that your respondents were very interested in the topic and appeared to give honest and thoughtful answers.

Evaluation

Finally, it is worth including a short section evaluating the effectiveness of your questionnaire, discussing which items worked well and which worked less well, and comparing the advantages and disadvantages of open and closed items. This will give you opportunities to gain marks by making 'reasoned judgements'.

Report on immunisation

Understanding immunisation

Immunisation is one of the most important tools in preventive medicine. Humans have immune systems that help them to resist diseases; nevertheless, there are some diseases that present a serious risk to life. For some of these diseases (caused by bacteria or viruses) people can be made immune by artificial means. This is called immunisation. The main principle behind immunisation is to ensure that **antibodies** to disease-causing organisms are present in the blood before exposure to the disease. If this is achieved, people will be unaffected, or only mildly affected, if they encounter the disease organisms.

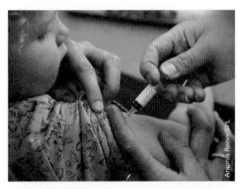

Immunisation protects the individual who has been immunised and reduces the risk of disease for others in the population who have not been immunised. For example, the MMR immunisation protects individual children against measles and reduces the chances of an epidemic, simply by reducing the number of people who can pass on the disease.

Immunisation prevents people from suffering from serious bacterial or viral infections

Active and passive immunity

There are two kinds of immunisation — that which creates active immunity and that which produces passive immunity.

Active immunity

Active immunity is achieved by giving the person a vaccine, either by mouth or, more commonly, by injection. A vaccine is a weakened (**attenuated**) culture of the disease-causing organism, or a sample of the organism that has been killed (**inactivated**).

The vaccine stimulates the immune system to produce **antibodies** against that particular bacterium or virus. The effect is the same as catching a very mild version of the disease that the immune system can easily overcome. The antibodies remain in the body, so subsequent exposure to the disease does not result in development of the disease.

This type of immunity is called 'active' because it relies on the immune system to produce antibodies. For this reason, vaccines with only weakened (attenuated) disease organisms are not given to people with damaged immune systems.

Some vaccines have to be given more than once, following a particular schedule. Others require only one treatment.

Passive immunity

Passive immunity cuts out the need for the body to develop its own antibodies. Blood is taken from a person who already has immunity. This blood contains antibodies. An extract of this blood (called immune serum) is injected into the person who needs to become immune. Note that the person is not given a vaccine in this case.

Key points

+ Active immunity is longer lasting than passive immunity because the antibodies remain in the blood and protect against future infections.
+ Passive immunity gives immediate protection, which is only temporary.
+ Immunisation has saved many lives — especially those of children.
+ Some immunisations have risks or side effects. Normally, these risks are greatly outweighed by the benefits.

Presenting the report

To meet the assessment criteria relating to this report, you have to:

+ describe immunisation procedures and the scientific principles underlying them
+ describe most of the associated risks, including those from the diseases named in the specification and the risks of immunisation itself
+ support your statements with evidence from a variety of sources

Suggested structure

The first section of the report should:

+ outline the principles behind immunisation, including active and passive immunity and the differences between them
+ outline the process of immunisation, including the method and schedules used for immunising babies and children against diphtheria, pertussis, tetanus and MMR
+ describe immunisations used to protect people before they travel to countries with known health risks, including those against cholera, hepatitis A, typhoid, malaria and rabies

The more of these diseases you consider, the better.

The second section should outline the causes (i.e. whether the disease-causing organism is a bacterium or a virus), main symptoms and long-term effects of the diseases covered. This could be in the form of a table.

The final section should be a general evaluation of the benefits and disadvantages of immunisation. This should be illustrated with reference to some of the immunisation procedures you have outlined. It could include a consideration of the physical-health effects, together with emotional impact, such as increasing or decreasing anxiety. It could also include the effects of immunisation on the individual and on the population as a whole.

In order to gain marks for use of evidence, you should use several sources of information — not just one textbook.

Report on the value of screening

Screening is another important tool in preventive medicine. Like some immunisations, it is applied to the whole population, or at least to the whole of a vulnerable section of the population. For example, breast cancer screening is available to women aged over 50.

Screening involves a variety of techniques that are designed to find out whether or not people have the early stages of a disease or disorder.

The principle behind screening is that by detecting a disorder early, the chances of successful treatment are increased. This not only reduces suffering but, because early treatment is usually much less expensive than treatment of a disease at an advanced stage, can also save money.

It is important to detect disorders early, so many screening tests are carried out on infants and children.

Presenting the report on the value of screening

To meet the assessment criteria relating to this report, you have to:

+ describe the full range of screening tests covered by the specification and the scientific principles underpinning each test
+ describe the value and importance of different screening tests to different client groups (e.g. children, tourists)

Your report should cover antenatal tests and screening tests for infants, children and adults. It should be supported by evidence from a variety of sources.

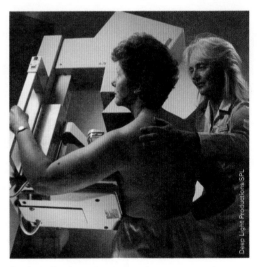

By detecting breast cancer early, mammography screening can lead to early treatment

Antenatal tests

Your report should include antenatal tests for:

+ the genetic disorders Duchenne muscular dystrophy, haemophilia and sickle-cell disease — amniocentesis and chorionic villus sampling
+ spina bifida — AFP test to measure the presence of alpha-fetoprotein in the blood of the mother
+ anaemia — blood cell count
+ blood group — cross-matching for ABO and rhesus types

Infant and child screening tests

Your report should describe screening tests for infants and children, including those for:

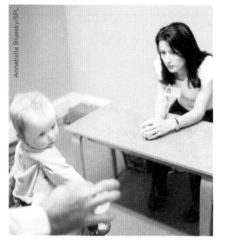

Annabella Bluesky/SPL

+ phenylketonuria — the Guthrie test
+ thalassaemia — blood test
+ developmental dysplasia of the hip (or clicky hip) — Ortolani–Barlow test (lying the baby down and gently moving the legs apart)
+ dental caries — visual examination, surface probing for softness, X-rays to detect cavities
+ visual defects — eye tests for visual acuity using a Snellen chart (wall chart with letters of decreasing size) and for colour vision; the use of behavioural response tests in infants — for example, seeing if they follow a moving object with their eyes.
+ deafness — hearing tests such as audiograms to measure the conduction of sound through the air and through bone; the use of behavioural response tests in infants (e.g. ringing a bell and seeing if the infant turns towards the sound).

A health visitor uses a simple behavioural response test to check an infant's hearing

Adult screening tests

Your report should describe screening tests for adults, including those for:

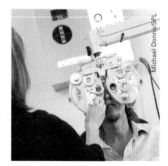

Michael Donne/SPL

+ hypertension — blood pressure test using a sphygmomanometer
+ cervical cancer — smear test
+ breast cancer — mammography
+ testicular cancer — physical examination
+ tonometry (pressure test) for glaucoma and tests for other visual defects (e.g. short sight, long sight and astigmatism)

An ophthalmologist will use a range of tests to check vision

Suggested structure

The first section should outline the importance of screening for the client groups given above.

The second section should contain a brief description of each test, which includes:

+ how the test is carried out
+ when it is performed
+ what is being looked for
+ how a positive result (i.e. showing the disorder is present) is different from a negative result
+ the scientific basis of the test

This section could be presented in the form of a table.

Your report should be supported by references to your sources of information, which should be included in the text, as illustrated in the example below.

Glaucoma occurs when the amount of aqueous humour in the eye increases (according to the *Harvard Medical School Family Health Guide*, 2003).

This raises pressure in the eye, which can hurt and lead to blurred vision. It can also cause permanent damage to the optic nerve, leading to blindness.

The test can be carried out by an optician using a machine (tonometer) that blows a tiny jet of air at the cornea. The machine measures the resistance to this jet of air as it bounces back off the cornea. A positive result is obtained if the resistance is high. This means that the cornea is under pressure and the person probably has (or is starting to develop) glaucoma. If the resistance is normal, the person does not have glaucoma.

The glaucoma test is aimed at people over 40 years old, especially if they have close relatives with the disorder. Afro-Caribbean people are more likely to suffer from glaucoma, so it is more important for them to be tested regularly. The reason for these groups being screened is that some types of glaucoma are caused genetically and these groups are more likely to have that gene. Glaucoma usually develops quite slowly, so the test needs to be carried out only every 2 or 3 years. It is important for people to be screened regularly so that the disorder is detected before it does permanent damage to the person's vision.

The description in the example is very detailed; for some tests, much briefer descriptions would be adequate.

Answers to 'Try it out' questions

Page 82

Answer A: the negative concept of health
Answer B: the positive concept of health
Answer C: the holistic concept of health

Page 84

Answer A: ill health as disorder or malfunction
Answer B: ill health as disease symptoms
Answer C: ill health as a subjective sensation of illness

Page 86

Example 1

(a) The holistic concept
(b) Ill health as illness — a subjective sensation ('I don't feel right')

(c) The negative concept —absence of disease

(d) Ill health as disease — observable symptoms

Example 2

(a) Ill health as illness — a subjective sensation ('he doesn't feel ill')

(b) Ill health as disorder — malfunction of body systems

Further reading

The British Medical Association (2004) *The British Medical Association A–Z Family Medical Encyclopedia*, Dorling Kindersley.

Komaroff, A. L. (ed.) (2003) *The Harvard Medical School Family Health Guide* (UK edn), Cassell.

Websites

Department of Health:

  www.dh.gov.uk

Family patient notebook (US site):

  www.fpnotebook.com

GP notebook (UK site):

  www.gpnotebook.co.uk

Medical Advisory Services for Travellers Abroad (MASTA):

  www.masta.org

The Merck Manual of Medical Information:

  www.merck.com/mmhe/

Patient website:

  www.patient.co.uk

Child development

4

This chapter provides relevant material to prepare you for the examination of **Unit 4: Child development.**

Between birth and 8 years, the average child changes from a helpless individual, with very little understanding of its surroundings, into a person at least twice as tall who is self-aware and can talk, run, dance, make friends and influence other people.

In this chapter, the term 'infant' is used for children aged 0 to 2 years, 'toddler' means 2–3 years, 'pre-school child' means 3–5 years and 'school age' means 5–8 years.

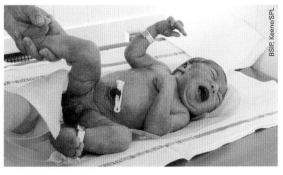

A 'helpless individual' — but not for long

Factors and processes influencing development

Two kinds of factor influence development. These are genetics (sometimes called **nature**) and the environment (sometimes called **nurture**).

Genetics

The genetic make-up of a child (called the **genotype**) is acquired at the moment of conception when 23 chromosomes from one of the father's sperm cells combine with 23 chromosomes from an ovum produced by the mother. This makes a set of 46 chromosomes (23 pairs), which is the normal number for each body cell in humans.

The genes contained in each chromosome code for information that guides the growth of body cells. Much of the genetic information is the same in almost all humans — for example, the information that leads us to develop organs such as the heart and kidneys, to grow two eyes and to form five digits on each hand and foot. Some genetic information differs from person to person, which partly explains why people differ in hair and eye colour, susceptibility to disease, and personality.

Although a child receives half its genetic material from the mother and half from the father, this does not mean that the child will be very similar to either. Only people with exactly the same genetic material are very similar. These are identical twins.

The genotype explains why people are similar to each other in anatomy and physiology – we have much genetic information in common. It also partly explains why people are different from each other in height, build, personality and abilities – we each have a unique set of genes.

Some children have genetic conditions that significantly affect their development, causing disorders such as cystic fibrosis and haemophilia.

Maturation

The key process linked to genetics that leads to development is called **maturation**. This is the process by which genetic information acquired at conception leads to growth and development throughout life. A simpler definition is that maturation is genetically programmed development.

The effect of maturation is that at various times in the growth of a child, a genetically predetermined development is triggered. A striking example is the development of sexual maturity at puberty. The genetic information to enable this to happen is present at conception, but the genetic instructions include a mechanism to trigger puberty around 12 or more years after conception.

Some people confuse the word maturation with 'becoming mature'. People often talk about 'maturity' meaning being grown-up or behaving sensibly and responsibly. However, maturation is a technical term and does not mean the same as 'getting older', 'becoming more sensible and confident' and so on.

Environment

The '**environment**' is a rather broad term that, when talking about child development, means 'those non-genetic factors that influence development'.

Direct environmental influences

For most children, the main environmental influence is the behaviour of their parents towards them. Parents can significantly influence their child's development because what they do influences the child's quality of life. For example, parents can provide psychological security, social approval and support, stimulation and choice.

Other significant direct environmental influences are other children and adults (especially in education), disease and nutrition. In Britain today, children are normally healthy (because of, among other things, immunisation programmes and infant screening) and well nourished. In some other countries, disease and malnutrition have significant negative effects on development, slowing down growth and limiting achievement.

Indirect environmental influences

There are other factors, such as culture, social class and housing, that have indirect effects on development.

+ An example of the effects of **culture** — some cultures are tolerant of a wider range of behaviours than others. For example, in some cultures, boys might be discouraged from dancing and girls might be discouraged from rough-and-tumble play. In other cultures, these behaviours are more accepted.
+ An example of the effects of **social class** — one social class of families might value education more than another. This might affect a child's development indirectly. A parent in this class might buy the child more books, spend more time reading and encourage the child to work hard at school.
+ An example of the effects of **housing** — a child growing up in a crowded flat might have few opportunities to play, partly because there is not enough floor space for toys and also because there might not be access to outdoor play space, such as a garden.

Note that in connection with child development, 'the environment' does not have its usual meaning of the physical, geographical world. It mainly refers to the social world of the child — in other words, the people the child spends time with.

Learning

One of the most important processes by which the environment influences development is **learning**. Learning is the acquisition of behaviours and ideas by direct experience and from other people, particularly parents, other children and teachers.

There are several ways in which learning can take place in infants and young children. One way is by the **reinforcement** of behaviours. Reinforcement refers to some rewarding stimulus that makes a behaviour more likely. For example, if a child says something interesting and a parent responds by smiling and giving attention, the child is more likely to say similar things in future.

Another way in which learning can take place is by **observation** and **imitation** (also called **modelling**). For example, a child might see someone spitting on the pavement and start doing the same.

Learning can also take place by direct experience — by children trying things out for themselves. For example, infants can learn by trial and error that a dropped wooden block can be easily picked up, but spilt milk cannot. This type of learning is called **discovery learning**.

The first few years of life are a period of intense learning. Note that this takes place without teaching. Only when children are older can they learn by being taught.

Some aspects of growth and development are strongly influenced by genetics, while others are more influenced by the environment. In almost all development, both genetics and the environment operate together. These two influences are sometimes referred to as nature and nurture.

Physical growth

Physical growth is the increase in size and complexity that takes place during the earlier stages of an individual's life, especially during infancy and childhood.

Physical growth involves three types of change that happen to cells in the body:

+ **Cell expansion** – cells absorb nutrients and become larger, gaining weight and volume
+ **Cell division** – each cell has the ability to split in two, producing two so-called 'daughter cells' that are genetically identical to the original cell. This leads to an increase in the overall number of cells during periods of growth.
+ **Cell differentiation** – genetic material in each cell enables that cell to develop into a specialised type (e.g. a cell in bone, a red blood cell, a nerve cell). This enables the body to grow different types of tissue – for example, muscle, connective tissue and nervous tissue.

Absolute growth

During childhood, the processes of cell expansion, division and differentiation lead to increases in height and weight. This is sometimes called **absolute growth**. These increases in height and weight are shown in Figures 4.1 and 4.2. Note that the graphs show ranges of height and weight for each age.

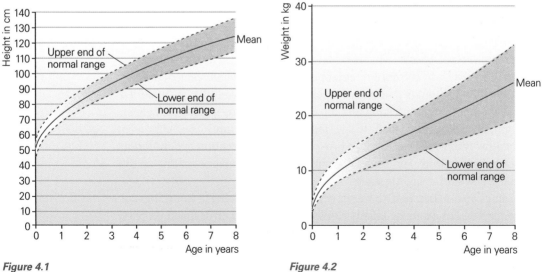

Figure 4.1
Normal height range for children from birth to 8 years

Figure 4.2
Normal weight range for children from birth to 8 years

Growth norms and individual differences

Paediatricians and health visitors need to have some way of assessing whether the growth of a child is within the normal range or not. When making **developmental assessments** they refer to data on growth norms.

There are two ways of collecting information to obtain growth norms. One way is by undertaking a **cross-sectional study**. This studies a large group of children of different ages. For example, you could record the length and weight at birth of 200 children selected at random. You could find the same information about a group of 1-year-olds, 2-year-olds and so on.

An alternative way of collecting this information is a **longitudinal study**. The lengths and weights of a large sample of newborn babies are measured. The heights and weights of these same children are measured as they grow up. To collect data about the first 16 years of life will, therefore, take 16 years, so this method does not give the instant results that the cross-sectional method does.

A mean weight and height can be found for each age. However, it is important to understand that the height or weight of an individual can be much greater or lower than the mean.

If a child's weight or height is outside the normal range (usually below in the case of children with developmental disorders; above in weight for obese children), then there is a need for investigation and possible treatment.

Allometric growth

Growth begins at conception. However, growth of different parts of the body before and after birth is not uniform. The term **allometric growth** refers to the fact that different parts of the body grow at different rates during infancy and childhood.

For example, at birth, the head takes up one-quarter of the length of the body. The legs also take up around one-quarter of the length (see Figure 4.3). In other words, the lengths of the head and the legs are nearly the same. In contrast, by adulthood, the legs take up nearly one-half of the length of the body, while the head takes up only about one-seventh.

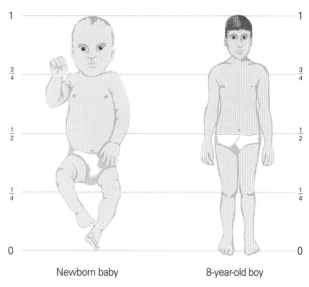

Figure 4.3
Allometric growth

Newborn baby   8-year-old boy

A newborn baby has a very large head in proportion to the rest of the body. This is partly because the human brain is large and complex, and is highly developed before birth. During infancy and childhood, all parts of the body grow, but the head grows at a slower rate than the limbs.

To get an idea of allometric growth, try to imagine what your legs would be like if they were the same length as your head is now.

Ask some friends to hold their arms up, hands clasped together high above their heads, making large oval shapes. Now try to imagine your friends' heads so large that their arms only just fit round them. That's how big their heads would be if growth were uniform, i.e. not allometric.

Factors influencing growth

Growth is influenced by maturation and by environmental factors, such as the presence of disease and the quality of nutrition. Disease and inadequate nutrition in childhood can both slow down the rate of growth and restrict overall growth to below that of the full genetic potential. Extreme stress, for example caused by neglect and/or abusive parenting, can also lead to restricted growth.

In countries such as Britain, in which child health is usually good, maturation is the main factor that influences growth. This means that differences in the heights of children at different ages (and variation among children of the same age) are mainly caused by the genotype. Nutrition is also usually adequate and often very good for children in Britain. The main exception is overeating, leading to a surplus of food energy, which makes some children obese.

Try to find photographs showing adults from different generations of your family — for example, of you with your parents and grandparents, or your parents with their parents and grandparents. Is there any trend or pattern in the heights of the adults of different generations?

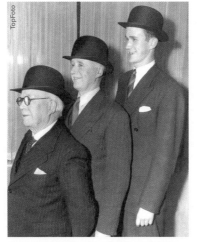

TopFoto

As health and nutrition improved during the last century, successive generations in many families became taller

If you find a trend, it is likely to show that people born before around 1930 were significantly shorter than those born around 1950. Those born around 1970 are likely to be significantly taller, but they might not be as tall as you. This sort of trend has nothing to do with genetics because the genetic make-up of populations does not change so quickly. It has much more to do with improvements in health and nutrition, particularly after the introduction of the Welfare State in the 1940s.

If you do not find a trend, it might be that your recent ancestors were better nourished and healthier than most.

Development

Development refers to the acquisition of new behaviours and skills that occurs during childhood. It depends partly on growth.

Several kinds of development take place between birth and 8 years. These include:

+ motor development
+ cognitive development (including the development of thought and language)
+ social and emotional development

Motor development

Motor development is the development of the ability to make controlled movements. This ability depends partly on the development of muscles and partly on the development of the motor areas in the brain, which send the nerve impulses needed to move muscles.

Newborn babies have very little intentional control over their movements. Effective actions tend to be reflex rather than controlled. By the age of 8 years, the child has excellent control of voluntary movements.

Gross and fine motor skills

Motor skills can be subdivided into gross motor and fine motor skills. **Gross motor skills** are those that involve large muscles to make large movements, for example in moving the whole body. Examples of gross motor skills include rolling over, sitting up, picking up large objects, walking and running.

Fine motor skills are those that tend to use smaller muscles to make small, precise, movements. Fine motor skills include peeling fruit, fastening buttons, drawing and drinking through a straw.

The achievement of a new motor skill (such as starting to walk) is called a **motor milestone**. By observation of the development of many children, the mean ages at which different milestones are reached have been determined. Some children develop faster than others, so there is usually quite a range of ages between which each milestone is reached. As with measures of growth, this knowledge can be used to assess whether the development of a child is within the normal range. Developmental problems can then be detected in those children whose development is significantly behind that of the average child.

Infant reflexes

At birth, the infant shows a number of reflex responses. These include:

+ the **rooting reflex**. If the infant is touched on the cheek, he or she turns the head towards the point of touch. This reflex is important for feeding, because it helps the baby to find the nipple.
+ **coordinated sucking and swallowing**. This reflex is also present at birth to enable the infant to feed.

+ the **grasping reflex**. The infant's hand can grasp a person's finger, or a pencil, surprisingly strongly. Touching the palm of the hand can trigger this reflex.
+ the **plantar** or **Babinski reflex**. When the sole of the foot is stroked, the toes spread open and the foot turns inward.
+ the **startle reflex**. With the infant supine, a loud noise is made (e.g. a hand clap). The infant is likely to blink or screw up the eyes, cry and extend the arms and legs. (Supine means lying on the back; prone means lying face down.)
+ the **Moro reflex** (Figure 4.4). With the infant held supine in the hands and the head supported, the head is allowed to suddenly drop a small amount. The response is usually for the arms to be extended rapidly, and then withdrawn again.

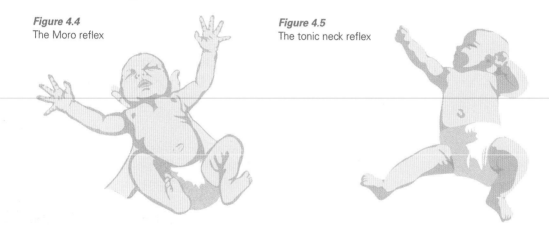

Figure 4.4
The Moro reflex

Figure 4.5
The tonic neck reflex

Did you know ?

Reflexes are simple, often involuntary responses to particular stimuli. This means that they happen automatically, sometimes whether we like it or not. They are not learned, but genetically in-built.

Reflexes are genetically in-built in humans and other species because they have survival value. Some reflexes remain throughout life. They are often extremely quick responses. The blinking reflex is an example of one such reflex. This helps to keep the surface of the eye clear and moist. It also helps prevent damage from objects. Imagine you are walking along a road and a car passes throwing up a small stone, which is likely to hit your eye. The stone is approaching so quickly that you are not even aware of it until it hits you. However, the blinking reflex will have closed your eye before the stone hit, preventing serious damage.

Other reflexes that have survival value are coughing, sneezing and vomiting. These reflexes help to remove irritants or toxins from the body. The salivation reflex, in which saliva floods into the mouth on the sight, smell or taste of food, helps digestion.

+ the **tonic neck reflex** (Figure 4.5). With the infant supine, the head is turned to one side, rotating the neck. The infant then straightens the arm and leg on the side that the head is facing. The other arm and leg are bent.
+ the **walking reflex**. The infant is supported with the feet just touching a flat surface. The infant then makes stepping or walking movements.

Tests

Most of these reflexes are lost after a few weeks. Newborn babies are tested for some of these reflexes. The presence of these reflexes indicates that parts of the nervous system are working properly.

The continued presence of the Moro and tonic neck reflexes at 8 months is regarded as a sign of impaired development.

Motor milestones during infancy

Gross and fine motor milestones during infancy are outlined below.

At 6 weeks

Gross motor milestone:

+ head control (Figure 4.6) — when gently pulled from a supine to a sitting position, infant holds own head upright, without wobbling.

Fine motor milestone:

+ in supine position, tracks an object steadily by moving head and eyes

At 3 months

Gross motor milestone:

+ from a prone position, raises chest taking own weight on the forearms

At 6 months

Gross motor milestones:

+ sits with support, keeping back straight and head steady
+ rolls over

Fine motor milestones:

+ stretches out to reach for objects
+ transfers an object from one hand to the other and holds objects to mouth
+ grasps objects with whole hand (i.e. fingers, thumb and palm — the palmar grasp)

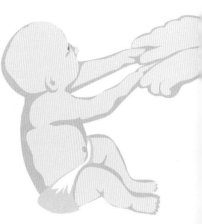

Figure 4.6
Test for head control

At 9–10 months

Gross motor milestones:

+ crawls
+ sits without support, and without wobbling
+ pulls self into a standing position
+ stands while holding onto some support, such as a chair

Fine motor milestones:

+ explores or inspects objects by touching or poking them with the index finger
+ begins to pick up small objects between thumb and fingers

At 12 months

Gross motor milestones:

+ crawls quickly
+ walks if one or both hands are held by an adult
+ stands briefly without support

Fine motor milestones:

+ repeatedly drops objects on purpose — 'casting'
+ grasps small objects between the index finger and thumb, in a pincer grip
+ points to objects, using the index finger

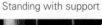
Standing with support

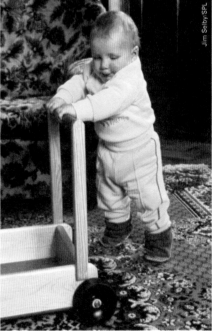

Jim Selby/SPL

At 15 months

Gross motor milestones:
+ walks unaided
+ crawls upstairs

Fine motor milestone:
+ can pick up more difficult small objects (e.g. string) with pincer grip

At 18 months

Gross motor milestones:
+ climbs onto a chair
+ walks backwards
+ climbs upstairs
+ carries toys while walking

Fine motor milestones:
+ scribbles
+ turns pages
+ shows hand preference, i.e. is clearly either left- or right-handed

Motor milestones in toddlers and pre-school children

Gross and fine motor milestones in toddlers and pre-school children are outlined below.

At 2 years

Gross motor milestones:
+ runs
+ kicks a ball
+ climbs downstairs (with both feet coming to rest on each step)

Fine motor milestones:
+ builds a tower of six blocks
+ turns door knobs
+ uses spoon to eat

At 3 years

Gross motor milestones:
+ dresses and undresses unaided
+ runs fast
+ rides a tricycle
+ climbs upstairs (with only one foot coming to rest on each step)

Fine motor milestones:
+ threads beads
+ uses spoon and fork to eat

At 4 years

Gross motor milestones:
+ climbs a ladder

+ can hop on one foot
+ can balance on one foot

Fine motor milestones:

+ draws recognisable pictures
+ copies a drawing of a square or cross
+ can use blocks to copy a simple construction, e.g. a three-block bridge

Motor milestones in school-age children

Gross and fine motor milestones in school-age children are outlined below.

At 5 years

Gross motor milestones:

+ walks downstairs with only one foot resting on each step
+ bounces and catches ball

Fine motor milestones:

+ copies a drawing of a triangle
+ colours pictures neatly

At 6–8 years

Gross motor milestones:

+ rides bicycle
+ rollerskates

Fine motor milestones:

+ writes
+ ties and unties laces

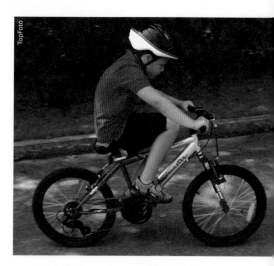

A gross motor milestone for an 8-year-old

Usefulness of motor milestones

The motor milestones listed above are only a small sample of the developments that occur. There are several reasons why it is useful to know about these motor milestones.

Paediatricians and health visitors can use the milestones to assess whether the development of an individual child lies within the normal range. As with growth, there are quite large individual differences. For example, some infants walk at the age of 11 months, while others might not start until 15 months. Some children do not go through a crawling stage at all, but move about by sitting and shuffling on their bottoms.

It is also useful for parents to know about these milestones, so that they can understand their child's behaviour. For example, if parents know that 'casting' objects is very common at 12 months, they will not make the mistake of interpreting this as naughty behaviour.

Factors influencing motor development

Motor development follows a maturational pattern. In other words, new developments take place because they are triggered by genetic information. Although poor nutrition and disease delay motor milestones, the sequence of development follows a similar pattern in all children. Reflexes present at birth are clearly genetic in origin, because the child has had no opportunity to learn them.

Learning and practising both play a part in motor development, but they are not the whole story. People often talk as if children 'learn to walk' in a similar way to young adults learning to drive. This is misleading. Maturation plays a greater role than learning. A famous piece of early research from the USA illustrates this. Wayne and Marsena Dennis (1940) compared the ages at which two different groups of children started to walk. One group were traditionally reared children of Hopi Indians, who were kept swaddled and bound to cradle boards for the first nine months of their lives. The other group were normally reared American infants.

You might think that having restricted movement would make the Hopi Indian children start to walk much later — they had less practice. In fact, there was no difference in the mean age of walking of the two groups. This suggests that maturation had more influence than the environment.

In an earlier experimental study, Gesell and Thompson (1929) observed a pair of identical twins. One of the twins was allowed access to the stairs; the other twin was not allowed near the stairs. When the first twin was competent at using the stairs, the other twin was allowed access to them and very soon reached the same level of competence. The lack of practice did not have a lasting effect on this twin.

Cognitive development: understanding concepts

Cognition includes abilities such as memory, perception and language. For Unit 4, you need to know about the development of the ability of children to understand concepts and about language development.

Early work in the development of the ability to understand concepts was carried out by the Swiss psychologist Jean Piaget. He devised a number of simple tests of this ability.

Object permanence

Object permanence means knowing that objects exist independently from us in the world and continue to exist when we are not observing them. An alternative behavioural definition is the ability to react to the disappearance of a previously present object, for example by searching for it.

You might think that everyone would grasp this, but young infants often act as though they have no knowledge or awareness of objects that are out of sight.

Piaget's test of object permanence

This test requires a small toy, such as a teddy bear, and a blanket. First, the child is encouraged to play with the toy. Then, when the child's attention is distracted, the toy is surreptitiously hidden under the blanket.

If the child looks round, and appears to be searching for the toy, he or she has object permanence. If, on the other hand, the child appears to forget about the toy and starts playing with something else, he or she might not have object permanence.

Piaget found that most children began to show object permanence at the age of about 8 months.

Conservation

Conservation is the ability to understand that redistributing material does not affect its mass, number or volume. (Conservation literally means 'keeping things the same'.)

Here is an everyday example of conservation. Take two identical unopened tins of beans and bash one of them against a hard object, such as a brick, to leave a big obvious dent. The tins now look different, but the contents must still be the same, assuming nothing has leaked out. Now ask someone whether there is about the same amount of food in the two tins or more in one than in the other. Someone who says there is less in the dented tin does not understand the concept of conservation. This example illustrates a common feature of conservation tests – that they involve some aspect that looks different, but is not.

Piaget's test of the conservation of liquid volume

The best known of Piaget's many conservation tests is about the **conservation of liquid volume**. It is popularly called the 'three beakers test'.

For this test, two identical tall, thin, transparent plastic beakers and a third transparent beaker with a much wider cross section are required, together with a jug of water, squash or similar liquid.

Water is poured into the two identical beakers, up to the same height in each. The child is asked: 'Is there the same amount of water in these two beakers or is there more in one than in the other?' The child is likely to say that the amount is the same.

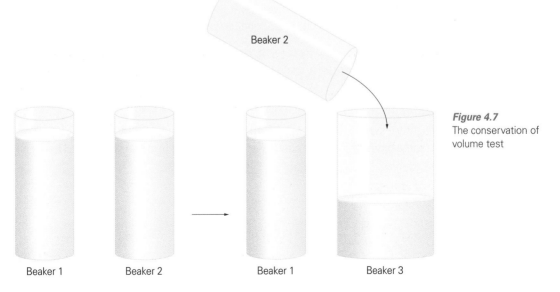

Beaker 2

Beaker 1   Beaker 2   Beaker 1   Beaker 3

Figure 4.7
The conservation of volume test

Next, the water in one of the beakers is poured into the third, wider beaker while the child watches. The third beaker is placed beside the tall, thin beaker of liquid and the same question is asked: 'Is there the same amount of water in these two beakers or is there more in one than in the other?' Using the same wording is very important, to avoid biasing the answer.

A child who can conserve will understand that just pouring the water from one beaker to another does not make any difference to the volume and will say that the amounts are the same. However, a child who cannot conserve is likely to say that there is more in the tall, thin beaker.

What seems to happen is that the child who cannot conserve relies on judging by appearances. The liquid is higher in the tall, thin beaker, so the child thinks there must be more in it.

Most children under the age of seven cannot conserve on this test. Those of seven and over usually can.

Although this is a simple test, many people do not carry it out properly. For example, some people make the mistake of asking a different second question. After pouring the liquid from one beaker to the other they might ask, 'Which beaker has got more in?' or 'Is there more in one beaker than the other now?' Such leading questions prompt the child to give an answer that indicates that they cannot conserve. Asking the second question this way makes the test meaningless.

Try it out

You could try out this test with a 5- or 6-year-old child. However, you should do this ethically. Only try it out with a child who already knows you and with the parents' full knowledge and permission. Do not tell the child that he/she has got the answer wrong or has 'failed' the test. Do not carry out, or continue with, the test if the child seems uninterested, unwilling or upset. Treat the child with the respect you would give an adult. Try to make it into a bit of fun for the child. For safety reasons, do not use breakable glass beakers. Do not give parents the impression that their child is unintelligent or not normal developmentally.

If the child is interested by the test, and did not conserve, you might like to repeat it, asking, 'Shall we try it again?' and getting the child to do the pouring this time.

Figure 4.8
The conservation of mass test

Other conservation tests

Slightly less messy is the **conservation of mass** test (Figure 4.8). All that is needed is some modelling clay or play dough. This is rolled into two equal-sized balls that

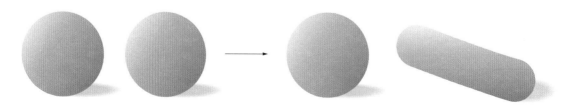

are placed in front of the child. The child is asked, 'Is there the same amount of clay in these two or is there more in one than the other?' The child is likely to say, 'The same'.

One of the balls is now rolled into a sausage shape and the same question is repeated.

A child who can conserve will again say, 'The same'; a child who cannot conserve is likely to say that the sausage shape has more.

Conservation of number can be shown by counting out two sets of eight beads and placing them in two parallel lines of equal length. The child is asked whether one row has more beads than the other or whether they are the same. The child is likely to say 'The same'. One row is now spread out so that it is longer. A child who cannot conserve is likely to respond that there are more beads in the longer row.

Egocentrism

Egocentrism means being unable to see a situation from the point view of another person. According to Piaget, the egocentric child assumes that other people see, hear and feel exactly the same as the child does. For example, a little girl might cover her eyes up and say, 'You can't see me, can you, Mummy?'

This is different from the everyday meaning of the term egocentrism, which means self-centred or selfish.

Piaget's mountains test of egocentrism

Piaget's mountains test of egocentrism used a board on which were placed three mountain shapes. The mountains were different, with snow on top of one, a hut on another and a red cross on top of the third (Figure 4.9). The child was allowed to walk round the model, to look at it and then to sit down at one side. A doll was seated at another side. The child was given ten pictures representing the scene from different angles and asked to pick out the card that showed the scene as the

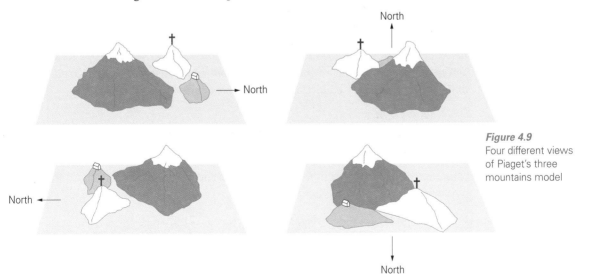

Figure 4.9
Four different views of Piaget's three mountains model

117

doll would see it. Piaget assumed that if the child correctly picked out the card showing the doll's view, then the child was not egocentric. Egocentrism would be shown by the child who picked out the card showing the view he or she saw.

Piaget found that 4-year-olds always chose the card that showed the view from their own position. The 6-year-olds often chose a different perspective, but not always the correct one. Only 7- and 8-year-olds consistently chose the correct picture.

Decentring

The problem with the word '**decentring**' is that it has two meanings.

A child who can pick out the right cards in the mountains test has decentred, because the child can see things from other people's point of view and is no longer egocentric. The child can decentre.

The other meaning of the term decentring is 'being able to take more than one feature of a situation into consideration at the same time'. Think back to the three beakers test. A child who fails to conserve seems to be judging by the height of the water in the beaker. If a child could take into account not only the height but also the cross section (or width) of the beaker, the child might be able to conserve. Being able to consider the height as well as the cross section is an example of this kind of decentring.

Nature and nurture in cognitive development

Nature: genetics and maturation

According to Piaget, all children go through the same sequence of stages of cognitive development. This suggests that maturational processes underlie cognitive development.

Nurture: environmental factors, especially parental behaviour

However, Piaget also believed that environmental influences were important for cognitive development. Piaget described a child's learning through play as 'discovery learning'. For this to happen, the child needs to have access to a range of stimulating toys and play opportunities. The emphasis on learning through play that features in nursery education was influenced by Piaget's work.

Cognitive development: language

Stages of language development

Language development can be divided up into several stages, according to the type of vocalisation the child produces.

Pre-linguistic stage (0–12 months)

This is the period before the child begins to speak. During this stage, the child produces various vocal sounds. In the first weeks of life, the main sound is crying, which is produced when the infant is hungry, tired, in pain or in discomfort.

At around 6 weeks, an additional cooing sound is produced. This seems to correspond with feelings of pleasure. From about 6 months, most babies start to produce more varied sounds, called **babbling**. Babbling is the production of recognisable speech sounds (**phonemes**). These speech sounds (such as 'ba' and 'ada') will be used later to produce words. However, at this stage the sounds are disjointed and do not appear to have any particular meaning. Babbling has another speech-like feature called **intonation**. This means the variation in pitch or tone of voice that speakers use. This can be heard when the infant babbles in a 'sing-song' voice. Late in this stage, infants often produce strings of repeated phonemes, such as 'dadadadada'. This repetition of phonemes is called **echolalia**.

At the end of this stage, some infants produce their first recognisable words.

Holophrase speech stage (12–18 months)

At around 10 to 14 months, most infants produce their first distinct words and use these words with meaning.

The term '**holophrase**' means a single word is used to represent a sentence. For example, a child might say 'doggy' to mean that the dog has just walked into the room.

The child's pronunciation is likely to be impaired by an inability to make some speech sounds. This can sometimes make it difficult to decide what the child means, although usually the context makes this clear because the child is likely to talk only about the situation at the time. A child who says 'dink' probably means 'I would like a drink'. A child who has just been tickled and says 'gain' is probably asking to be tickled again.

Telegraphic speech stage (18–24 months)

At this stage, infants begin to combine words into sentences. Usually these are two- or three-word combinations — for example, 'More bikkit', 'Where car go?' and 'Ball gone'. These are not the same as true sentences in adult speech because 'function words' (words not completely essential to the meaning of the sentence) have been missed out. For example, an adult might say, 'The ball has gone'.

The term '**telegraphic speech**' refers to a time when telegrams were used to send messages. These were charged according to the number of words used, so to save money, people used to write messages with non-essential words missed out, such as 'Back Tuesday. Paul'.

A characteristic error at this stage is called **overextension**. This means that a child applies a word to a wider range of objects than it actually denotes. For example, a child knows the word 'peas'. On seeing sweetcorn for the first time, the child may say 'yellow peas'. Similarly, some infants make the mistake of using the word 'dada' to mean all adult males.

Fully developed speech (2 years onwards)

From the age of about 2 years, the child begins to use longer strings of words and also complex sentences. For example, the child might say, 'I'm going to play with Teddy, 'cos Teddy likes to play it as well'.

Vocabulary develops rapidly. The child often actively seeks new words, for example by pointing at objects and asking, 'What's that?'

A characteristic error early in this stage is **overregularisation**. This refers to situations in which a word has to be made plural or changed into a different tense. For example, children in this stage soon grasp the grammatical rule that to make a word plural, the letter 's' is added. They apply this to all cases. Therefore, when they come across words to which this rule does not apply, they make mistakes. For example, they might say, 'furry mouses', or 'three mans'. Irregular verbs also cause problems. In regular verbs, the past tense is formed by adding '–ed'. For example, 'I look' becomes 'I looked'; 'I walk' becomes 'I walked'. When a child does the same with irregular verbs, such as 'to go' and 'to sing', the result is 'I goed' and 'I singed'.

Children usually have fluent speech with few errors, by the age of 5 years.

Factors influencing language acquisition

People tend to assume that language is acquired entirely by learning. This is an oversimplification. For most people, acquiring a language by learning is quite laborious. If you tried to learn a new language now, you would probably find it difficult. Imagine how much more difficult it would be if you did not speak any languages to start with. The fact that almost all infants acquire language with little apparent effort suggests that something other than just learning is going on.

Language development involves both maturation (nature) and the environment (nurture) — especially learning from others.

Maturation

There is plenty of evidence to suggest that language acquisition, like other developments, is driven by maturation:

+ Deaf infants produce a similar pattern of babbling to hearing infants and at the same age. This suggests that babbling is not learned by copying adult speech sounds, but is genetically programmed.
+ The pattern of speech in infants is the same all over the world. For example, telegraphic speech occurs in children using different languages. Children all over the world go through the stages described above.
+ Infant speech is strikingly different from adult speech. Adults do not usually say such things as 'gooses goed away', showing that language acquisition is more than just copying.
+ Infants seem to have the ability to acquire languages easily. For example, a child who regularly hears both English and Urdu spoken at home quickly becomes competent in both languages. However, later in childhood, the ability to acquire languages easily is lost by most people. This suggests that children go through a critical maturational period during which language acquisition is easiest.

The above suggests that the ability and tendency to produce speech is genetically in-built in humans. The human throat is constructed in such a way as to make speech possible; while in our closest relatives, the chimpanzees, the structure of the voicebox means that speech is not possible. The human brain contains structures involved in the production and comprehension of speech.

Learning

It is clear that learning also plays an important part in language acquisition. For example, children acquire vocabulary by hearing words applied to particular objects, actions and situations. In the fully developed speech stage, children learn whole phrases by observation and imitation — for example, '...and they all lived happily ever after'.

Children also acquire speech accents by observation and imitation of those around them.

Role of social factors in language acquisition

Language-learning opportunities are provided by:

+ contact with adults — especially parents, but also nursery and childcare staff
+ contact with other children
+ the mass media, particularly television and books

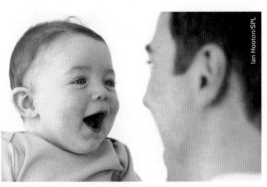

Face-to-face interactions with a parent can aid a child's development during the prelinguistic stage

These are sometimes called the **agents of socialisation**. Parents are usually the most important and contribute to language acquisition by their children in several ways:

+ During the prelinguistic stage, parents sometimes have face-to-face interactions with their infants. Typically, parents sit the child on their knees and have 'conversations' in which they respond to the child's changes of expression and to babbling. These responses are both verbal and non-verbal. This kind of interaction often features 'turn-taking', which is essential in conversations.
+ Parents also produce speech, which infants observe and sometimes imitate. In everyday situations, parents talk about objects and people who are present. The infant recognises which words go with which objects and so learns vocabulary.
+ Parents of infants often use a simplified version of speech (sometimes called 'baby talk' or 'motherese'). This involves using simple sentences and speaking slowly and clearly in a high-pitched voice. This gives the infant the best chance of hearing and understanding speech.
+ Parents read books to children. The combination of words and pictures aids the development of vocabulary.
+ Parents also often feed back improved or corrected versions of their children's speech. For example, if a child says, 'I runned all the way', the parent might say, 'You *ran* all the way'.
+ Parents can encourage speech and language development by listening to their children, taking what they say seriously and by having conversations about topics the children want to talk about. During the pre-school stage, parents can also help by talking to the child as an equal, i.e. by using adult speech and vocabulary.

Although parents sometimes imagine that they are teaching their young children to talk, the learning that takes place involves very little teaching. An important part of the role of the parents is to be a language resource that the children can use whenever they want. The best example of this is the tendency of children to ask their parents 'what?' and later 'why?' questions. The frequent repetition of the questions 'What's that?' and 'But why...?' can be frustrating for parents, but makes a major contribution to language and cognitive development.

Try it out

Read the following examples of conversations and then answer the questions.

1 *Child*: Him go away.
   Parent: Yes, the postman's going away. He hasn't got any letters for us today.
   Child: Back again?
   Parent: Yes, I expect he'll come back tomorrow.
2 *Child*: That car and that car and that car and all them cars. Put 'em in the garage.
   Parent: (No response)
   Child: Now it's the morning. Cars coming back out.
   Parent: Your nanna's coming this afternoon.
   Child: And one drives out, voom. And the other he drive out.
   Parent: Will you shut up about them cars?
3 *Parent*: Was that a smile?
   Child: Oooooo, awa.
   Parent: Ooh, yes that was a smile.
   Child: Awa, aduh.

Question 1
In which stage of language development are the children in each of examples (**1**), (**2**) and (**3**)?

Question 2
Identify two ways in which the parent in example (**1**) is helping the child's language development.

Question 3
Briefly evaluate the parent's behaviour in example (**2**).

Question 4
In what physical position are the parent and child most likely to be in example (**3**)?

Social and emotional development

Attachment

Attachment is a strong and long-lasting relationship between two people that leads to grief on separation. The term is particularly used to describe the relationship an infant has with another person (most often the mother).

Within the first few weeks of life, infants show no signs of attachment. Between about 3 months and 7 months, infants behave differently towards familiar and unfamiliar people. For example, they tend to smile more at familiar faces. However, they still show no specific attachment and are happy to be looked after by a stranger. From about 7 months to 9 months, infants begin to show a marked change in behaviour. They begin to seek contact with one familiar person (usually the mother) and to protest when separated from that person. For example, if the mother moves away across the room, the infant will try to follow (e.g. by crawling). If the mother leaves the room, the infant is likely to start crying loudly (showing **separation anxiety**). At about the same time, the child begins to show **stranger anxiety** — a dislike of being in the presence of unfamiliar people — for example, crying when talked to by a friendly stranger in the street.

This development often takes parents by surprise. They might think that the child has suddenly become more anxious and clinging than before. In fact, it is a sign of normal development. Even so, it can be inconvenient for parents, for example, if an infant will not tolerate separation for the short time it takes the mother to go to the toilet. Furthermore, the child can no longer be looked after by unfamiliar baby-sitters and will only tolerate familiar adults. There are quite large individual differences between infants — some are much less tolerant of brief separations than others.

Very soon after the onset of this specific attachment, the child begins to show multiple attachments to other familiar people, such as the father, brothers and sisters and grandparents that they see frequently.

Attachment behaviour remains at approximately the same level until about 3 years of age, when most children become able to tolerate short separations and the presence of strangers. For example, the child is able to attend nursery school for a morning. Even so, some children show signs of separation anxiety and stranger anxiety up to the age of five, and this can make starting school an upsetting ordeal.

Attachment is seen as a very important first step in social and emotional development. It sets the pattern for later relationships and (if satisfactory) gives the child a feeling of security. For this reason, it is sometimes called primary (i.e. first) socialisation.

The word 'attachment' is usually used to refer to the infant's attachment to the carer (usually the mother). However, parents usually form attachments to their infants too. This is more often known as **bonding**. One difference between the attachment of infants and the bonding of parents is that bonding is present very soon after birth, whereas a child's attachment develops later.

Factors influencing the development of attachment

Genetics

The fact that the onset and pattern of attachment are similar in infants all over the world suggests that maturation is involved. One possible explanation is that attachment behaviour has become genetically in-built because it has survival value. Just as infants are becoming mobile (crawling and walking), they begin to develop specific attachments. The result is that they stay close to a familiar adult. This reduces the chances of the infants wandering off and getting into danger.

Environment

It is clear that experiences a child has during the first 3 years of life influence the development of attachment. For example, if the child has regular contact with several adults, he or she will form multiple attachments. If the child only has contact with one adult, a single attachment will develop.

Other environmental factors are situations that might cause separation, such as those described below.

Consequences of separation

Separation means the loss of contact between a child and familiar people. If a child has only a single attachment (usually to the mother), the chances of this happening are much greater than if the child is attached to several people.

Separation can take place for a variety of reasons, for example:

+ a parent could become ill or die
+ a child might need hospital treatment
+ a child might have to be taken into the care of a local authority social-services department to protect the child from abuse or neglect
+ a child might be left with strangers when parents take up work

In the last case, separation is for a short period. In the case of the death of a parent who was the only familiar figure in the child's life, the separation is permanent. The consequences of separation for a child between 1 and 3 years of age can be emotionally devastating and more unpleasant for the child than some better-known causes of suffering in children. Even children who have been neglected or abused by their parents form attachments to those parents and suffer when separated.

Attachment was not well understood until the 1950s, when John Bowlby published the results of research carried out by himself and others. Bowlby reported that separation had negative short-term and long-term consequences.

Short-term consequences

When a child is first separated from familiar people, he or she is likely to protest, crying and screaming for long periods, evidently in great distress. Because of stranger anxiety, the child cannot be comforted by other people.

Within a few hours, the child's behaviour becomes quieter. Soon the child becomes apathetic and unresponsive to other people. This stage is called despair.

If the separation lasts a few days or more, the child is likely to show detachment when reunited with the parent. This means that the child is not so clinging and might even resist contact with the parent for a while.

These effects of protest, despair and detachment are regarded as potentially harmful to the child, partly because of the distress caused and partly because of the loss of attachment, emotional security and trust. Following the work of Bowlby and others, attempts were made to reduce separation during the first 3 years of life. For example, parents of infants and pre-school children who had to go to hospital were encouraged to stay with them, and mothers who gave birth while in prison were allowed to keep their infants with them.

Long-term consequences

Bowlby claimed that separations of a few days or more could have several damaging effects on children in the long term, including:

+ **delinquency** – disruptive and low-level criminal behaviour, including stealing and violence
+ **affectionless psychopathy** – an inability to have feelings for other people
+ **retardation of cognitive development** – a slowing down of a child's intellectual (i.e. cognitive) development.

The consequences of separation as described by Bowlby are summarised in Table 4.1.

Short-term consequences	Long-term consequences
Protest	Delinquency
Despair	Affectionless psychopathy
Detachment	Retardation of cognitive development

Table 4.1
Consequences of separation

Later research into separation

Bowlby's work seems to imply that children up to 3 years of age should never be separated from their mothers. In fact, this is what Bowlby himself believed. However, later research suggests that separations can be harmless if they are properly managed. For example, a child could start attending a day nursery from the age of 6 months. As the child begins to attach, he or she will form attachments to some of the staff at the day nursery. Provided there is always a familiar member of staff around, the child will not suffer from separation anxiety. This enables mothers and fathers to return to work before their children start attending school.

This type of arrangement does not seem to weaken the attachments that children form with their parents. In fact, provided that the quality of childcare is good, the arrangement can benefit the child.

In contrast, if a child starts attending a day nursery at the age of 1 year when attachment has developed, he or she is likely to experience separation anxiety. In this case the child should be accompanied by a familiar adult for several sessions until he or she has formed attachments to nursery staff.

Socialisation

Socialisation is the process by which an individual acquires behaviours, beliefs and attitudes that influence the way they act with other people. This is mainly a learning process. **Agents of socialisation,** such as parents and peers (children of similar age, such as school-friends), provide opportunities for social learning. These agents of socialisation act as 'models', showing behaviour that the child can copy.

+ **Pro-social behaviour** means positive behaviour, such as helping other people, sharing and cooperating.

✦ **Antisocial behaviour** is behaviour that tends to harm other people, or society as a whole, such as bullying, showing hostility and various kinds of crime.

If a child sees parents and friends acting violently, the child is more likely to develop this kind of antisocial behaviour. In contrast, if a child has parents, brothers and sisters who are mainly helpful, affectionate and cooperative, the child is more likely to develop this sort of pro-social behaviour. Other agents of socialisation, such as the media, have significantly less influence. Television shows plenty of pro-social behaviour as well as antisocial behaviour, but has much less influence than does parental behaviour.

Development of self

In the first year of life, infants show no real awareness of a sense of self. By the age of 2 years most infants show evidence of being able to recognise themselves. A famous demonstration of this was devised by Lewis and Brooks-Gunn (1979).

The test requires a mirror, a cloth and some red face-paint. It works as follows. During the course of wiping a child's face, a dab of red face-paint is placed on the child's nose, in such a way that the child does not notice it being done. The child is observed looking into a mirror. Some children reach their index fingers out towards the mirror; others touch the spot on their noses.

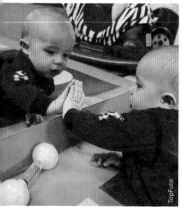

This toddler does not show self-recognition

Children who touch their own nose appear to recognise the image in the mirror as being of them. This shows that they have a sense of self. Children who reach out towards the mirror seem unaware that the image is in fact of them.

Over the next few years, the children develop a **self-concept** – knowledge or belief about what they actually like. For example, a child might become aware of being a boy, of being good at running and not liking cabbage.

Self-concept includes **self-esteem**. Self-esteem means knowledge and beliefs about your own value. People with high self-esteem will tend to think of themselves as good people – as likeable and skilled. People with low self-esteem will tend to think of themselves as bad people who are not likeable and who are no good at anything.

Factors influencing the development of self

Self-concept, including self-esteem, is influenced by several factors, including the reactions of others and social comparison.

Reactions of others

If people seek your company, say nice things about you and appear to like you, this tends to lead to high self-esteem and a belief in your own competence and attractiveness. If people ignore and avoid you, this tends to lead to a more negative self-concept.

In childhood, it is the reactions of parents that are probably the most important. Parents who show affection and approval towards their children and are interested in what they do and say are likely to produce more positive self-concepts in their children. In contrast, parents who show hostility or a lack of respect, ignore or frequently criticise their children are likely to produce more negative self-concepts in their children.

Social comparison

Children are able to compare themselves with their peers. For example, children soon find out whether they can run as fast as their peers or own as many toys and games. The children's self-concept can be influenced by these comparisons.

Importance of play

Play is an enjoyable activity that people (especially children) engage in for its own sake, i.e. without any useful goals in mind. Infants and young children spend a lot of time playing and put more effort and attention into their play than some adults put into work.

Play and development

Psychologists believe that play in childhood is more than just pleasant time-filling. They believe that play can contribute to development in various ways.

Play and cognitive development

Jean Piaget believed that play could contribute to cognitive development. The kind of play that can do this is that which makes cognitive demands on a child. Examples include construction toys and 'shape sorters', where a child has to select the correct shape to fit into or post through a hole.

Piaget thought 'pretend play' was important, because it showed that the child had developed the ability to use symbols. For example, a child plays with wooden blocks, pretending that they are a herd of horses.

Play and social development

Mildred Parten (1932) observed that, in terms of how social it is, children's play changes as they get older. She used the following descriptions to categorise the play she observed in children aged from 2 to $4\frac{1}{2}$ years. The categories are listed starting with the least social and going on to the most social types of play:

+ **Solitary play** – playing alone without paying attention to what others are doing
+ **Parallel play** – playing alongside other children, probably with a similar activity (e.g. painting), but without watching or talking to them
+ **Onlooking play** – watching others play, but not joining in with them
+ **Associated play** – playing in connection with another child – for example, two children with ride-on toys, one following the other around. Another example is playing at different activities, but occasionally talking to each other.
+ **Cooperative play** – play activities that are only possible when two or more children join in and play expected roles. A simple example is playing catch with

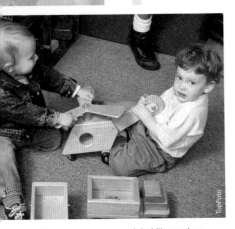

Play can increase social skills, such as learning to share, take turns and manage conflict

a ball. Cooperation is necessary because the game works only if each child throws the ball back in a catchable manner. Another example is role-play in the house-corner of a day nursery or playgroup, where children can adopt different roles, such as parent and child.

Parten found that the more social types of play occurred more often with the older children in her sample. It is reasonable to assume that children's play reflects their growing interest in other people and also contributes to their increasing social skills. For example, playing with others soon gives rise to situations where children have to learn to share, to take turns and to manage conflict.

Note that Parten's categories are not stages. For example, solitary play does not stop as children get older, it just becomes less frequent.

Try it out

Decide which of the above categories of play best fits each of the examples below.

1 Two children are side by side, each one painting a picture of Father Christmas. One asks the other, 'What colour are you doing for his socks?' The other replies, 'You can't see mine's socks 'cos he's in the chimney'.

2 Three children, Janine, Sonya and Anwar, are playing in the house-corner. Janine says,

'I'm the mummy and Sonya's the daddy, so you're the baby Anwar'. Anwar says, 'I'm always the baby'. Janine says, 'Go to bed this instant, you naughty boy,' and Anwar does so.

3 A few minutes later, Janine and Sonya have forgotten about Anwar. He is absorbed in watching other children playing on the climbing frame.

Play and motor development

The development of gross motor skills might be helped by play activities involving running, climbing, balancing and riding. Toys such as climbing frames, slides and seesaws, and also ride-on toys, are suitable for this.

The development of fine motor skills is aided by toys that require careful manipulation. Examples include beads for threading and construction toys in which small pieces have to be assembled together precisely.

Creative play

Creative play includes drawing, painting and building objects or models designed by the children. With this sort of activity, children can express their own feelings and personalities. Creative play is sometimes used to help children who have experienced some upsetting life event, such as a serious accident, the death of a

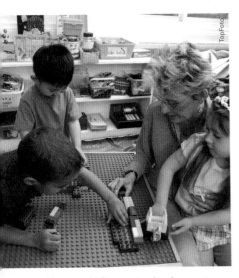

Play can aid fine motor development

parent or physical abuse. Children often show their distress through drawings and paintings, even when they are unable to talk about the distressing event.

Play resources

Play resources include equipment, space and human resources.

Play equipment includes purpose-made toys, play materials such as modelling dough, and equipment such as swings and slides. Children frequently use other materials in their play. For example, a large cardboard box (provided it has no metal staples) provides an excellent and versatile resource, especially if windows and doors are cut out.

Play space includes safe areas within the home where children can spread toys out and move about. Outdoor space, such as a garden or park where children can kick a ball and ride a tricycle, is particularly important for gross motor development.

The most important resource is the human one — other children to play with and adults to supervise play. Playing alongside infants and pre-school children enables parents to form good relationships with their children, as well as aiding their development. Parents (and childcare workers) can also set challenges to stimulate development — for example, 'Try to see what other things will sink or float'.

Health and safety

The following risks can occur with toys, play apparatus and play spaces:
+ choking on small objects
+ suffocation
+ strangulation
+ cuts or puncture wounds
+ poisoning by toxic materials (including some plants)
+ infection from dirty toys and animal faeces
+ falls
+ drowning
+ burns and scalds

Health and safety precautions depend on the age of the child. Infants are likely to put toys in their mouths, so balls, construction bricks and so on must be large enough to avoid the risk of swallowing or choking. Play materials must also be non-toxic because infants are quite likely to eat the modelling clay and lick the paint. Toys should, as far as possible, be unbreakable and should not have sharp edges or points, such as stiff metal wire. Cords or ribbons longer than 30 cm should be avoided because of the risk of strangulation. Infants like to play with packaging, so it is important to remove plastic bags, which pose a suffocation risk, and to remove any staples. Toys should also be washable, to minimise the risk of spreading infections.

With toddlers and pre-school children, the risks of eating or swallowing are lower, but the risk of falls increases. Play apparatus, such as swings and climbing frames, must be secured to the ground or otherwise designed so that they cannot tip over. Surfaces beneath and around apparatus should be shock-absorbent to minimise injuries caused by falls.

In the home, to reduce the risk of slipping, floors should not be highly polished. Loose rugs, which can cause trips and slipping, should also be avoided and stairs should be gated to prevent falls. Toys should not be left where they are likely to cause trips — for example, on the stairs. The risk of burns and scalds should be reduced by using fireguards, keeping matches out of reach and turning the handles of cooking pans away from the reach of toddlers. The risk of poisoning can be reduced by keeping household cleaning chemicals and medicines locked away or otherwise out of reach.

To minimise the risk of diseases carried by cats and dogs, parks and gardens should be free from their faeces. Ponds should be covered with mesh if children are to play outside with minimum supervision. Garden plants that are highly toxic should also be avoided — for example, laburnum trees produce chewy but poisonous seeds.

The single most important safety precaution is to supervise children while they are playing.

Figure 4.10
CE and Lion marks

Safety standards

The packaging on toys often includes guidance on the age range, or the minimum age, for which the toy is intended.

Toys and equipment are labelled to show that they meet the relevant safety standards (Figure 4.10):
+ A CE mark indicates that the toy meets European Community standards of safety.
+ A Lion mark is used on British-made toys that meet British safety standards.

Toys without appropriate safety labelling and information should be avoided.

Sample examination questions with model answers

The model answers given would score full marks. In some cases, alternative answers would be acceptable.

1 Gill has a 1-year-old daughter. She lives next door to her friend Naomi, who has a son aged 6 months. One afternoon, the two mothers and infants are in Gill's house. Gill says that her daughter is very clinging and screams if she is left alone. Naomi says that her son is quite happy to be left alone.
 (a) Outline the most likely explanation for the difference in behaviour between the two infants. (3 marks)

Gill's daughter has formed an attachment with her, which causes her to want to stay close to her mother. Naomi's son is not yet old enough for this kind of attachment to have developed.

(b) The same afternoon, Gill's sister comes to visit. She has not seen Gill or her daughter for nearly a year. Gill's daughter screams, clings to her mother and seems frightened of the visitor. Explain why Gill's daughter is frightened by the visitor, but not by Naomi. (4 marks)

Gill's daughter has formed an attachment, so she shows stranger anxiety towards people she does not know well. She has not seen her aunt since she was very young, so the aunt is a stranger. She probably sees Naomi quite often, as she lives next door and is a friend of the family. Therefore, Naomi is not a stranger.

(c) Outline one short-term and one long-term consequence of separation. (4 marks)

One short-term effect is despair. This is when, after the initial period of protest, a child becomes quiet and apathetic.

One long-term effect is affectionless psychopathy. An affectionless psychopath is a person who does not seem to have any feelings for other people.

(d) Explain how one agent of socialisation can influence the development of pro-social behaviour. Illustrate your answer with an example of pro-social behaviour. (4 marks)

Television is one agent of socialisation. It can influence children's behaviour because they observe people on television and can imitate that behaviour. For example, a children's programme could show a child helping another child to catch up on schoolwork.

Total: 15 marks

2 (a) Describe *two* behaviours that are present at birth. (4 marks)

Behaviours present at birth include reflexes. One reflex is rooting, in which an infant moves its head towards something touching its cheek. This helps the child to find the nipple to breastfeed. Another reflex is grasping. If an infant's palm is touched (e.g. with a pencil), the child's fingers curl round and grip the object.

(b) What is meant by the term 'maturation'? (2 marks)

Maturation is development that is programmed by genetics – for example, babbling in infants.

(c) The table shows the ages in months at which each of a representative sample of toddlers first walked unaided.

Child's name	Age in months at which the child first walked unaided
Ali	12
Barry	15
Ceri	15
Dawn	13
Edward	14
Fiona	24
Gemma	14

(i) Explain why most children start walking at about the same age. (2 marks)

The onset of walking is mainly influenced by maturation. The environment does not have much effect.

(ii) Explain the purpose of checking the age at which children achieve motor milestones, such as walking unaided. (2 marks)

The purpose is to find out whether the child is developing normally. If the child is late in reaching a milestone, there might be something wrong that requires treatment.

(iii) From the table, identify one child whose development might not be normal and give one possible reason for this. (2 marks)

Fiona's development is a long way behind that of the other children. It could be that she has a genetic disorder that is affecting her development.

(d) Briefly describe the language behaviour likely to be produced by most of the children in the table. (3 marks)

Most of the children are likely to be in the holophrase speech stage. This means that they speak in single words. One word is used to mean a whole sentence. An example is a toddler saying 'Teddy!' to mean 'Where is Teddy?'

Total: 15 marks

Further reading

Bee, H. and Roberts Boyd, D. (2003) *The Developing Child* (10th edn), Allyn and Bacon.

Bruce, T. and Meggitt, C. (2002) *Child Care and Education*, Hodder Arnold.

Smith, P. et al. (2003) *Understanding Children's Development*, Blackwell.

Websites

GP notebook:

www.gpnotebook.co.uk

Royal Society for the Prevention of Accidents:

www.rospa.com

Nutrition and dietetics

This chapter provides information to prepare you for the examination of **Unit 5: Nutrition and dietetics**.

Nutrients in food

Food supplies us with chemical energy that is used to do 'work', such as moving about or thinking. It is also needed to maintain and repair body structures. Most organs in the body are continually being repaired. For example, red blood cells live for only a few weeks and new cells are being produced continuously. Bone tissue is regularly replaced too. Damage caused by injury (for example, a broken bone or a tear in the skin) also makes demands on nutrients for repair.

Growing children, pregnant women and athletes in training need nutrients to grow body tissues.

Nutrients are substances in food that can be digested and absorbed into the body. The body digests food by extracting nutrients, some of which have to be changed into another form before they can be absorbed.

Food components are divided into two major groups:

+ **Macronutrients** are those nutrients that are needed in relatively large quantities. They include fats, carbohydrates and proteins.
+ **Micronutrients** are food components that are needed in small (sometimes very small) amounts. They include minerals and vitamins.

Macronutrients and their functions: fats

Fats are found in many foods derived from animals. The highest fat levels are found in foods such as bacon, salami, crisps, cream and cheese. Most fruits and vegetables contain little or no fat. The exceptions are nuts and seeds that are high in unsaturated fats (called oils). For example, sunflower seeds are used to make cooking oil. Cooking oil, butter, margarine and lard contain very little apart from fat. Low-fat butter substitute spreads contain mainly oils made into an emulsion with water.

Chemical composition

+ Fats are solids or liquids (also called **oils**) that do not mix with or dissolve in water.
+ Fat molecules are made up almost entirely of carbon and hydrogen atoms, with a small number of oxygen atoms.
+ Each fat molecule is built up from one molecule of glycerol and three molecules of fatty acids. It is because of this arrangement that fats are also known as **triglycerides** (Figure 5.1). When digested, fats break down into free fatty acids and glycerol, which enter the bloodstream. The fatty acids are taken up by a range of body tissues as well as the blood, while glycerol is taken up by the liver.

Fatty acids are long chains of carbon atoms combined with hydrogen and oxygen atoms. There are many different fatty acids.

Saturated fatty acids have carbon chains in which the carbon atoms are bonded to as many hydrogen atoms as possible (Figure 5.2). There are no double bonds between the carbon atoms. This is why they are called saturated — they could not possibly contain any more hydrogen.

Saturated fatty acids:

+ are solid at room temperature
+ are found in large quantities in the fat on meat, butter, lard, whole milk and cheese
+ raise the level of cholesterol in the body and, therefore, increase the risk of coronary heart disease

Unsaturated fatty acids can be divided into monounsaturated and polyunsaturated fatty acids. They are usually liquid at room temperatures.

A **monounsaturated fatty acid** molecule has one link in the carbon chain that is a double bond (Figure 5.3). Therefore, the molecule contains two fewer hydrogen atoms than it would if it were saturated. Monounsaturated fatty acids are:

+ found in oils such as olive oil and groundnut oil and in soft margarine
+ are useful in building cell membranes in the body

A **polyunsaturated fatty acid** molecule has several double bonds at different places in the carbon chain (Figure 5.4). Therefore, the molecule contains several fewer hydrogen atoms than it would if it were saturated.

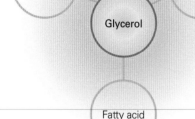

Figure 5.1
Basic structure of a triglyceride fat

Figure 5.2
A saturated fatty acid

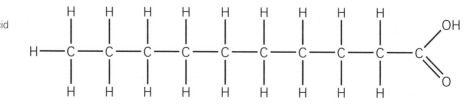

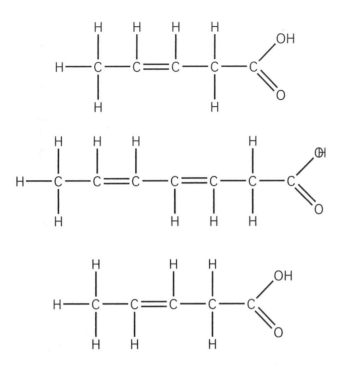

Figure 5.3
A monounsaturated
cis-fatty acid

Figure 5.4
A polyunsaturated fatty
acid

Figure 5.5
A *trans*-unsaturated
fatty acid

Polyunsaturated fatty acids perform the same function as monounsaturated fatty acids and are found in the same types of food.

Trans-unsaturated fatty acids (also called *trans*-fats) are unsaturated fatty acids that have been partly saturated by adding hydrogen, in a process called hydrogenation. During this process, some of the hydrogen atoms attached to carbon atoms that are joined by double bonds change position from the normal *cis*-position (same side of the carbon chain) to the *trans*-position (opposite sides of the carbon chain), producing a *trans*-unsaturated fatty acid (Figure 5.5).

This monounsaturated fatty acid has the same chemical composition as the fatty acid shown in Figure 5.3. The difference is in the position of the hydrogen atoms attached to the carbon atoms in the double bond.

The purpose of hydrogenation is to make a liquid fat into a solid fat — for example, when making margarine from sunflower oil. Hydrogenation also prolongs shelf-life, because saturated fats become rancid more slowly than unsaturated fats.

Trans-fats occur naturally in small quantities in beef, butter and milk and in much larger quantities in margarine and deep-fried foods. Recent evidence suggests that *trans*-fats probably raise cholesterol levels in a similar way to saturated fats, which they closely resemble. Therefore, excessive consumption of saturated and *trans*-unsaturated fats leads to health risks.

Consumption of *cis*-unsaturated fats is either beneficial to health or harmless.

Fats or fatty acids?

As stated above, a molecule of a fat is composed of a molecule of glycerol combined with three fatty acid molecules.

In practice, people often use the terms 'fat' and 'fatty acid' as if they were the same. Technically, it is the fatty acid rather than the fat that is saturated, mono-unsaturated or polyunsaturated. However, it is common for people to talk as if the fats were saturated or unsaturated. What people mean by a 'saturated fat' is a fat with high levels of saturated fatty acids, such as butter.

Actually, fats almost always contain a mixture of saturated, monounsaturated and polyunsaturated fatty acids. For example, fatty acids in a typical butter are 65% saturated, 32% monounsaturated and 3% polyunsaturated.

Functions

+ A key function of fat is as a supply of chemical energy to the body. Fats contain a great deal of chemical energy — more calories per gram than any other food.
+ Fats are useful because they can be stored in the body. By gradually converting stored fat to blood sugar, people can survive for a long time without much food.
+ Fat is important in body structures. For example, the eyeballs are cushioned by fat in the eye sockets. The kidneys are protected from damage (for example, from a sharp blow to the back) by fat.
+ Fat just below the dermis (the skin) acts as a heat insulator, increasing the ability of the body to maintain temperature. This fat is called subcutaneous (under the skin) fat. Women tend to have a thicker layer of subcutaneous fat than men.

Is fat essential in the diet?

The body can make fats from carbohydrates and proteins. In theory, a person who ate no fat but had an intake of carbohydrate and protein greater than the energy and growth requirements of the body would still get fat. However, the body can

Did you know

Why we get fat

Many species of animal eat as much food as they can while it is plentiful (usually during the summer) and store some of this as fat. In the winter, when food is scarce, they use up the fat to provide them with energy. A layer of fat under the skin also acts as a heat insulator to protect the body from cold.

For thousands of years, humans living in latitudes where there are warm summers and cold winters (i.e. outside the tropics) also needed to store up fat in their bodies. People living in the most northerly parts of the world are among the best at storing fats.

Within the last few hundred years (more recently in some countries), improved food-production methods and global transport have meant that many people have enough food and do not go hungry in the winter. However, our appetite for food has not changed. The result is that some people (especially those whose bodies are best adapted to store fat) have too much fat stored in their bodies, which can lead to obesity.

Cholesterol

Cholesterol is an important constituent of body cells. It is involved in hormone and bile salt formation and the transport of fats in the bloodstream.

Cholesterol contained in, or bound to, high-density lipoproteins (HDL) seems to protect against arterial disease. Cholesterol bound to low-density lipoproteins (LDL) increases the risk of atherosclerosis ('plaque' formation on inner arterial linings). The level of low-density lipo-proteins can be reduced by eating unsaturated, rather than saturated, fats.

only make saturated and monounsaturated fatty acids from carbohydrates. It cannot make polyunsaturated fats, so these have to be obtained in the diet.

Fats may contain fat-soluble vitamins, including vitamins A, D, E and K. This is a good reason for eating foods containing oils, such as mackerel and other oily fish.

Macronutrients and their functions: carbohydrates

Carbohydrates include sugars, starches and non-starch polysaccharides (NSPs):

+ The highest sugar levels are found in chocolate, honey, syrup, jam, cakes, sweet biscuits and puddings. Some fruits, such as grapes and apricots, also contain quite high levels.
+ Foods containing high levels of starch include bread, rice, potatoes, pasta and breakfast cereals.
+ High levels of NSPs are found in bran products, wholemeal bread, peas, beans, apricots and coconut.

Chemical composition

Carbohydrate molecules contain only the three elements carbon, hydrogen and oxygen. Each molecule has twice as many hydrogen atoms as oxygen atoms.

Sugars

Sugars are soluble in water. They are also known as saccharides. A simple sugar (monosaccharide) contains six carbon atoms linked to hydrogen atoms, hydroxyl groups (containing one hydrogen and one oxygen atom) and one other oxygen atom. Altogether, there are 6 carbon atoms, 12 hydrogen atoms and 6 oxygen atoms. The chemical formula of glucose is $C_6H_{12}O_6$.

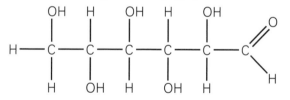

Figure 5.6
A monosaccharide (glucose)

There are three particularly important monosaccharides: glucose, fructose and galactose. The arrangement of atoms in each sugar is slightly different, although the number of each type of atom is the same. Glucose and fructose occur naturally in fruits.

Other sugars are combinations of these three simple monosaccharides. The disaccharides are combinations of two monosaccharides:

+ Sucrose molecules are made up of glucose and fructose.
+ Lactose molecules are made up of glucose and galactose.
+ Maltose molecules are made up of two glucose molecules.

Sucrose is the sugar people add to tea and coffee and use in baking. Lactose is a sugar found in milk.

Starches

Starches are **polysaccharides**. Polysaccharide molecules are large and made up of many linked glucose molecules. Although made up of many glucose molecules, the properties of starch are very different from those of glucose. For example, starch is not soluble in water. Starches (such as those in wheat flour and potatoes) are not easily digested and have to be chemically altered first, by cooking.

Non-starch polysaccharides

Non-starch polysaccharides (NSPs) include substances known as fibre. Some of these are insoluble and cannot be broken down by digestion. They pass through the body chemically unchanged. The main type of insoluble fibre is cellulose, the chemical that gives plant stems their structural strength. Soluble fibre includes gums and pectins that are not digested to any significant extent.

Wheat bran contains insoluble fibre. Oats, beans, peas and fruit contain soluble fibre.

Functions of carbohydrates

Functions of sugars and starches

The main function of sugars and starches is to act as energy supplies to the body. They are the easiest nutrients to convert into glucose. They produce the quickest increase in blood sugar levels and, therefore, the quickest 'energy boost' of any food.

Glucose is the main fuel for a chemical reaction that releases chemical energy and converts it to mechanical energy (to move muscles) and electrical/chemical energy (to drive nerve impulses from sense organs to the brain and spinal cord, or from the brain and spinal cord to muscles and glands).

Sugars and starches are the most important foods for providing energy for exercise. These foods can be used in the anaerobic production of energy in the lactic acid system.

Sugars and starches are also the most efficient form of food energy. Fats contain more energy per gram than these carbohydrates, but require more oxygen to metabolise. Sugars and starches already contain a significant amount of oxygen, so require less oxygen to release chemical energy. If people stop eating these carbohydrates, it does not mean that they will run short of energy, because fats and proteins can be converted to glucose by the metabolism.

Starch is digested and stored in the body (mainly in muscles) as **glycogen.**

Functions of fibre

Strictly speaking, fibre has no nutritional value because it passes through the body undigested. However, fibre does performs useful functions:

+ It adds bulk to the faeces, helping them move through the intestines more easily. This reduces the risk of constipation. Fibre adds bulk because it absorbs water during its passage through the intestines.

What is energy?

Energy is a word that is used in different ways in different contexts, so it is easy to get confused about it.

When talking about nutrition, the word energy has a scientific meaning. It means something that can do work. In connection with the body, work means moving muscles (e.g. in climbing stairs) and driving chemical processes such as digestion and the transmission of nerve impulses. Energy is used in all activities, including walking and reading.

You could think about energy in nutrition as being similar to the use of petrol or diesel fuel in a car. A car engine combines fuel with oxygen to release chemical energy and convert it into mechanical energy that turns the wheels. The car also converts some of the energy to electricity to power, for example, the lights and also to store in the battery. The human body combines the 'fuel' of blood sugar with oxygen to release chemical energy and convert it into mechanical energy in muscles and electrical energy in nerve cells. It also stores some of the energy (still as chemical energy) in the form of fat.

Some people talk about energy conversion in the body as 'burning'. For example, long-distance runners talk about endurance exercise as being 'fat-burning'. This is misleading, because the oxidation reaction in the body is rather different — there are no flames! However, the amount of available chemical energy in food can be measured by burning the food. For example, to measure the amount of chemical energy in a gram of bread, the bread is first dried, then placed in a container called a calorimeter and burned. The heat given off is measured in units called calories.

The energy contents of different foods are given in calories (or more usually kilocalories). An alternative unit is the joule (more usually kilojoule). The average energy content per gram of the three macronutrients is given in the following table.

Macronutrient	Energy (kilocalories per gram)
Carbohydrate	4.2
Protein	5.6
Fat	9.2

In practice, the body is not completely efficient in making use of the chemical energy in food, so when the energy contents of foods are calculated, slightly lower figures of 4, 4 and 9 kilocalories per gram respectively are used.

Energy is not a food component. It can be confusing when a food label indicates the amount of energy the food contains, as well as the amounts of the three macronutrients. The energy figure simply indicates how much chemical energy is contained in those macronutrients.

In everyday life, people often use the word 'energy' in a different way. For example, a person might say: 'I haven't got any energy'. This could mean a feeling of tiredness or a lack of motivation to do anything. People who complain of not having any energy probably have plenty of chemical energy (unless they have not eaten for several days). It is more likely that they lack stimulation and are feeling bored and lazy. After a big meal, the body has plenty of energy in the scientific sense. However, people do not feel like doing very much, as the body uses more resources to digest all that food.

The energy equation

For the body to function well, the energy intake should be about the same as the energy output. This is sometimes called the 'energy equation'. Taking in less food energy than the energy that is used results in weight loss, first from body fat and then from muscle tissue.

Taking in more food energy than is used results in weight gain, mainly in the form of fat.

People can balance the equation by altering their food intake, their energy output (e.g. by taking more exercise) or both.

+ Fibre-rich foods give a feeling of fullness. This means that a fibre-rich diet results in a smaller amount of nutrients being eaten. This helps to reduce the risk of not only over-eating and obesity but also related diseases such as heart disease.
+ By smoothing out the rate at which carbohydrates are absorbed, a diet high in fibre helps diabetics to control their blood sugar levels.
+ Fibre helps to reduce the risk of other diseases, such as heart disease.

Recent research suggests that soluble fibre is much more effective as an aid to digestion than insoluble fibre. Soluble fibre, such as pectin, also lowers the levels of cholesterol in the body. It does this by combining with the cholesterol in a gel. This gel is then excreted through the intestines.

Macronutrients and their functions: proteins

Proteins are mainly found in foods that are derived from animals, especially meat, fish, eggs, milk and cheese. Nuts also contain high levels of protein; peas and beans contain significant, though smaller, amounts. Proteins extracted from soya beans and fungi are often eaten by vegetarians.

Chemical composition

Protein molecules are very large and consist of chains of amino acids. Amino acids themselves are molecules containing a backbone of carbon atoms, together with hydrogen, oxygen and nitrogen atoms. There are about 20 naturally occurring amino acids. A protein molecule can be made up of around 1000 linked amino acids, although there are many smaller proteins. The human body can make some amino acids but others (essential amino acids) can be obtained only through the diet.

Functions

The main functions of proteins are to build, maintain and repair body tissue.

+ Body structure – proteins form an important part of the body structure. They are the main constituents of muscles. This is true of all vertebrates and is why meat (which is muscle) is such a good source of proteins.

Did you know ❓

Within the last century, most people in Britain have become well nourished. Before that time, many people suffered from dietary deficiencies, either because they could not afford to buy enough food or because they could not get access to the range of foods needed for good health. As a result, many people were underweight, children did not grow to their full potential and diseases caused by dietary deficiencies were common in some groups. For example, children reared with a diet low in calcium and vitamin D developed rickets (malformed bones and joints). Sailors developed scurvy owing to a lack of fresh fruit.

The problem of undernourishment was made worse by the fact that the lifestyles of many people had large energy requirements. People often walked to work, did strenuous jobs, such as mining and laundry work, unaided by machinery. Clothes were relatively expensive and had poor insulation properties, and houses were inadequately heated in winter. This meant that food energy was used in mechanical work and in generating body heat.

In recent decades this has changed. People use cars, buses and trains instead of walking; they have access to affordable, efficient clothes and central heating. Very few jobs require great physical effort and those that do (such as professional sport or ballet dancing) tend to employ very few people. More importantly, most people in Britain today are enormously wealthy compared with the past. Living standards have improved greatly. Most people can afford food of a quantity and quality that previously could only be obtained by the richest few. For many people, their energy output (meaning work and exercise) is less than their energy consumption in food.

The results of these changes include:

+ the disappearance of deficiency diseases such as rickets and scurvy
+ children growing to their full potentials
+ a rapid increase in obesity owing to taking in more energy in food than is used in work and exercise

+ Body movement — the proteins in muscles enable us to move when muscle fibres contract and relax.
+ Enzymes are proteins. They regulate and enable processes of chemical change in the body. Chemical changes are needed to digest food, build tissues, convert sugars to fats and to release chemical energy in muscles and nerve cells.
+ Some hormones, such as insulin, are proteins.
+ Antibodies, which fight infections, are proteins.

Proteins in the body break down over time, which is why they have to be replaced by eating proteins in the diet.

Protein is the most important macronutrient for survival. It is possible to survive on a diet rich in protein, with only small amounts of carbohydrate and fat. This is because protein can act as an energy source. However, there are practical and health advantages of eating a balanced diet containing all three macronutrients.

Ask people from the older generations of your family how they travelled to school, how their houses were heated and how often they and their parents ate meals in restaurants. Try to find photographs of people from earlier generations to see whether body shape has changed over the years.

Try it out

Summary

The sources and functions of macronutrients are summarised in Table 5.1.

Macronutrient		Main sources	Functions
Fat		Cooking oil, butter, margarine and lard, bacon, salami, crisps, cream, cheese, nuts, some seeds	As chemical energy Energy storage Cushioning body organs Heat insulation under the skin A source of fat-soluble vitamins
Carbohydrate	Sugars	Chocolate, honey, syrup, jam, cakes, sweet biscuits, puddings, grapes, apricots	Energy supply
	Starches	Bread, rice, potatoes, pasta, breakfast cereals	
	Non-starch polysaccharides (fibre)	Bran products, wholemeal bread, peas, beans, apricots and coconut	Digestion Cholesterol reduction
Protein		Meat, fish, eggs, milk, cheese, nuts, peas and beans	Body structure Body movements Body chemical processes involving enzymes, hormones and antibodies

Table 5.1
Macronutrients — their main sources and functions

Micronutrients and their functions: minerals

The minerals you need to know about are included below. There are others (not included) that you do not need to know about for this unit.

Minerals are chemical elements such as iron, calcium, phosphorus, iodine and zinc. They occur in food in the form of salts that contain the element. Minerals are needed to build some of the chemical raw materials for cell growth.

Iron

Iron is found in large quantities in liver and black pudding. It is found in rather smaller amounts in many other foods, including kidney, meat, fish, peas, beans, watercress, breakfast cereals and plain chocolate.

It is needed to make a substance called **haemoglobin,** which occurs in red blood cells. Haemoglobin takes up oxygen from the air we breathe and transports it round the body. Iron is also a component of **myoglobin,** which occurs in muscle cells.

For an average person, the daily iron requirement is about 10 milligrams (mg).

Effects of deficiency

A deficiency of iron is one of the causes of **anaemia**, a condition in which the red blood cells contain too little haemoglobin. The result is that the oxygen-carrying capacity of the blood is reduced. As a result, a person with anaemia might look pale, feel tired and be short of breath.

Calcium

Good sources of **calcium** include bread, milk, cheese, green vegetables and fish with edible bones, such as canned sardines.

Calcium is an important element in the construction of bones and teeth. It is also needed in such processes as muscle contraction, nerve transmission and blood clotting.

The daily requirement for calcium depends on sex and age:

+ For young children and mature adults it is about 500 mg (i.e. about half a gram) per day. Young children need this much because their teeth and bones are growing.
+ For adolescents and young adults, the daily requirement rises to almost 1000 mg (1 gram).
+ The average person needs around 800 mg of calcium per day.
+ Pregnant and breast-feeding women need more calcium than other adults (about 1200 mg per day) because they need calcium to build the bones of the unborn baby and to produce milk respectively.
+ Older people might benefit from a larger than average intake as their ability to absorb calcium from food is reduced.

Effects of deficiency

In children, calcium deficiency can cause **rickets**, which is a condition that leads to weakened bones and bone deformities, particularly in the legs (bow legs) and the spine.

In adults, calcium deficiency leads to low bone density. Normal bones are not solid; they contain small cavities or pores. A person who has low bone-density has relatively small amounts of solid bone tissue and relatively large pores. After the age of about 50 years, some adults begin to lose bone tissue faster than it can be replaced. This is particularly true of post-menopausal women. In severe cases (called **osteoporosis**), bone density is so low that there is a high risk of bone fractures. An adequate calcium intake throughout life reduces this risk.

Calcium deficiency can also lead to impairment of muscle and nerve functions.

Phosphorus

Phosphorus is found combined with oxygen as phosphates, in meat, milk, fish, cereals, peas, beans and fruit.

In combination with calcium, phosphates are important for the building and maintenance of bones and teeth. Phosphorus is also involved in the reactions that turn chemical energy from food into work, and in storing energy in muscles.

For an average person, the daily phosphorus requirement is about 800 mg.

Effect of deficiency

Phosphorus occurs in large enough quantities in most foods to ensure that deficiency rarely occurs. When it does, the effects are very similar to those of calcium deficiency.

Iodine

Iodine occurs as iodine salts in seawater, and seafood is a good dietary source. It is also found in small quantities in milk and green vegetables.

Iodine is needed by the body to produce hormones in the thyroid gland that control the rate of metabolism.

For an average person, the daily iodine requirement is about 0.15 mg.

Effects of deficiency

Iodine deficiency can result in a swollen thyroid gland, which produces a swelling in the neck called **goitre**. Another effect is **hypothyroidism**, in which thyroid activity slows down.

Zinc

Zinc is found in meat, eggs, shellfish, peas and beans, nuts, milk and cereals.

Zinc is involved with several processes including sperm production, growth, energy-producing reactions, healing of wounds, blood clotting and in the immune system. For an average person, the daily zinc requirement is about 13 mg.

Effects of deficiency

Zinc deficiency is rare except in some Middle-Eastern countries. Deficiency slows down growth in children and can cause loss of appetite, hair loss and skin inflammation. (Note that an excess of zinc is toxic.)

Summary

Important facts about minerals are summarised in Table 5.2.

Mineral	Functions	Recommended daily intake (mg)	Main sources	Effects of deficiency
Iron	Essential for haemoglobin production in red blood cells Involved in oxygen take up and oxidation reactions in the body	10	Liver, black pudding, kidney, meat, fish, peas, beans, watercress, breakfast cereals	Anaemia Tiredness Reduced resistance to infection
Calcium	Bone growth Enzyme activity Nerve transmission Muscle contraction	800	Bread, milk and cheese, green vegetables, and fish containing edible bones, such as canned sardines	Osteoporosis Rickets Muscle weakness and cramps
Phosphorus	Bone growth Cell membrane structure Activity of B vitamins	800	Meat, milk, fish, cereals, peas, beans and fruit	Deficiency is very rare Restricted bone growth Muscle weakness
Iodine	Production of thyroid hormones	0.15	Seafood	Goitre Hypothyroidism
Zinc	Involved in enzyme activity connected with energy release and protein building Involved in immune system and sexual maturation	13	Meat, eggs, shellfish, peas and beans, nuts, milk and cereals	Weak immune system Poor wound healing Failure to grow Skin inflammation

Table 5.2
Minerals — their functions, daily requirement, main sources and effects of deficiency

Micronutrients and their functions: vitamins

The vitamins you need to know about are included below. There are others (not included) that you do not need to know about for this unit.

Vitamins are chemicals that enable chemical reactions in the body to take place:

+ Some vitamins act as part of enzymes, which control chemical processes (such as digestion) in the body.
+ Some vitamins are antioxidants. This means that they help to reduce damage to cells caused by free radicals (containing oxygen) produced by chemical

reactions in the body. These vitamins are said to 'mop up' unwanted free radicals.

Most vitamins cannot be produced by the human body, so must be taken in with food. An exception is vitamin D, which is made in the body if the skin is exposed to sunshine.

Some vitamins are soluble in fat; others are soluble in water. If a vitamin is soluble in fat, it will be found only in foods that contain fats and oils, such as the tissues of oily fish. Water-soluble vitamins are found in foods containing watery tissue, such as fruit.

Fat-soluble vitamins

Fat-soluble vitamins include vitamins A, D, E and K.

Vitamin A

+ **Vitamin A** occurs in liver, eggs, cheese, milk and carrots.
+ It has a function in the growth and maintenance of cells, particularly in the skin and eyes. It is needed for night vision. It aids the development of cell structure, bones and teeth.
+ The main effect of deficiency is poor night vision.

Vitamin D

+ **Vitamin D** is found in oily fish and vitamin-fortified foods such as margarine. It is also produced by the action of sunlight (containing ultraviolet light) on the skin.
+ It helps chemical reactions involved in absorbing the mineral calcium from food. Therefore, it is important in building and maintaining bones and teeth. It helps absorption of calcium in the intestines and maintains the balance of calcium and phosphates in the body. It also helps nerve tissue and muscles to work.
+ Effects of deficiency include rickets and osteomalacia (a softening of the bones).

Vitamin E

+ **Vitamin E** is found in vegetable oils, nuts and whole-grain foods.
+ It is an antioxidant that slows down damage to cells and so reduces cell ageing. It helps to build red blood cells.
+ Deficiency occurs very rarely. One effect is anaemia.

Vitamin K

+ **Vitamin K** is found in cabbage, broccoli, spinach, eggs and pork. It is also produced by the action of bacteria in the intestines.
+ It helps to produce blood-clotting proteins.
+ Deficiency occurs very rarely, although sometimes in newborn babies. The effect is a failure of blood clotting.

Fat-soluble vitamin	Functions	Daily requirement (mg)	Main sources
A	Maintains skin health Aids night vision Aids bone development	0.65	Liver, milk, cheese, eggs carrots
D	Promotes growth of bones and teeth	0.01	Fish oils, vitamin-fortified processed foods (e.g. margarine); also formed by the action of sunlight on skin
E	Antioxidant	9	Vegetable oils, nuts, whole-grain foods
K	Necessary for blood clotting	0.07	Cabbage, broccoli, spinach eggs, pork; also formed in the intestines by bacteria

Table 5.3
Fat-soluble vitamins — their functions, recommended intake and main sources

Water-soluble vitamins

Water-soluble vitamins include vitamins B_1, B_2, B_3, B_9 and C.

Vitamin B_1

+ **Vitamin B_1** (also called **thiamine**) is found in liver, kidney, whole-grain foods, peas, beans and cereals.
+ It helps the reaction that releases energy from carbohydrate in muscles and nerve cells.
+ A deficiency can cause the disease **beriberi**, the symptoms of which include numbness and heart failure.

Vitamin B_2

+ **Vitamin B_2** (also called **riboflavin**) is found in milk, dairy products, meat and leaf vegetables.
+ It helps the reaction that releases energy from carbohydrates, regulates hormone production and helps to maintain nerve cells, eyes and skin.
+ Deficiency is rare, and causes mouth sores.

Vitamin B_3

+ **Vitamin B_3** (also called **niacin**) is found in meat, poultry, fish, peas, beans and whole-grain foods.
+ It helps the enzyme reactions that release energy from fats and carbohydrates, helps nerve function and the production of sex hormones.
+ Deficiency causes **pellagra**, a condition in which the skin darkens and becomes scaly.

Vitamin B_9

+ **Vitamin B_9** (**folic acid**) is found in liver, leaf vegetables, peas, beans and nuts.
+ It helps to build body cells, including red blood cells. It helps to build nucleic

acids, including DNA. In the first 3 months of pregnancy, it reduces the risk of birth defects such as spina bifida.

+ Deficiency can cause **anaemia**, and **spina bifida** in a fetus.

Vitamin C

+ **Vitamin C (ascorbic acid)** is found in citrus fruits (oranges, grapefruits and lemons) and green vegetables.
+ It is an antioxidant. It is involved in producing adrenaline and in the maintenance of healthy bones, teeth, gums and blood vessels. It contributes to wound healing.
+ Deficiency leads to **scurvy**, a disease featuring bleeding under the skin and poor wound healing. This often used to be fatal for sailors on long voyages because of the lack of fresh food, particularly fruit.

Water-soluble vitamin	Functions	Daily requirement (mg)	Main sources
B$_1$ (thiamine)	Involved in enzyme action to release energy from carbohydrates Aids nervous system functions	0.9	Liver, kidney, whole-grain foods, peas, beans, cereals
B$_2$ (riboflavin)	Involved in enzyme action to release energy from carbohydrates and fats Maintains healthy skin	1.5	Milk, dairy products, meat, leaf vegetables
B$_3$ (niacin)	Involved in enzyme action to release energy from carbohydrates Helps to synthesise fats in the body	17	Meat, poultry, fish, whole-grain foods, peas, beans
B$_9$ (folic acid)	Involved in enzyme action for growth of red blood cells and DNA production	0.2	Liver, leaf vegetables, peas, beans, nuts
C (ascorbic acid)	Helps to build collagen (connective tissue), for example, in skin Aids iron absorption Helps to form adrenaline Antioxidant	40	Citrus fruits, green vegetables

Table 5.4
Water-soluble vitamins — their functions, recommended intake and main sources

The daily requirement figures given in Tables 5.3 and 5.4 are Reference Nutrient Intakes. The figures given are approximate. Individual requirements are linked to body mass, so women and children tend to need less than men. Some people will need more than the amounts given, others less.

Other important substances in food

Water

The body is made up of many different molecules — some simple, some complex. One of the simplest molecules in the body is water. It is also the most common, making up about 70% of the body by weight.

The water consumed in drinks and food:

+ is an aid to digestion
+ is a medium for chemical reactions
+ is a lubricant for joint surfaces and between cells
+ helps to regulate body temperature by sweating

Non-nutrients in food

Phytochemicals

Phytochemicals are found in plants, including fruit and vegetables. The name means 'plant chemicals'. They give plants colour, flavour, smell and texture. Some phytochemicals help protect against disease, including cancer, diabetes, cardio-vascular disease and hypertension. Useful sources of beneficial phytochemicals include raspberries and strawberries, broccoli, cocoa beans, green tea and red wine.

Phytochemicals are described as **non-nutrients** because they do not serve the main functions of energy supply, repair and maintenance.

Beneficial phytochemicals include:

+ **astaxanthin**, which is the pink pigment found in seafoods, such as salmon and lobster. (It is obtained by them from algae, through the food chain.) It acts as a powerful antioxidant and anti-inflammatory.
+ **flavonoids**, which are antioxidants that help prevent the growth of cancer cells. Onions contain more flavonoids than most other plants, with the strongest-smelling onions containing the most effective flavonoids.

Phytochemicals that are known to have health benefits are sometimes called 'nutraceuticals'.

Toxins

Some of the naturally occurring chemicals in food are slightly toxic — for example, lectins in red kidney beans. These chemicals would not be allowed as food additives. However, they usually occur in quantities too small to be harmful, or are reduced by cooking.

Food additives

Food additives are substances that are added by manufacturers and food processors to improve food in some way.

The main types of additives are preservatives and antioxidants, texture enhancers, flavour and appearance enhancers and micronutrients. You need to know the purposes of these additives, but you do not need to know their names.

Preservatives and antioxidants

Preservatives keep food from deteriorating over time.

The addition of preservatives to food started several thousand years ago. The commonest method was by adding salt (sodium chloride) — for example, in producing bacon. However, an excess of salt in the diet can be harmful, increasing the risk of hypertension and strokes.

The preservatives approved by the EU have the benefit of reducing the risks of bacterial infections and toxins in food. These preservatives are labelled using E-numbers. Preservatives given E-numbers do not have harmful effects.

Some preservatives are designed to kill or reduce the growth of bacteria and moulds in food. These include nitrates and nitrites in bacon and other processed meat products, and propanoic acid in bread and cakes.

Other preservatives (called **antioxidants**) are designed to prevent food from reacting with oxygen in the atmosphere. This oxidation reaction spoils the taste of foods and makes oils go rancid. Antioxidants also slow the rate at which vitamins in food, such as A and C, break down.

Texture enhancers

Texture enhancers are added to improve or maintain food texture. For example, pectin (E440) is a form of soluble fibre added to jams and marmalade to stop them being liquid.

Emulsifiers and **stabilisers** are chemicals that help to form and maintain food emulsions, giving a creamy texture. An emulsion is a mixture of water and oil. Examples of food emulsions are mayonnaise and low-fat (butter substitute) spreads. Without stabilisers, these foods would separate out into water and oil.

Flavour and appearance enhancers

Flavour can be enhanced by adding **sweeteners**, such as aspartame (E951). One benefit of such sweeteners is that they are low-energy substitutes for sugars.

Colourings are used to improve appearance. For example, tartrazine (E102) is an orange colouring that is added to soft drinks.

Micronutrients

Vitamins and minerals are added to maintain or improve the nutritional quality of processed foods such as breakfast cereals and low-fat spreads. These additives reduce the risk of deficiency diseases.

Look at the nutritional information provided on the packaging of two kinds of foods — one a meat product, such as sausage or ham; the other a bakery product such as biscuits or cake. List the minerals, vitamins, preservatives and other additives present.

A recent advertisement showed the contents of two brands of spread.

Spread 1 contained:

+ sunflower oil (36%)

+ buttermilk (5%)

Try it out

+ salt (1.5%)
+ water
+ emulsifier
+ preservatives E202 and E330
+ vitamins A, D, E, B_6, B_9 and B_{12}
+ colour
+ flavouring

Spread 2 contained:

+ butter (60%)
+ vegetable oil (31%)
+ salt (1.3%)
+ water

The advertisement was aimed at selling only one of these spreads (the other spread was made by a market competitor). The advertiser believed that people reading the lists would assume that one of the products was much better than the other.

Question 1

Decide which of these spreads is likely to be better for health, and why. You might need to look again at the description of fats on pages 134 and 135.

Question 2

Decide whether the advertiser was trying to sell spread 1 or spread 2.

Answers to these questions can be found at the end of the chapter (see p. 164).

Try it out

Did you know

Are food additives beneficial, harmful or neither?
Some people believe that food additives are harmful and prefer to eat food that has had nothing added to the basic foodstuff. For a time during the last century, there was a popular belief that additives such as food colourings and flavour enhancers caused hyperactivity in children. Controlled studies demonstrated no clear connection between food additives and hyperactivity, although a small number of people show allergic reactions to some additives.

Modern food additives are usually either harmless or actually beneficial. Benefits include:

+ reducing the risk of bacterial contamination
+ providing low-fat alternatives
+ enhancing vitamin content

Modern food additives have to be tested for safety and if found to pose even a slight risk to health are banned. In 2005, a banned food colouring (called Sudan 1) was found in a range of processed foods. Foods containing this additive were removed from sale, even though the health risk was extremely small. The main risk to health comes from traditional additives, especially salt and sugar.

However, one indirect harmful effect of additives is that they can make food so appetising and attractive that people are tempted to eat to excess.

Apart from obesity, the main health risk associated with food is food poisoning. This occurs most often in foods that do not have preservatives added to them — for example, fresh and frozen meats.

A balanced diet

Maintaining a balanced diet

A balanced diet is one that contains adequate amounts of macronutrients and micronutrients for the energy requirements, maintenance and repair of the body. These amounts are indicated in tables of Dietary Reference Values (DRVs), such as those on page 155.

Dangers of deficiency and excess

If some key nutrients are missing from the diet, these dietary deficiencies can cause problems:

+ A lack of fats and carbohydrates can result in low body weight and the conversion of muscle tissue into chemical energy. This lack of macronutrients means that energy supply can be maintained only at the expense of maintenance and repair.

+ A lack of minerals and vitamins can cause other deficiency diseases such as pellagra, beriberi, scurvy and rickets.

Excesses of macro- and micronutrients can also cause problems:

+ An excess of carbohydrates and fats can lead to obesity (excessive amounts of fat in the body). Obesity increases the risk of diabetes, heart disease, hypertension and some cancers.

+ An excess of some vitamins causes damage to the liver, kidneys and nerve tissue. Excesses of vitamins A and D in the diet are very unlikely and usually only occur in people who take supplementary vitamins.

The effects of dietary deficiency and excess are summarised in Table 5.5.

Dietary component	Effects of deficiency	Effects of excess
Fat	Lack of energy Deficiencies associated with lack of fat-soluble vitamins	Coronary heart disease Obesity
Carbohydrate	Lack of energy	Obesity
Protein	Restricted growth in children Impaired growth of muscle	Minimal
Fibre	Constipation	Minimal
Water	Headaches Constipation	Minimal
Vitamin K	Increased bleeding	Clot formation (thrombosis)
Folic acid	Diarrhoea Anaemia Deficiency during pregnancy can lead to spina bifida in the fetus	Minimal
Ascorbic acid	Scurvy Bleeding gums Weakness	Diarrhoea
Niacin	Pellagra (skin disease)	Headache Liver damage
Calcium	Osteoporosis Rickets	Constipation Kidney stones
Iron	Anaemia	Liver damage

Table 5.5
Dietary deficiency and excess

Importance of variety

Although it is possible to devise a diet, using only a small range of foods, which on paper seems to meet most dietary requirements, there are several reasons why eating a wider variety of foods is beneficial, including the following:

+ The diet might contain plenty of protein, but if it is not varied it might not contain the full range of proteins required.
+ Some micronutrients might not be present.
+ A varied diet is likely to be more appealing. One important aspect of nutrition is the pleasure of different flavours and textures.

Dietary planning

Planning a balanced diet involves considering several factors, including:

+ the **nutritional value** of each food. This means the energy content and amounts of different nutrients.
+ **palatability**. This means the extent to which the food appeals to the person for whom the diet is planned.
+ **cost**. Food high in micronutrients and phytochemicals (such as fresh fruit) tends to be expensive.
+ **ease of preparation**. Some processed foods are ready to eat or are easy to prepare (such as microwave-ready meals). However, these foods tend to contain excessive amounts of salt (sodium chloride).

Why some people do not have a balanced diet

In practice, it can be difficult to achieve a nutritionally ideal balanced diet. This relates particularly to those people:

+ who cannot afford fresh fruit
+ who have little time to prepare meals
+ who are restricted to a narrow range of foods by what they find palatable
+ who by lifestyle choice can find it difficult to achieve a balanced diet

Organisations such as hospitals, schools and residential homes can ensure that they supply the elements of a balanced diet, but they cannot ensure that their clients actually choose those foods that together make up a balanced diet.

Nutrition tables

Much information about nutrition is presented in the form of tables. You should be able to extract information from such tables, although you do not need

Food	Water (g)	Protein (g)	Fat (g)	Carbohydrate (g)	Fibre (g)	Energy (kcal/100 g)
White bread	37.3	8.4	1.9	49.3	1.5	235
Wholemeal bread	38.3	9.2	2.5	41.6	5.8	215
Skimmed milk	91.1	3.3	0.1	5.0	0.0	33
Whole milk	87.8	3.2	3.9	4.8	0.0	66
Cheddar cheese	36.0	25.5	34.4	0.1	0.0	412
Boiled eggs	75.1	12.5	10.8	0.0	0.0	147
Bacon	40.5	14.2	41.2	0.0	0.0	428
Roast chicken	68.4	24.8	5.4	0.0	0.0	148
Grilled fishfingers	56.2	15.1	9.0	19.3	0.7	214
Tinned sardines	58.4	23.7	13.6	0.0	0.0	217
Potato chips	56.5	3.9	6.7	30.1	2.2	189
Tinned baked beans	71.5	5.2	0.6	15.3	3.7	84
Brussels sprouts	86.9	2.9	1.3	3.5	3.1	35
Frozen peas	78.3	6.0	0.9	9.7	5.1	69
Raw tomatoes	93.1	0.7	0.3	3.1	1.0	17
Bananas	75.1	1.2	0.3	23.2	1.1	95
Oranges	86.1	1.1	0.1	8.5	1.7	37
Roasted salted peanuts	1.9	24.5	53.0	7.1	6.0	602
Milk chocolate	2.2	8.4	30.3	59.4	0.0	529
Marmalade	28.0	0.1	0.0	69.5	0.6	261

Source: Food Standards Agency

Table 5.6
Nutritional composition
of selected foods

to learn the data contained in them. You should also be able to compare nutrient intake with Dietary Reference Values (see page 155) to make judgements about how balanced a particular diet is.

Table 5.6 shows the nutritional composition (macronutrients, water, fibre and energy content) of selected foods.

Studying Table 5.6 reveals a number of interesting facts:

+ Many foods contain high proportions of water.
+ Only foods that are plants (or are wholly or partly derived from plants) contain fibre.
+ Foods containing relatively high proportions of fats and/or carbohydrates contain the most energy per 100 g.

Note that Table 5.6 does not include micronutrients. Some foods that have a fairly low energy content are beneficial because of their vitamin and/or mineral contents — for example, Brussels sprouts, oranges and tomatoes.

Dietary and nutritional needs of client groups

The Department of Health publishes tables of Dietary Reference Values (DRVs). DRVs give an indication of the quantity of each nutrient required by people, according to their sex and age.

Included in the DRVs are Reference Nutrient Intake (RNI) values. The RNI for any one nutrient is the amount that is enough for most individuals in a particular age and sex group. RNIs are higher than the nutrient needs of the average person because they are set so as to be sufficient even for people with particularly high nutrient needs. For example, the RNI for protein for an adult female is 45 g.

DRVs also include Estimated Average Requirements (EARs). These are average values, so some people will need more and others less. For example, the EAR for food energy for an adult male is 2550 kcal per day.

To understand tables of DRVs, you need to know about the units of measurement used:

+ Quantities of macronutrients are given in grams (g).
+ Quantities of micronutrients are given in smaller units (because far less of these nutrients is needed). The units used are sometimes milligrams (mg) or micrograms (μg):
    + A milligram is one thousandth of a gram.
    + A microgram is one millionth of a gram.
+ Energy is measured in kilocalories (kcal). A kilocalorie is one thousand calories.
+ An alternative measure of energy is the kilojoule (kJ). A kilojoule is one thousand joules.
+ 1 calorie = 4.184 joules

You do not need to remember actual DRVs for different client groups. However, you should understand what they are and you should be able to interpret and draw conclusions from DRVs (e.g. given in tables) in the examination.

Variation in DRVs

DRVs are usually given according to a person's age, sex and (in the case of women) whether or not they are pregnant.

Note that some tables showing DRVs do not list fats and carbohydrates separately, but simply indicate 'energy', most of which is provided by these two food components.

Age in years	Energy requirement for males (kcal/day)	Energy requirement for females (kcal/day)
1–3	1230	1165
4–6	1715	1545
7–10	1970	1740
11–14	2220	1845
15–18	2755	2110
19–50	2550	1940
51–59	2550	1900
60–64	2380	1900
65–74	2330	1900
75+	2100	1810
19+ and pregnant		2140

Table 5.7
Estimated average energy requirements in the UK

Source: Food Standards Agency

Group	Age in years	Protein (g/day)	Reference nutrient intake Calcium (mg/day)	Iron (mg/day)	Vitamin B_9 (µg/day)
Children	1–3	14.5	350	6.9	70
	4–6	19.7	450	6.1	100
	7–10	28.3	550	8.7	150
Males	11–14	42.1	1000	11.3	200
	15–18	55.2	1000	11.3	200
	19–50	55.5	700	8.7	200
	50+	53.3	700	8.7	200
Females	11–14	41.2	800	14.8	200
	15–18	45.0	800	14.8	200
	19–50	45.0	700	14.8	200
	50+	46.5	700	8.7	200
	19+ and pregnant	51.0	700	14.8	300

Table 5.8
Reference nutrient intakes for protein and three selected micro-nutrients for the UK

Source: Food Standards Agency

Age

Tables 5.7 and 5.8 show that DRVs tend to increase during childhood and adolescence. They then tend to remain steady during adulthood and decline with the approach of old age. A major reason for this pattern is the change in body mass of the individual, on which the requirement for nutrients partly depends. For example, a person with a larger body mass requires more energy to run and climb stairs than a lighter person.

Level of physical activity

Energy requirements are also influenced by activity levels. This is one reason why the EAR for energy is higher in young adults than in people over 50 years of age. However, there are large variations in energy requirements between different people. For example, a 60-year-old marathon runner will have a larger energy requirement than a 16-year-old who takes no exercise. Remember that EARs are only average figures across the population.

Gender

The sex of a person influences dietary requirements. This is because, on average, males have larger, heavier bodies than females, particularly from adolescence onwards. They also tend to build more muscle than females during adolescence. Another important sex difference is that from puberty until the menopause, girls and women have a much larger requirement for iron and vitamin B_6 than boys and men. This is because these girls and women lose significant amounts of blood through menstruation every month. Iron and vitamin B_6 are needed to make haemoglobin — an important constituent of blood.

Pregnancy also increases the requirement for some nutrients, as does lactation (the production of milk in breastfeeding mothers).

Pregnancy

Pregnancy increases the requirement for some nutrients, including protein, vitamin B_9 and iron, as well as increasing the requirement for food energy. This is partly because of the increased combined body mass of woman and fetus, and partly because of the requirements for the chemical raw materials (especially proteins) needed to grow the baby.

State of health

Illness can influence dietary requirements in several ways:

+ People whose illness makes them immobile (for example, confined to bed) will have a lower energy requirement than others of the same age, sex and body mass.
+ Those suffering from anaemia will require higher levels of iron and vitamin B_6.
+ People who have a very low body mass for their age and sex, possibly because of anorexia or cancer, will need to gain weight by increasing their intake of macronutrients.
+ Obese people are likely to benefit from a period with a reduced intake of the main energy-providing macronutrients, i.e. fats and carbohydrates.

Try it out

Answer these questions by referring to the tables of Dietary Reference Values.
Question 1
Which age range in males shows the highest average energy requirement?
Question 2
Give one reason why the energy requirement for males of this age is higher than for males 10 years older.

Question 3
In which two age groups is the RNI for calcium highest?
Question 4
Give one reason why the calcium requirement for these age groups is higher than that for people 10 years older.

Answers to these questions are given at the end of the chapter (see p. 164).

Try it out

Dietary variations

People's diets can be influenced by several factors, including their religious beliefs, lifestyle choices, health needs, food allergies and food intolerances.

Religious beliefs

Some religions require their followers to avoid certain foods:

+ Hindus are not permitted to eat beef. The usual diet is mainly, but not entirely, vegetarian.
+ Muslims are not permitted to eat pork, blood products or shellfish, or to drink alcohol. These forbidden foods are called 'haram'. Any meat eaten should be 'halal', i.e. dedicated to God by a Muslim present at the slaughtering.
+ Jews are not permitted to eat pork. Any meat eaten should be 'kosher'. Kosher meat is from animals that have cloven hoofs, such as cows and sheep. To be kosher, this meat should come from animals slaughtered by someone who has a special religious licence to do so, and then salted. Dairy products, such as milk and cheese, must not be consumed together with meat. Non-kosher foods are called 'treifa'.

These religious requirements do not create particular difficulties in providing a balanced diet.

Lifestyle choices

Vegetarian

Vegetarians do not eat meat, poultry and fish — in other words, any animal that has to be killed to provide food. However, vegetarians (sometimes called lacto-vegetarians) will eat animal food products, such as eggs, milk, cheese and butter because animals do not have to be killed to obtain these.

Vegan

Vegans do not eat meat, poultry, fish or any other animal food products, even if obtaining the food does not involve killing the animal. This rules out eggs and dairy products. All these foods are good sources of proteins, vitamins and minerals, so vegans (and to some extent vegetarians) have to take particular care to ensure that they have sufficient sources of these nutrients in their diets.

Health needs

Diabetes

Diabetes mellitus is a disease affecting the hormone **insulin**. Insulin is important because it enables body cells to take up glucose (blood sugar) from the blood. The disease can happen either because the pancreas stops producing enough insulin (Type 1 diabetes) or because the cells of the body become resistant to this hormone (Type 2 diabetes).

Normally the pancreas releases insulin after a meal is eaten. Digestion converts some of the food into blood sugar. As the level of sugar in the blood rises, more insulin is secreted. If the blood sugar level begins to fall, for example if someone has not eaten for a long time, blood sugar stored in the liver is released, keeping the level in the blood fairly steady.

In diabetics, however, the sugar is not taken up by body cells and this has two results:

+ First, the body cells do not get enough energy. This means that the person feels weak and in severe cases might lose consciousness, fall into a coma and possibly die. The person also feels hungry and tends to eat more.
+ The level of sugar in the blood increases and the excess is eliminated from the body in the urine.

Type 1 diabetes is controlled by the sufferer injecting insulin into the body each day. Type 2 diabetes can sometimes be controlled by diet.

To prevent large rises in blood sugar, diabetics have to limit the amount of carbohydrate they eat. This means that they should avoid sugar-rich foods, eat low-sugar alternatives such as diabetic chocolate, monitor their food intake and avoid overeating. It is also best to eat about the same amount of food each day and to take meals at about the same time each day.

Food allergies

Some foods can cause allergic reactions, which can vary from mild inflammations to death from **anaphylactic shock**. Anaphylaxis involves the release of large amounts of histamine into the bloodstream, which lowers blood pressure and constricts the airways. It can result from a nut allergy. Other foods that can trigger allergies include shellfish and eggs.

Hives (otherwise known as urticaria or nettle rash) can result from a food allergy. The symptoms are raised rashes of itchy red patches.

Asthma can be caused by food allergies. The symptoms include breathlessness, a feeling of tightness in the chest, wheezing and a dry cough.

Food intolerance

Food intolerance is an inability to digest certain foods. It is not an allergy, because no allergic reaction is produced.

Gluten intolerance

Gluten is a protein found in cereals such as wheat and rye. Some people cannot digest gluten, so they are intolerant of flour-based foods such as bread and pasta. The condition, called coeliac disease, runs in families. The 'gluten reaction' damages the small intestine, leads to vomiting and diarrhoea and an inability to absorb vitamins and minerals from food.

Milk or lactose intolerance

Lactose is a sugar found in milk and milk products. It is digested by an enzyme called lactase. Some people produce very little lactase, meaning that lactose in their diet is not digested properly. Lactose intolerance produces symptoms including stomach pains, bloating, flatulence and diarrhoea.

Food preparation

Food poses a significant risk of causing infection. Large numbers of bacteria, viruses, mould or fungal spores are taken into the body in food and water.

Common illnesses associated with poor food hygiene

Common illnesses associated with poor food hygiene are various types of food poisoning. The symptoms of food poisoning are stomach cramps, diarrhoea and vomiting. Depending on the cause of the food poisoning, symptoms may develop within a few hours of eating the infected food or may take over a day to appear.

Microorganisms causing food poisoning

+ *Salmonella* and *campylobacter* are bacteria that frequently occur in chicken, turkey and eggs.
+ *Clostridium* is a bacterium that can infect warm stews and gravies that have been left to cool. The bacteria can multiply in the warm conditions.
+ *Escherichia coli* (better known as *E. coli*) is carried by cattle and can be transmitted to humans in undercooked beef, in milk and also by contamination of fruit and vegetables with cow manure. Small numbers of the bacteria can cause serious infections.
+ *Staphylococcus* bacteria live on the skin. If people do not wash their hands before preparing food, this bacterium can infect the food. Cuts in the skin are likely to be infected by this organism. Preparing food whilst having infected cuts that are not covered up is a common cause of food poisoning. To prevent this infection being passed on, it is important that people who prepare food cover any cuts or wounds.

+ Viruses can also cause food poisoning. The most common causes are rotavirus and the Norwalk virus (which is often found in shellfish).

Client groups most at risk

Vulnerable groups include pregnant and breastfeeding women, infants, elderly people and those whose immune systems have been weakened either by disease (such as AIDS) or by medical treatment for cancer.

Health and safety precautions applying to food storage and preparation

Storing food

The following applies most to foods that are called 'perishable' — that deteriorate rapidly if kept at room temperature. These include meat, poultry, fish and milk. Other foods, such as dry cereals, uncooked pasta, biscuits, cakes, raw fruit and vegetables can be kept safely at room temperature.

Perishable foods provide excellent places for disease-causing organisms to live and multiply. Most such foods contain small numbers of disease-causing organisms, but at levels too low to be harmful. The danger occurs if these organisms have the opportunity to multiply.

Keeping perishable foods in a refrigerator slows down the rate at which bacteria and other organisms multiply. However, it does not completely stop their growth. For this reason, most perishable foods should not be kept for more than a few days in a refrigerator before being consumed. 'Sell by' and 'use by' dates on food are designed to let consumers know how long food may be safely stored.

Freezing food is an effective way of stopping the growth of disease-causing organisms, although it does not kill them.

Perishable food should not be left at room temperature for more than 2 hours before cooking (or if ready to eat, before eating). Perishable food that has been stored at room temperature should not be subsequently frozen. This is because disease-causing organisms are likely to have multiplied during room-temperature storage, and freezing the food will not kill them. When the food is thawed again, the disease-causing organisms will continue to multiply. The result will be the same as if the food had been stored at room temperature for a much longer time.

Preparing food

People who prepare food should follow the principles of good hygiene. Most importantly, they should wash their hands. The purpose of this is to reduce the population of disease-causing organisms on the skin, so that as few of these as possible are transferred to food.

+ Hands should be washed:
  + before handling food
  + between preparing different food items

+ after visiting the toilet
+ after any contact with a potential source of infection (such as a pet, or a baby's nappy)

+ Hand jewellery, such as rings, should not be worn because it can collect dirt that harbours large populations of microorganisms that could easily be transferred to food.
+ Cuts on the skin should be covered with a waterproof wound plaster. Plasters (coloured blue for easy visibility) are normally used in the catering industry.
+ Hair should be covered by a cap to prevent hair or dandruff from falling into the food. Hair and flakes of skin also carry disease-causing organisms.
+ Clothing should be clean.
+ Food should not be handled unnecessarily.
+ Coughing and sneezing should be avoided near food.
+ Smoking should be avoided. It can cause contamination of food by ash, and increases the probability of coughing.
+ Work surfaces should be cleaned with hot water and soap or washing-up liquid. Food spills should be cleaned up.
+ Dishcloths, sponges and non-metallic scouring pads used in washing up and cleaning work surfaces are often warm and damp and contain fragments of food, thus providing ideal habitats for bacteria. They can be decontaminated by heating in a microwave for 1 minute.

Cooking

Cooking is the most effective way of destroying disease-causing organisms in food. They are killed by temperatures above 65°C. Large pieces of food, such as whole chickens, must be cooked for longer, because it takes time for the heat to penetrate into the centre.

Cooking at high temperature is only effective if there is enough time for the heat to penetrate right into the food. The key points are to cook at a high temperature and thoroughly.

Undercooking can sometimes occur when food is cooked from frozen. Parts of the food might not reach the required temperature during cooking.

Microwave ovens sometimes heat food unevenly, so it is important to stop and change the position of the food during cooking — for example, by stirring a stew.

Other hygiene measures

+ Fruits in which the skin is eaten (such as apples, strawberries, grapes and peaches) should be washed before eating.
+ Vegetables contaminated by soil (such as potatoes and carrots) should be washed before peeling.
+ Raw and cooked foods should be kept separate, and different utensils should be used for each of them. For example, it would be a mistake to cut up some raw chicken on a chopping board and then use the same board and knife to slice some cooked pork. Disease-causing organisms from the chicken could be

transferred to the pork. (This is also the reason why the hands should be washed between preparing different food items.)

+ Frozen food should be allowed to defrost in a refrigerator or be defrosted by microwaving.

+ Prepared food that is not refrigerated should be covered or kept in airtight containers. Leaving prepared food exposed to the air increases the risk that airborne microorganisms will contaminate it or that flies will land on it. Flies carry disease-causing organisms on their legs and leave their excreta on food.

+ If foods such as stews and gravies are prepared in order to freeze for later use, they should be cooled down as soon and as quickly as possible. Cooling can be speeded up by stirring and by using a wide, shallow pan.

+ Waste food should be removed from the premises as soon as possible, to reduce the risk of infestation by vermin such as rats and cockroaches, which can carry bacteria and spread disease. Sealing waste food in bags and placing in a vermin-proof bin helps to avoid this problem.

Sample examination questions with model answers

The model answers given would score full marks. In some cases, alternative answers would be acceptable.

1 Ryan is 16 years old. The table below shows Ryan's daily intake of selected nutrients, together with Dietary Reference Values (DRVs).

	Ryan's daily diet	DRVs for males aged 15–18
Energy (kcal)	3150	2750
Protein (g)	65	55
Iron (mg)	11.5	11
Vitamin B_9 (µg)	150	200

(a) Use the information in the table to analyse Ryan's daily diet.   (6 marks)

Ryan is eating food containing more energy than is recommended for his age. Part of this excess might be because he is eating more protein than the recommended figure, but it is likely that he also eats more carbohydrate and fat. Ryan's intake of iron is at the required level, although his intake of vitamin B_9 (folic acid) is low.

(b) Suggest *one* food that could be added to improve Ryan's diet.   (1 mark)

Liver would increase his intake of folic acid.

(c) Despite his diet, Ryan is not overweight. Give *one* likely
explanation for this. (2 marks)

One explanation is that Ryan balances his energy equation by taking a lot of
exercise. Perhaps he plays a lot of sport.

(d) Explain three ways in which the DRVs for 15–18-year-old girls
would be different from those shown in the table. (6 marks)

The energy requirement would be less because, on average, girls have less
body mass than boys at this age. The requirement for protein would also be
less because girls are less likely to be growing muscles to the same extent as
boys. The iron requirement would be higher because girls of this age lose
iron during menstruation.

Total: 15 marks

2 (a) Explain how a person's diet can be affected by:
(i) religious beliefs
(ii) health needs (6 marks)

Religious beliefs can affect a person's diet because some religions forbid
people to eat certain foods. For example, Muslims are forbidden by their
religion to eat pork or shellfish or to drink alcohol. They might also have to
go without food (fast) for some periods.

Health needs can affect diet if eating a certain food is harmful to a person.
For example, a person who has a nut allergy cannot eat nuts. Eating nuts
might make them develop allergic symptoms such as asthma or even go
into anaphylactic shock.

(b) (i) Explain why a person who is a vegan might have difficulty
in eating a balanced diet. (4 marks)

Vegans do not eat meat or fish. They also do not eat other animal products,
such as eggs, milk and cheese. These foods are high in proteins and some
vitamins (e.g. vitamin D in oily fish), so a vegan must take care to eat
enough alternative foods that are high in these nutrients.

(ii) Suggest a range of foods a vegan could eat, which would
help to provide some of their requirements for macronutrients
and micronutrients. (5 marks)

Vegans could eat plenty of nuts, peas and beans, because these contain
proteins. They could eat fungal protein too, such as Quorn™. The peas and
beans will also provide them with a range of B vitamins. They could get some
of the fat-soluble vitamins from vitamin-enriched spreads and breakfast
cereals.

Total: 15 marks

Answers to 'Try it out' questions

Page 150

(1) Spread 1 is better for health, because it contains more unsaturated fats and vitamins. Spread 2 contains more saturated fats and fewer vitamins.

(2) You might be surprised to find out that the advertiser was selling spread 2. The advertiser is probably assuming that consumers are prejudiced against foods containing additives and ignorant about the health benefits of vegetable oils compared with animal fats.

Pages 156–57

(1) In males, the age range with the highest average energy requirement is 15–18 years.

(2) They are more active.

(3) In males aged 11–14 and 15–18 years.

(4) Their bones are still growing.

Further reading

Bender, A. E. and Bender, D. A. (1999) *Food Tables and Labelling* (Combined Schools edn), Oxford University Press.

Food Standards Agency (1995) *Manual of Nutrition* (10th edn), London TSO.

Sprenger, R. A. (2000) *Hygiene Sense, Hygiene Awareness*, Highfield Publications.

Websites

The British Nutrition Foundation:
  www.nutrition.org.uk/

Nutrition Matters:
  www.nutrition-matters.co.uk

Common diseases and disorders

This chapter provides information to prepare you for the examination of **Unit 6: Common diseases and disorders.**

Infectious diseases

General introduction to infections

Infectious diseases are caused by tiny living organisms. These organisms are specialised to live in and on people. They rely on us for food and also to enable them to reproduce. This means that they are **parasites**. For example, a type of bacterium that causes pneumonia lives and multiplies in body tissues and is spread to other people in droplets on sneezing.

A human being is a host to many bacteria. Some of these bacteria are useful. For example, some live in the intestines and help to digest food. In return, they have a warm, wet place to live and plenty of food.

How do disease-causing organisms enter the body?

Some organisms live on the skin (e.g. those causing some fungal infections), but most have to enter the body before they cause problems. The ways in which they enter the body include:

+ being breathed in
+ getting into the eyes
+ being swallowed in food or drink
+ through the penis and vagina during sex
+ through wounds in the skin as a result of accidents or surgery

Do they always lead to diseases?

Just because a disease-causing organism enters the body, it does not mean that the person will necessarily suffer from the disease. Most of the time, the immune system acts to destroy the organisms or to prevent them from multiplying. Occasionally, however, the organisms enter the body and reproduce rapidly until they reach the level needed to make the person ill. This is most likely to happen with organisms to which we have not already developed immunity.

The symptoms we feel when we are ill are largely due to the body defences.

Immune response

The human body has effective systems for dealing with disease — in particular, the **immune system**. When disease-causing organisms, such as bacteria and viruses, are detected in the blood, skin or other tissues, the body starts attacking them. White blood cells (**leucocytes**) are important in this process.

When disease-causing organisms enter the body, white blood cells called **phagocytes** engulf and deactivate them. There are different types of phagocyte:

+ **Monocytes** circulate in the blood to attack disease-causing organisms in the bloodstream.
+ **Macrophages** are found within body tissues.
+ **Neutrophils** circulate in the blood, but when body tissue is affected by a disease-causing organism, blood flow to the infected part of the body increases and fluid rich in neutrophils diffuses into the tissues.

As part of the immune response, cells release **histamine**. This causes swelling and redness (inflammation). In respiratory infections, mucus production in the respiratory system increases and this helps to flush out the disease-causing organisms. For example, the raised temperature and runny nose that are typical of the common cold are caused by the body's defence mechanism. In fact, many of the symptoms of infectious diseases are caused by the body's own defence and repair mechanisms.

Once an attack by an organism has been defeated, the body often develops a specific immunity to that particular strain of organism. **Lymphocytes** (another type of leucocyte) recognise the disease-causing organism and divide and swell into plasma cells that produce **antibodies.** Antibodies neutralise the toxins produced by disease-causing organisms and attack bacteria and viruses.

It is because of specific immunity that diseases can sometimes be fought off before the development of symptoms.

Diseases caused by bacteria

Bacteria are tiny organisms. Each consists of a single cell (the human body is made up of many millions of cells). Bacteria have simple shapes, such as spheres or straight rods. They reproduce by growing and then splitting into two. A bacterium can reproduce itself about every half an hour. Some bacteria are adapted to living in human tissues, such as on the skin, in the blood, or in the intestines or lungs.

Why are people at risk from so many diseases?

Humans can suffer from a great variety of diseases. During most of the time humans have existed, they lived in small groups as hunter-gatherers. In these conditions, humans evolved to resist the limited range of diseases each population encountered.

Comparatively recently — during the past few thousand years — human lifestyles changed. Humans started living in larger groups and they started keeping animals instead of merely hunting them. Domesticated animals were sometimes kept very close to where people lived — even in the same house. In rural parts of eastern Asia (such as China and Vietnam), this still happens. Living in close contact with pigs and chickens has enabled disease-causing organisms, which used to affect only those animals, to adapt to humans. New strains of the influenza virus keep developing, partly because of the ability to infect humans and other animals. Now humans can catch diseases that used to affect only other species, such as 'bird flu'.

Keeping domestic pets, such as cats and dogs, causes allergies in some people.

Living in large groups, such as in cities, has enabled diseases that used to be restricted to small local populations to spread more widely. Living in cities also enables the spread of disease through water supplies contaminated by faeces.

When humans migrated from the warm parts of the world where they first evolved, they began to make and wear clothes. Very recently, humans have begun wearing more tight-fitting clothes and shoes. One result is that parts of the body such as the feet, groin and armpits are damper and less well ventilated than they used to be. This has increased the risk of some skin diseases.

The ease of air travel means that new infectious diseases can now spread very rapidly across the globe.

Keeping animals, wearing clothes, living in cities and frequent travel have exposed humans to a wider range of diseases. However, despite these 'unnatural practices', human health is better and life expectancy probably much greater than it was 20,000 years ago — at least in the most developed countries. This is partly because:

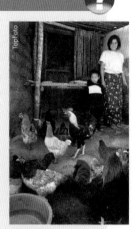

+ people are much better nourished thanks to more effective food production methods
+ of improvements in urban sanitation
+ modern scientific medicine has led to the effective treatment and prevention of diseases that only a century ago were often fatal

Some human diseases result from living in contact with domestic animals

Evolution of microorganisms

Like other living organisms, disease-causing organisms evolve. Compared with humans, they evolve very quickly. This means that new strains sometimes occur that can overcome the immune system and resist drug treatments. An example is a strain of Staphylococcus aureus. The antibiotic drug methicillin (similar to penicillin) used to be an effective treatment against this bacterium. However, some strains of the bacterium managed to survive and these have evolved into bacteria that are almost unaffected by the antibiotic. The newly evolved strain — called MRSA (methicillin-resistant Staphylococcus aureus) is extremely dangerous to people who are already ill. It has caused serious illness in, and death to, some hospital patients.

Reproduction in bacteria

Start with one bacterium. Assume that it takes half an hour to split into two daughter cells. Assume that each daughter cell also takes half an hour to split into two (i.e. after 1 hour there will be four cells, after 1 hour 30 minutes there will be eight cells) and so on. Work out to the nearest hour how long it would take for 1 million bacteria to be produced. Assume that none of the bacteria die during this time (which is a bit unlikely). Use a calculator — it won't take long.

The answer is given at the end of this chapter *(see p. 202).*

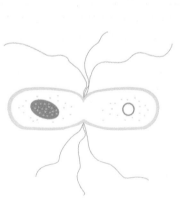

Figure 6.1
Diagram of a *Salmonella* bacterium

Try it out

Bacteria cause many diseases. The specification for Unit 6 covers three: meningitis, pneumonia and gonorrhoea.

Meningitis

The **meninges** are three layers of tough membrane surrounding and protecting the brain and spinal cord. In the skull, they form a sort of rubbery bag that contains the brain. The meninges are called the *dura mater*, *arachnoid mater* and *pia mater* (see Figure 6.2). (You do not have to learn these names.)

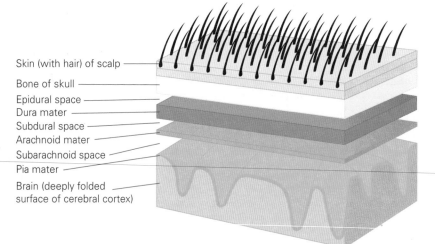

Figure 6.2
Small section of a head showing the layers that protect the brain

Skin (with hair) of scalp
Bone of skull
Epidural space
Dura mater
Subdural space
Arachnoid mater
Subarachnoid space
Pia mater
Brain (deeply folded surface of cerebral cortex)

Meningitis is an inflammation of the meninges. The problem is that, like other tissues, the meninges swell up when they are inflamed. However, because there is little room for expansion inside the skull, this puts pressure on the brain, which may cause permanent damage or even death.

What causes meningitis?

Bacterial meningitis is caused by meningococcal and pneumococcal bacteria and Hib (*Haemophilus influenzae*). These bacteria usually live in the throat. If the person has a sore throat, the bacteria may enter the bloodstream and be carried to the meninges. The infection can spread from the ear or sinuses directly to the brain.

Meningitis can also be caused by viruses. Viral meningitis is less harmful than the bacterial form. It usually clears up without treatment after about a week.

How is it transmitted?

Meningitis is spread by close physical contact, such as kissing, and in droplets resulting from coughs and sneezes. It can also be transmitted in the birth canal from mother to baby.

What are the symptoms?

The symptoms of meningitis include fever, nausea, vomiting, drowsiness, a painful headache, a dislike of bright lights and a stiff and painful neck. This last symptom is very noticeable when the sufferer tries to bend the head forward. The symptoms develop rapidly and the condition soon becomes much more serious. Sufferers become confused or disorientated, lapse into unconsciousness and, if untreated, die. The speed with which the disease develops is what makes it particularly dangerous.

In babies, the symptoms are slightly different, featuring fever, vomiting, fits, a skin rash, irritability and a dislike of being handled. Another sign in babies is bulging of the skin of the scalp over the fontanelles (two small gaps in the bones of the skull which close later in infancy). This bulging is caused by the pressure resulting from the inflamed meninges just beneath.

Who is most vulnerable?

People at risk include:

+ children. This group is the most at risk. While bacterial meningitis is fatal in only a small number of cases overall, in newborn babies it is fatal in over 25% of cases. Newborn babies who survive an infection might have permanent brain damage, resulting in hydrocephalus, cerebral palsy and other conditions.

+ young adults. Cases of meningitis often occur when people from different parts of the country spend time together — for example, at university.

+ people with impaired immune systems (e.g. those with AIDS or who are being treated for cancer)

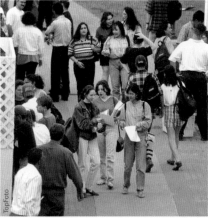

Outbreaks of meningitis can occur when young people from different areas meet at university

How can it be prevented?

Immunisation against some strains of bacteria (including meningococcal A and C groups, and Hib) can be provided by vaccination. Ideally, everyone up to the age of 25 should be vaccinated.

Pneumonia

Pneumonia is a disease that affects the lungs. The lungs enable us to absorb oxygen from the air we breathe and to get rid of waste carbon dioxide. These gases diffuse through the alveoli, which are the tiny air sacs that make up the lungs. There are many millions of alveoli in each lung, so the surface area for diffusion is very large. Alveoli are only one cell thick, so the diffusion path for the gases is short.

What causes pneumonia?

The symptoms of pneumonia are caused by the body's own defences against the disease-causing organisms. Mucus production is increased, to flush out the organisms from the lungs. The result of this is that the alveoli become filled with fluid, which makes gas diffusion more difficult.

Pneumonia often develops following an infection higher up in the respiratory system — for example, in the throat.

The most dangerous of the organisms that cause pneumonia are bacteria, such as *Streptococcus pneumoniae* (also called *pneumococcus*), *Pseudomonas aeruginosa* and *Staphylococcus aureus*.

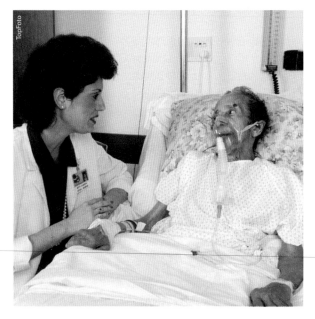

People with weak immune systems who are bedridden are most at risk from pneumonia

How is it transmitted?

The most common way the disease-causing organism is transmitted from person to person is in the tiny droplets that spray from the nose and mouth on coughing or sneezing. These droplets can be breathed in by other people nearby.

What are the symptoms?

The symptoms of pneumonia are coughing, shortness of breath, feeling tired and ill, a high temperature and aches in different parts of the body. The shortness of breath is a result of the fluid in the alveoli. Coughing is a reflex designed to remove excess fluid from the lungs. However, sometimes people with pneumonia have dry coughs and do not cough up any phlegm from the lungs.

Who is most vulnerable?

People at risk include:

+ elderly people, because their immune systems are weak and they are more likely than others to be poorly nourished
+ people who already have another lung disorder (e.g. emphysema or bronchitis) or heart disease. This is especially true of smokers.
+ people with diabetes, because this disease weakens the ability of white blood cells to fight the disease
+ people with weakened immune systems, such as AIDS sufferers and those who have received chemotherapy and/or radiotherapy (e.g. to treat cancer)
+ people who are bedridden. They tend to suffer most because the cough reflex becomes weaker and they are unable to clear infected sputum from the lungs. People in hospital following surgery are particularly at risk from MRSA (methicillin-resistant *Staphyloccocus aureus*).
+ infants, because their immune systems are not fully developed

How can it be prevented?

The risk can be reduced by keeping away from people who are coughing and sneezing, especially in confined spaces such as in cars or on public transport. If contact with an infected person cannot be avoided, it is important to wash the hands afterwards. Sufferers can help to reduce the spread of the disease by covering the nose and mouth when sneezing.

People known to be at a high risk (e.g. those in hospital after major surgery) are sometimes given antibiotics to prevent the development of pneumonia. However, some strains of bacteria (such as MRSA) are resistant to antibiotics.

Vaccines can be used to immunise people against *pneumococcus* and Hib.

Gonorrhoea

Gonorrhoea is an infection of the male and female sexual organs.

What causes gonorrhoea?

It is caused by the bacterium *Neisseria gonorrhoeae*. The body's defence mechanism against this bacterium leads to inflammation of the urethra in males and of the vagina in females. (The urethra is the tube that in males leads from the bladder and out through the penis.)

How is it transmitted?

The infection is almost always spread from an infected person to another person during sexual intercourse. It can also be transmitted when clothing and towels used by an infected person are shared by another person.

What are the symptoms?

The symptoms include a discharge of pus from the penis or vagina and pain or a burning sensation when urinating. The urine is often cloudy. As the disease progresses, other organs become inflamed. In men, the testicles, prostate gland and bladder are affected, which, in severe cases, can make urination impossible. In women, bacteria can spread to the Fallopian tubes and uterus, where they cause scarring and pelvic inflammatory disease. This can lead to infertility.

One problem with gonorrhoea is that some sufferers (about half of infected women and a third of infected men) do not develop any symptoms. This means that infected people can pass on the disease without realising it.

Who is most vulnerable?

Sexually active people especially in the age range 15–25 years are most at risk, particularly those who have sex with a series of different partners and those who do not use condoms.

How can it be prevented?

Using a condom for any penetrative sex act is a sensible precaution. Only having sex with one partner, who does not have sex with any other partners, greatly reduces the risk. The surest way to avoid the disease is by not having sex at all.

Diseases caused by fungi

There are many varieties of fungus. Most are much smaller than the familiar mushrooms and toadstools. Some are specialised to live on humans, usually on the skin surface.

Athlete's foot and ringworm (which together are known as *tinea*) and thrush (also known as candidiasis) are common fungal infections.

Athlete's foot

Athlete's foot is an infection of the skin of the feet, particularly between the toes. The infection can spread to the toenails.

What causes athlete's foot?

It is caused by the fungus *Tinea pedis*, which feeds on dead cells on the skin surface, particularly in warm, dark, moist areas. Waste products from the fungus cause itching.

How is it transmitted?

The fungal spores that cause infection are present all the time. Infection occurs when spores enter the body through a graze on the skin or if the warm, damp conditions they need are present.

Athlete's foot can be transmitted by physical contact with a person who has the infection, by sharing towels with an infected person, or by walking barefoot in a changing room or swimming pool and picking up spores left by an infected person.

What are the symptoms?

Athlete's foot presents as patches of white, cracked skin between the toes. The cracking or flaking of the skin surface exposes an inflamed layer of new skin below, which is very itchy.

If untreated, the fungus can spread to the toenails, which become thickened, brittle and chalky in texture.

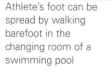

Athlete's foot can be spread by walking barefoot in the changing room of a swimming pool

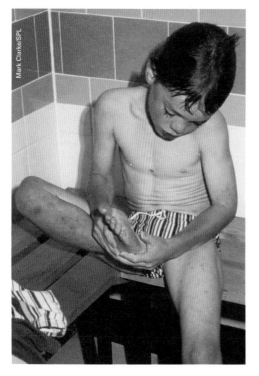

Mark Clarke/SPL

Who is most vulnerable?

Lifestyle is a key factor in contracting athlete's foot. People who often visit sports facilities and take showers there are at a higher risk of contracting the infection than others. The warm damp conditions that favour the fungus are created both by sweating during exercise and by frequent showering.

How can it be prevented?

Athlete's foot can be prevented by:

+ wearing protective footwear in moist areas, such as around swimming pools
+ drying carefully between the toes after a bath or shower
+ not sharing towels
+ not wearing shoes without socks or tights
+ changing socks, stockings or tights every day
+ wearing woollen or cotton socks, to reduce dampness

Also, for people who often take part in sports, it is a good idea to spend some time each day without shoes or socks.

Ringworm

Ringworm has nothing to do with worms. It is a fungal infection that starts as small, round, itchy red patches on the skin, which gradually get bigger.

What causes ringworm?

It is caused by the *Tinea corporis* fungus, which feeds on dead cells on the skin surface in various parts of the body, including the scalp. Waste products from the fungus cause itching.

How is it transmitted?

Ringworm can be transmitted by contact with infected people, by sharing combs or towels with an infected person and by contact with infected household pets.

What are the symptoms?

Ringworm causes an itchy round rash. The centre of the rash sometimes heals, leaving a surrounding ring of infection. Scratching the rash can break the skin surface, making the person more likely to contract other infections through the wound.

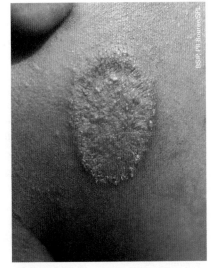

Ringworm causes an itchy round rash

Who is most vulnerable?

Ringworm is most common in young children and often spreads through contact with other children at school.

Taking antibiotic drugs can also increase the risk of fungal infections. This is because antibiotics do not kill only disease-causing bacteria. They can also destroy useful bacteria that live on the skin and prevent the growth of fungi.

How can it be prevented?

Ringworm infections can be prevented by:
+ keeping the body clean and dry
+ by avoiding contact with infected people
+ by not sharing towels or combs
+ by treating pets that have ringworm, so as to avoid transmission to humans

Thrush (candidiasis)

Thrush, which is also known as candidiasis, is a skin infection that causes itchy rashes, especially around the groin.

What causes thrush?

It is caused by the *Candida albicans* fungus. Like other fungal infections, the fungus feeds on dead skin cells. The waste products cause inflammation.

How is it transmitted?

Candida albicans occurs in the mouths of healthy people, where it usually causes no trouble. This is because bacteria living in the mouth keep the fungus under control by feeding on it. A person who develops thrush might not have caught it from another person. However, the fungus can spread from person to person by close contact, such as kissing and sexual intercourse.

What are the symptoms?

Thrush is characterised by itchy, deep red rashes on the skin in moist parts of the body, especially in women where they may occur under the breasts, in the armpits, around the vagina and groin area, around the anus and in the mouth. In the mouth, infection often produces raised, pale cream-coloured rashes. Infection occurs in the parts of the body where the skin is most likely to be moist, therefore creating the conditions the fungus needs to thrive.

Who is most vulnerable?

The infection affects more women than men. It tends to develop when something happens that kills bacteria, such as the hormonal changes during pregnancy. Since women experience more frequent hormonal changes than men, this might explain why women are more vulnerable.

People who have taken antibiotics, or who use antibacterial mouthwash, are also at risk. This is because these treatments kill the useful bacteria that provide protection against the fungus.

How can it be prevented?

Thrush can be prevented by wearing loose-fitting clothes and cotton underwear, so that the skin is kept as dry as possible.

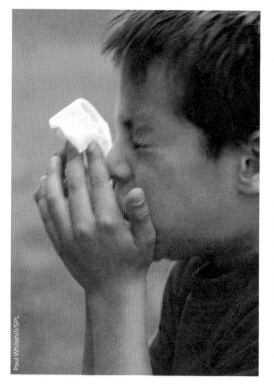

Colds and flu are often spread by sneezing

Paul Whitehill/SPL

Diseases caused by viruses

Viruses are tiny organisms, many times smaller than bacteria. Unlike bacteria, they live inside human body cells. They cause a wide range of diseases, the commonest of which are colds and flu.

The common cold

The common cold is a mild viral infection of the respiratory system that mainly affects the nose and throat.

What causes the common cold?

The common cold has nothing to do with being exposed to draughts, cold weather or getting wet. It is caused by many different viruses (at least 200 different kinds) which infect the respiratory tract. The main symptoms are caused by the body's defence mechanism against the virus.

How is it transmitted?

Colds are spread by:

+ breathing in droplets containing viruses that have been coughed or sneezed out by an infected person

+ rubbing the eyes or nose with fingers that have picked up the virus by touching hands with an infected person or touching virus-contaminated surfaces

What are the symptoms?

Mucus production in the nose and throat is increased. This mucus traps the virus, which is then expelled by coughing, sneezing and nose blowing. The resulting symptoms include a runny or blocked nose, sneezing, a dry cough, sore throat, tiredness, sore eyes, headache, earache, sinus pain and mild fever.

Who is most vulnerable?

Most people suffer from colds. However, some groups of people catch colds much more frequently than others. These are people who have weak immune systems. They include:

+ children who have not yet built up immunity. When people catch a cold and then recover, they develop some immunity to the virus that caused the cold. As a result, children's immunity to the common cold increases as they grow older.
+ elderly people
+ people suffering from a disease that damages the immune system, such as HIV (human immunodeficiency virus)
+ people whose immune systems have been weakened by medical treatment, such as chemotherapy to cure cancer

How can colds be prevented?

In practice, it is very difficult to avoid catching colds. There is no way of immunising people against colds at present. One precaution is to try to keep away from people who are coughing and sneezing. People with colds should cover their mouths and noses when sneezing and wash their hands regularly.

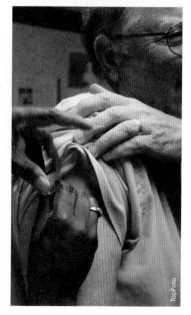

Vulnerable people, such as the elderly, are offered flu jabs

Influenza

Influenza is a more serious viral infection of the respiratory system. It is more commonly known as 'flu'.

What causes influenza?

It is caused by a virus, of which there are three types — A, B and C. The A-type virus is the most common. There are many different strains of each type of flu virus and new strains are continually emerging. These new strains are particularly dangerous if they spread before there is time to develop vaccines against them.

How is it transmitted?

Flu viruses are spread by:

+ breathing in droplets containing viruses that have been sneezed out by an infected person
+ rubbing the eyes or nose with fingers that have picked up the virus by touching hands with an infected person or touching virus-contaminated surfaces

Influenza is a highly infectious disease. Worldwide outbreaks (pandemics) occur. Although many people recover quickly, the weakening effect on the body of fighting the flu virus can lead to other opportunistic infections, such as pneumonia. For this reason, flu can be fatal to people in vulnerable groups. During the last century, millions of people died in flu pandemics.

What are the symptoms?
The symptoms, which develop very quickly, vary according to the strain of virus. The most common symptoms are headaches and muscle aches, tiredness, a raised temperature (fever), a feeling of being chilled, sore throat and cough.

Who is most vulnerable?
People at risk include:
+ those with weak immune systems (see page 175)
+ those who already have respiratory disorders, such as chronic bronchitis

How can it be prevented?
Immunisation (a 'flu jab') reduces the risk of suffering from some strains of the virus but does not provide protection against them all. The flu jab is usually given in the autumn, because the winter months are the time of highest risk. Usually the flu jab is given only to the most vulnerable groups, i.e. those suffering from serious disease conditions and the elderly.

Otherwise, the precautions are the same as for the common cold.

Infection with other parasites
At the beginning of this chapter, it was pointed out that disease-causing organisms are parasites. However, most people think of parasites as much larger, usually visible, organisms such as head lice, scabies mites and tapeworms. This section is about such parasites.

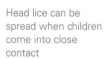
Head lice can be spread when children come into close contact

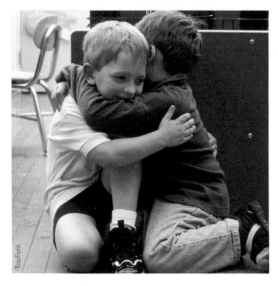

Head lice
Head lice (*Pediculus*) are small insects that live on the scalp. They bite into the scalp and feed on blood. Their waste products make the skin of the scalp itchy.

How are they transmitted?
Head lice can spread from an infected person to other people by physical contact, especially among children playing together. They can also be spread by sharing hats or combs or by sharing a bed with an infected person.

What are the symptoms?
The symptoms are an itchy scalp and small red bites on the scalp, neck and shoulders. These bites can

ooze, leading to the hair becoming matted. The insects lay tiny white eggs (nits), which can be found attached to hairs.

Who is most vulnerable?

Young children are most affected, probably because of the ease with which the parasite spreads in schools.

How can the spread of head lice be prevented?

The best way of preventing the spread of head lice is to avoid contact with infected people – for example, by not sharing clothes, towels or a bed with them.

Scabies

What causes scabies?

Scabies is a painful infection of the skin caused by the scabies mite (Figure 6.3), which is an arachnid about half a millimetre long. (The arachnid group of animals includes spiders.) The pregnant female mites burrow into the skin of the buttocks, genitals, wrists, hands, feet and armpits. They lay eggs under the skin that hatch in about two weeks. The young mites then spread the infection. The itching is caused by the toxic waste products (excrement) of the mites.

How is scabies transmitted?

Scabies is transmitted by close contact with an infected person, including sexual contact, and by contact with shared bed linen and clothing.

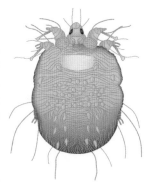

Figure 6.3
A scabies mite

What are the symptoms?

The symptoms are a painful itching of the skin, which is marked by dark wavy lines, each ending in a round lump. The wavy lines are burrows and the lumps are eggs. The skin around the burrow is often inflamed. An allergic reaction occurs when the eggs hatch.

People with scabies tend to scratch their skin, which becomes grazed and crusty.

Who is most vulnerable?

Scabies is most common in children and young adults and occurs most often among people who live in overcrowded conditions, which allow the mite to spread more easily.

How can scabies be prevented?

The spread of scabies can be reduced by regularly washing the clothes and bed linen of infected people and by not sharing a bed, clothing or towels with an infected person.

Tapeworms

A tapeworm is a ribbon-shaped, segmented flatworm that can grow up to 10 metres in length. It lives in the intestines.

The parasite enters the body when people eat food containing tapeworm larvae. The young worm attaches itself to the side of the intestine. Some types of tapeworm have hooks; others attach themselves by means of suckers. The tapeworm grows by absorbing nutrients from the intestinal contents. It eventually produces segments that contain eggs.

How are tapeworms transmitted?
Tapeworms are spread by eating beef, pork or fish that contains tapeworm larvae and which has not been properly cooked.

They can also be spread by contact with faeces of an infected person, which might contain eggs.

What are the symptoms?
Tapeworms can cause diarrhoea and stomach pains. Sometimes the end of the worm protrudes from the anus. Segments break off from the body of a tapeworm and are found in the faeces. These segments contain eggs.

Pork tapeworms sometimes produce cysts in various parts of the body. These can cause serious illness if they occur in the brain or liver.

Who is most vulnerable?
Tapeworm is quite rare in the UK. Lifestyle is a factor. In some cultures, raw fish is a popular food. This exposes people to a higher risk.

Also at risk are people with poor hygiene practices, such as not washing their hands after visiting the toilet.

How can infection be prevented?
The risk can be reduced by cooking meat and fish thoroughly and by effective personal hygiene practices.

Table 6.1
Summary of infectious diseases

Summary
Infectious diseases are summarised in Table 6.1.

Disease	Causal agent	Transmission	Main symptoms	Most vulnerable groups	Prevention
Meningitis	Bacteria — *Meningococcus*, *Pneumococcus* and Hib	Physical contact Coughs and sneezes	Fever Vomiting Headache	Children and young people	Immunisation Avoid contact
Pneumonia	Bacteria — *Streptococcus* (*Pneumococcus*), *Pseudomonas* and *Staphylococcus*	Coughs and sneezes	Coughing Shortness of breath	Those with reduced immunity (e.g. elderly, infants, diabetics)	Avoid contact Immunisation Antibiotics
Gonorrhoea	Bacterium — *Neisseria*	Sexual intercourse	Discharge of pus Burning sensation on urination	Sexually active people aged 15–25	Use condoms Restrict number of partners

Disease	Causal agent	Transmission	Main symptoms	Most vulnerable groups	Prevention
Athlete's foot	Fungus — *Tinea pedis*	Contact with spores in changing rooms and pools	Itchy, broken skin between toes	Sportspeople	Wear socks Protective footwear Dry feet thoroughly
Ringworm	Fungus — *Tinea corporis*	Contact with infected people	Itchy round rash	Young children and people treated with antibiotics	Keep clean and dry Avoid contact
Thrush	Fungus — *Candida albicans*	Physical contact, especially kissing and sexual intercourse	Itchy red or cream rashes	Women and people treated with antibiotics	Keep dry Wear loose-fitting clothes
Common cold	Virus — many types	Coughs and sneezes	Increased mucus production	People with reduced immunity	Avoid contact with coughing, sneezing people
Influenza	Virus — influenza viruses A, B and C	Coughs and sneezes	Head and body aches Tiredness Fever	People with reduced immunity	Immunisation Avoid contact
Head lice	*Pediculus*	Contact with infected people	Itchy scalp Bites, nits	Young children	Avoid contact
Scabies	Scabies mite	Contact with infected people	Itchy skin marked by wavy lines	Children and young people in overcrowded conditions	Wash clothes regularly Avoid contact
Tapeworm	Various species	Eating raw/under-cooked infected meat and fish Contact with faeces of infected person	Diarrhoea, stomach pain Excretion of worm segments	People who eat raw/undercooked infected foods	Cook food thoroughly Good hygiene practices

Table 6.1
continued

Allergies

An **allergy** is an abnormal response or overreaction of the immune system to irritant substances called **allergens**.

Allergies develop when the body has been stimulated to produce an **immune response** to otherwise harmless substances, such as pollen.

Allergens are first mistaken for harmful substances and absorbed by B-lymphocytes (a type of white blood cell). After a few days, the lymphocytes start to produce a large number of **antibodies (immunoglobulins)** designed to match the allergens. These are released and attach themselves to special cells called mast cells and another type of white blood cell called basophils. Allergens are then captured and bind to the antibodies. This process sensitises the person to the allergen so that the next time they are exposed to the allergen, the mast cells and basophils release histamine, which produces the inflammation. This inflammation is the main feature of allergic symptoms. While it is useful in resisting bacterial and viral infections, it is unnecessary with allergens because no disease-causing organisms are present. In the case of airborne allergies, the result is rather like having a cold.

Airborne allergens

These are allergens that are breathed in and which can cause inflammation of the mucous membrane lining the nose (Figure 6.4) and the nasal sinuses (cavities in the bones of the face, behind the nose). In some cases, the symptoms of asthma are produced, including narrowing of the airways, leading to breathing difficulties and wheezing.

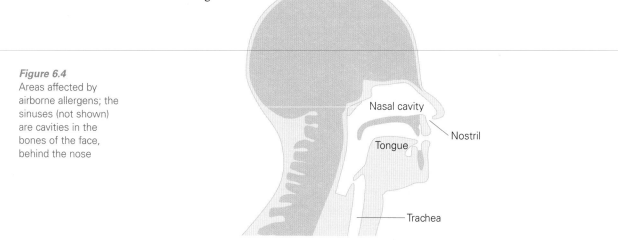

Figure 6.4
Areas affected by airborne allergens; the sinuses (not shown) are cavities in the bones of the face, behind the nose

Most people can breathe air containing large quantities of these allergens and suffer no reaction at all. Those who suffer from this type of allergy experience a blocked or runny nose, sneezing, watering and red, itchy eyes, and tickling in the throat. This set of symptoms is called allergic rhinitis. About one person in five suffers from airborne allergies.

Common airborne allergens include pollen, animal dander or feathers, dust mites and spores from moulds. People who are allergic to all or most of these suffer from allergic rhinitis for all or most of the year.

Pollen

Pollen is a dust-like substance produced by flowering plants. Some pollen is carried by the wind to fertilise other plants of the same species. Grasses produce large quantities of pollen, which is why an allergy to pollen is commonly called 'hay fever'.

People who are allergic to pollen develop seasonal allergic rhinitis, mainly from spring to early autumn. Most pollen in the spring comes from trees; in the summer most pollen comes from grasses. Winds spread the pollen over a large area. Dry conditions allow large quantities of pollen to build up in the air; wet weather washes the pollen out and reduces the problem. Weather forecasters predict the amount of pollen as a pollen count or index.

Animal dander and feathers

Dander is hair and skin cells shed from the skin of an animal. It is found at higher levels during the winter months when pets spend more time indoors and when wet weather and central heating produce a warm and humid atmosphere.

Feathers and dander cause similar allergic reactions.

Dust mites

Dust mites are tiny arachnids that live in most homes. They are found on carpets and bedding where they feed on dead skin cells shed by people and pets.

Spores from moulds

Moulds are fungi. Like other fungi, moulds reproduce by sending out masses of dust-like spores.

Moulds grow best in warm, damp conditions. They are often found on walls and windows in bathrooms and in other places in houses that are damp. The concentration of spores is greater in houses that are heated but not well ventilated.

Food allergens

About 1 in 100 people have a **food allergy**. A larger number of people – who sometimes believe they have a food allergy – have a **food intolerance**. Food intolerance is an inability to digest certain foods. It does not produce an allergic reaction.

Reaction to food allergens, like the reaction to airborne allergens, results from the body producing antibodies to the allergens.

The symptoms are different from those of allergic rhinitis. They include swelling of the airways and mouth, which can cause wheezing and more severe breathing difficulties, swollen lips and rashes. Among the most common allergenic foods are strawberries, eggs, shellfish and nuts. An allergic response can be produced by very small quantities of the allergen and usually develops within half an hour of eating the food. In rare cases, people have a very severe reaction (called anaphylaxis) to allergens. This reaction can restrict the airways and decrease blood pressure – both of which can be life-threatening. Shellfish and nuts can cause anaphylaxis in allergic individuals.

Skin allergy testing

People who suffer from food allergies often do not know which particular food is causing the problem. If they develop an allergic reaction after a meal containing several types of food, they will not know which food is the allergen.

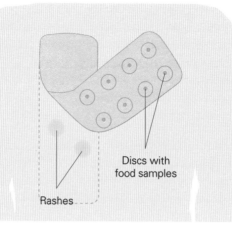

Figure 6.5
Skin allergy testing

Discs with
food samples

Rashes

Skin allergy testing is a scientific procedure designed to find out which foods cause an allergic reaction in a person, and which do not. The person can then avoid eating the allergenic foods in future.

The principle behind skin allergy testing is that if a person is allergic to one or more types of food, this will show up when a very small amount of the liquidised food is placed in contact with the skin. This is not dangerous and produces only a very mild reaction, compared with actually eating the food. If the person is allergic to that food, the skin will swell up or develop a rash at the point of contact. By marking out different areas on the skin (usually on the back), allergies to several different foods can be tested at once. A placebo is also used, to ensure that any reaction is really caused by an allergy. The procedure is as follows:

+ Prepare separate, small, liquidised samples of the food to be tested and place them on different discs attached to a strip of sticky tape.
+ Leave one or more discs blank, i.e. without a food sample. Such discs act as placebos.
+ Stick the tape onto the person's skin, so that the discs make contact.
+ After two or three days, remove the tape and observe the skin for swelling or inflammation.
+ An inflammation reaction under a disc shows that a particular food is an allergen for that person — unless the placebo test is also positive.

Disorders of the eye and ear

Anatomy of the eye

The human eye is spherical. The eyes are retained and moved within sockets of cushioned bones (the orbital bones) by means of several muscles.

The anatomical features of the eye are as follows (see Figure 6.6):

+ The central front surface of the ball is the transparent **cornea**, which lets light in.

+ Behind the cornea there is a space filled with a transparent watery liquid (called the **aqueous humour**).
+ Behind the aqueous humour there is a ring of coloured muscle called the **iris**. This ring of muscle can contract. The **pupil** is the hole in the middle of the iris.
+ Immediately behind the iris is the **lens**, which is a transparent, fat, squashy disc, suspended in a transparent capsule.
+ The almost spherical area behind the lens is filled with the **vitreous humour,** which has the texture of jelly.
+ On the curved inside rear surface of the eyeball is the **retina** (a layer of light-sensitive cells), which is supported on a layer of tough tissue. Nerve fibres from all over the retina converge and leave the eye in a bundle called the **optic nerve**. The two optic nerves (one from each eye) enter the brain.
+ The **conjunctiva** is a thin membrane that covers the white part of the eyes and the inside of the eyelids. It helps to ensure that unwanted substances, such as grit and disease-causing organisms, cannot get behind the eye.
+ Very little light gets into the eye, which is why the pupil looks black.

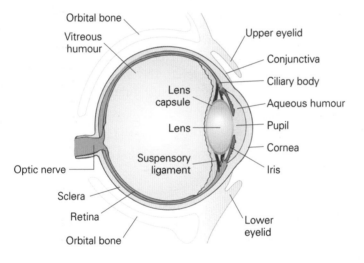

Figure 6.6
Anatomy of the eye

Functions of the eye

The eye is designed to allow light to enter and then to focus it into a clear, sharp image on the retina. The retina contains cells that absorb light energy and convert it into nerve impulses that travel along the optic nerve to the brain. The brain decodes these impulses and produces the experience of seeing objects. The eye can detect information about colour, brightness and movement, and the distance, shape and size of objects.

Focusing

Some **focusing** is done by the cornea, which can be seen as a distinct bulge in the front of the eye. However, most focusing is done by the lens, which works in a similar way to a glass convex lens. A convex lens can be used to focus light from a lamp onto a piece of paper. The image produced by a convex lens is upside down. It is the same with the lens in the human eye. The image produced on the retina is upside down. The world is seen the right way up because the brain decodes the signals from the optic nerves and corrects this.

One way that the lens in the eye is different from a glass lens is that it is made of living cells. It is also flexible, which enables it to focus light coming from different distances.

The lens sits in a transparent bag called the **lens capsule**. This is held in position by many tiny ligaments all round the edge that anchor it to a ring of muscle called the ciliary body. (Think of the springs holding a circular trampoline tight.) When the ligaments are tightened, the lens becomes flatter and distant objects can be focused. When the ligaments are slack, the lens becomes more rounded and close objects can be focused.

Role of the iris

The human eyes have an amazing range of sensitivity — much greater than most cameras. We can see in very low light levels and in extremely bright conditions. This is possible because the iris controls the amount of light entering the eye. The muscles of the iris can contract to quite a narrow ring, leaving a large pupil. This happens automatically in low light levels. This is called **pupil dilation**. In very bright light, the iris extends, making the pupil shrink to a very small black hole. This is called **pupil contraction**.

Try it out

Here are three simple exercises to help you get to know the eye. To carry out these exercises you will need a partner. You should not touch your eyes or your partner's eyes.

The cornea

Your partner should close their eyes and then — keeping the head still — swivel the eyeballs from side to side as though watching the ball in a game of tennis. Watch the closed eyelids. You should be able to see a bump moving back and forth under each eyelid. This bump is the cornea.

Focusing

Get your partner to read out these instructions for you to follow:

+ 'Hold your thumb up, about 15 cm away from and level with one eye. Keep the other eye shut. Look at your thumb.'
  You will probably be able to see lots of detail of the skin and thumbnail.
+ 'Without switching your gaze, notice what has happened to your view of more distant objects, such as the wall.'
  They probably look quite fuzzy. That is because your eye is focused on your thumb — a near object.
+ 'Without moving your thumb, focus on what you can see in the distance — just past your thumb.'

Now the distant view should be clear. Without switching your gaze, you will probably see that your thumb looks blurred. In fact, most of the time, the majority of objects in our visual field are out of focus. However, we don't notice this, because we always focus on what we intend to look at.

Pupil contraction

Take an electric torch and go into a fairly dark room (e.g. with the curtains drawn). You should just be able to see your partner's pupils without using the torch. Stay there for at least 1 minute. By this time, the pupils should be quite large. Then shine the torch near (but not directly into) your partner's eyes. At the same time watch the pupils — they should visibly contract. Blink, and you might miss this rapid reaction.

Try it out

Dysfunctions of the eye

There are several ways in which the eyes can fail to work properly, including:

+ short-sightedness (myopia)
+ long-sightedness (hypermetropia)
+ astigmatism
+ presbyopia
+ conjunctivitis
+ cataract

Most of these conditions can be corrected by using spectacles or contact lenses. Often a person has the same condition in both eyes, but to different extents.

Short-sightedness

Short-sightedness (also called **myopia**) is a problem in focusing light from distant objects, which look blurred as a result (Figure 6.7). Objects nearby are seen more clearly. This condition causes severe problems in playing ball games and driving a car. Short-sightedness can be caused by a cornea that is too curved and so focuses the light too much or by an eyeball which is too long, so that the light is focused at a point in front of the retina. The length of the eye is partly determined by the shape of the orbital bones. This shape is influenced by a person's genetic make-up and short-sightedness tends to run in families.

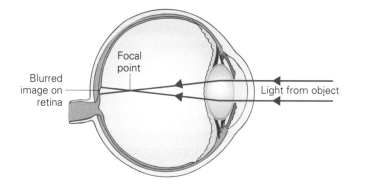

Figure 6.7
Short-sightedness

Long-sightedness

Long-sightedness (also called **hypermetropia**) is a condition in which objects in the distance are clearly seen but objects nearby are out of focus and look blurred (Figure 6.8). This can lead to difficulties in focusing on the written word. It can be caused by the eyeball being too short, so that light from near objects reaches the retina before it is brought to a focus.

Figure 6.8
Long-sightedness

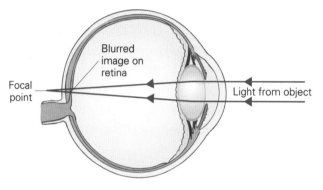

Astigmatism

Astigmatism is a condition in which some parts of the visual field are in focus while others are not. It is caused when the cornea or lens (or both) is unevenly curved — for example, if the corneal surface is more barrel-shaped than spherical. The result is that some parts of the visual field are more sharply focused than others. This is because different parts of the affected lens and cornea have different focusing power.

Presbyopia

Presbyopia is a condition in which the shape of the lens becomes progressively more difficult to change. The result is that nearby objects are out of focus. Distance vision is less affected. Presbyopia occurs because, as people grow older, the lens becomes stiffer, so the ciliary muscles cannot change its shape much. This is the reason why many older people have to use bifocal or reading glasses.

Conjunctivitis

Conjunctivitis is inflammation of the conjunctiva. The eye becomes pink or red and itchy, as though there is sand trapped inside the eyelid. It can be caused by bacterial and viral infections and by allergies.

Cataract

As a person gets older, the lens of the eye becomes stiffer and slightly thicker. Eventually, protein molecules form clusters that give the lens a cloudy, white appearance. This is called a cataract, and it makes the vision less clear and less sharp. In many people, the clouding does not affect vision seriously. However, some people need eye surgery to restore their vision.

The main factor in causing cataracts is ageing. However, the risk of developing cataracts that are severe enough to need treatment is increased by smoking, alcohol abuse, diabetes and some anti-inflammatory drugs. A simple surgical procedure is carried out to break and remove the lens, which is then replaced by a plastic one. Table 6.2 summarises these dysfunctions of the eye.

Dysfunction	Problem	Cause
Myopia	Distant objects blurred	Eyeball too long
Hypermetropia	Nearby objects blurred	Eyeball too short
Astigmatism	Some parts of visual field blurred	Barrel-shaped cornea
Presbyopia	Inability to alter focus	Stiff, hard lens
Conjunctivitis	Inflamed conjunctiva, 'pink eye'	Infection or allergy
Cataract	Blurred vision	Protein fibres in lens

Table 6.2
Dysfunctions of the eye

Anatomy of the ear

Outer ear

The **outer ear** is composed of cartilage, with a tube (the **ear canal**) leading inside the head (Figure 6.9). The outer ear collects sound and channels it towards the **eardrum**, which is a thin membrane that vibrates when sound reaches it. It also serves as a barrier preventing dust, insects or disease-causing organisms from getting further inside the ear.

Middle ear

Beyond the eardrum is the **middle ear**. This is a small, air-filled cavity with three delicate, linked bones: the **hammer**, **anvil** and **stirrup**. The hammer is in contact with the eardrum and it transmits vibrations through the anvil and stirrup to the **inner ear**. A thin tube, called the **Eustachian tube**, connects the middle ear with the throat. On swallowing, the end of this tube opens briefly and allows air in or out of the cavity. Going a long way uphill in a car or up in a plane sometimes causes the ears to 'pop'. This happens in order to equalise the air pressure inside the middle ear with the pressure outside (which is lower at altitude).

Inner ear

The inner ear contains the **cochlea**, a curled-up organ that resembles the shell of a snail. Lining the cochlea are many **hair cells** that pick up different frequencies of sound and convert them into nerve impulses, rather like a microphone converting sound into electrical impulses.

These impulses travel along the **auditory nerve** (one from each ear) into the brain, which interprets them.

The inner ear also contains three loop-shaped tubes, called the **semicircular canals**. These contain liquid and help us to sense our position. They are important for keeping our balance when standing or walking.

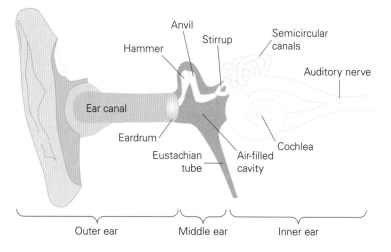

Figure 6.9
Anatomy of the ear

Functions of the ear

The auditory information received by the ears includes information on the loudness, pitch, tone and direction of sound. This is particularly useful when having a conversation in a room where several people are speaking. The ears also enable us to know our orientation in space (e.g. whether we are upright) and this helps us to balance – for example, when walking or running.

Dysfunctions of the ear

Glue ear

Glue ear is a condition of the middle ear that is common in children aged 2–5 years. A sticky fluid collects in the middle ear and can reduce hearing. Glue ear is more common in winter than summer and more common in boys than girls.

The usual cause is infection that leads to a blockage of the Eustachian tube, although it can also be caused by allergies and passive smoking. When the tube is blocked, air inside the middle ear is gradually absorbed by the lining of the middle ear. This results in a partial vacuum in the middle ear. Fluids from the walls of the inner ear then begin to seep into the space. Soon they become thick and sticky, which limits the movements of the bones of the middle ear.

The condition often clears up as the child grows older. However, the serious hearing loss that occurs in some children requires treatment because it could cause a delay in language development and education. One common treatment is to insert a 'grommet' into the eardrum. This is a tiny disc with a hole in it. The hole enables a practitioner to drain the sticky fluid from the middle ear.

Tinnitus

Tinnitus is a condition in which sounds are heard that are not coming from the environment. Sometimes described as 'ringing in the ears', tinnitus can be a range of sounds from humming and hissing to roaring. Some people hear tunes. The most common cause is damage to the hair cells in the cochlea. Hair cells can be damaged or killed by powerful vibrations transmitted from the middle ear. This type of hearing loss is much greater in people who listen to highly amplified music through speakers or headphones. Working in a noisy environment and using machinery such as pneumatic drills can also be a problem unless ear protection is worn. These damaged cells no longer detect real sounds but continue to send impulses to the brain, which the brain interprets as sounds. Other causes include infection of the Eustachian tube, a blockage (e.g. of wax) in the ear canal and high blood pressure. High blood pressure leads to turbulent blood flow and the sound of this is picked up by the ear. In this case, the sound is real.

Progressive deafness in the elderly (presbyacusis)

Most people gradually lose hearing sensitivity as they grow older. The main causes of this are progressive damage to, and natural degeneration of, the hair cells in the cochlea.

In most people, the ability to hear the highest-pitched sounds is lost earliest. Most children and teenagers can hear the very high-pitched squeaks that bats make, but most adults cannot. Some older people find it easier to hear deep or mid-range voices than high-pitched voices. This type of hearing loss cannot be reversed, though sensible precautions such as wearing ear protectors when working with noisy machinery can limit the damage.

Dysfunction	Problem	Cause
Glue ear	Fluid in the middle ear	Infection
Tinnitus	Perceived sound, originating inside the ear	Damage to cochlear hair cells
Progressive deafness	Reduced hearing acuity, particularly for high-pitched sounds	Damage to cochlear hair cells, natural degeneration

Table 6.3
Dysfunctions of the ear

Disorders of the teeth and gums

Anatomy of the teeth and gums

The primary (milk) teeth push their way through the gums between the ages of about 6 months and 3 years. Infants have 20 teeth — ten in the upper jaw and ten in the lower. The primary teeth are replaced by permanent teeth erupting below them at about age 6. There are 32 permanent teeth — 16 in the upper jaw and 16 in the lower jaw.

Teeth in different parts of the jaw have different functions, which is reflected in their shape. At the front of the jaws the teeth are designed for slicing through food (the **incisors**). Either side of the incisors are the **canines** (or cuspid teeth), which are designed to tear food. Behind the canines are the **premolars** and (at the back of the jaw) the **molars**. The premolars and molars of the upper jaw are designed to interlock with those of the lower jaw, so that pieces of food can be ground up using a side-to-side movement of the jaws.

A tooth consists of the **crown** (the part showing above the gums) and the **root** (which is the part embedded in the jawbone). The crown has a very hard shiny surface called the **enamel**. The main structure of the tooth, including the root, is made of another hard material, called **dentine**. Within the dentine is a space filled by tissue called the **pulp**, which contains the blood supply and nerves of the tooth. The blood supply and nerves enter the root through the **root canal**. The blood supply helps to repair the tooth and the nerve is needed so that we can feel what we are biting or chewing. The root (or, in the case of the molars, two or three roots) fits into a socket in the jawbone. Around the base of the root is a thin layer of bone-like tissue called the **cementum**. Between the jawbone and the tooth is the gum (Figure 6.10).

Figure 6.10
Longitudinal section of a tooth

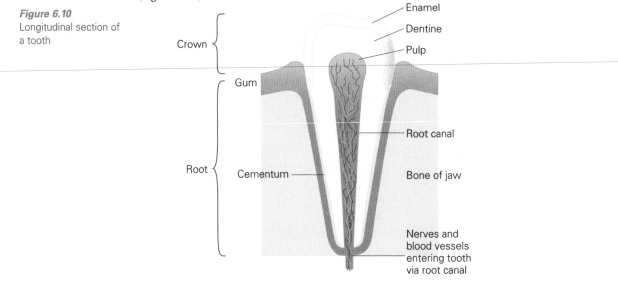

Dental caries

Tooth decay (**dental caries**) is caused by bacteria on the surface of the teeth that feed on sugar and produce acid waste. The bacteria live in a sticky coating of saliva and food remains called **plaque**. Plaque collects on the surface of the teeth and in the gaps between them.

The acid produced by bacteria feeding on the plaque dissolves the enamel of the tooth surface, leaving small pits. More plaque collects in these pits, which can become enlarged into cavities in the dentine. This process of dissolving is called **demineralisation**. The cavities can eventually expose the tooth pulp, which leads to sensitivity or pain (toothache). Eventually, the tooth may die. Cavities allow infections to penetrate deep into the roots, which can lead to painful abscesses inside and beneath the teeth.

A person who has a diet rich in sugary foods and drinks is more likely to suffer from dental caries. This is one reason why children should rarely, if ever, be given sweets. The risk of dental caries can be reduced by avoiding sugary foods and drinks. Regular brushing with toothpaste (also known as dentifrice) and the use of dental floss also help. Brushing dislodges food particles trapped between the teeth, and daily flossing is effective in removing plaque from the base of the teeth, where they enter the gums. Disclosing tablets can be used to show the presence of plaque. The addition of fluoride salts to the water supply in some parts of the UK has led to a significant reduction of tooth decay in children. Some toothpastes also contain fluoride salts.

Gingivitis

Gingivitis is an inflammation of the gums that gives them a red, shiny appearance. Like dental caries, it is caused by plaque. If untreated, the condition leads to the development of bleeding ulcers on the gums. The gums also shrink back to expose more of the teeth, increasing the risk of decay and abscesses. The gums become softer and bleed more easily.

The risk of gingivitis is increased in people who are experiencing changes in hormone levels, such as adolescents and pregnant or menopausal women.

Skin, spots and rashes

Skin

The skin is made up of layers of tissue (Figure 6.11). The outer layer is called the **epidermis**. The top layer of the epidermis consists of dead cells, which are continually replaced by cells dividing deeper inside the epidermis. The epidermis contains cells that produce the dark pigment melanin, which protects us from ultraviolet radiation from the sun. People with dark skins have more of these cells. Apart from providing this protection, the function of the epidermis is to seal the skin to prevent entry of disease-causing organisms. It is capable of resisting a lot of wear, caused by friction, without breaking. The parts of the body that have to withstand the most friction have the thickest layer of epidermis — particularly the palms of the hands and the soles of the feet.

Below the epidermis is a thicker layer called the **dermis**. This contains long fibres of **elastin** and **collagen**. Collagen is very strong and gives the skin its toughness. This helps the skin to resist tearing or being pierced and helps to protect organs such as blood vessels from damage. Elastin is stretchy, and makes the skin elastic. This elasticity helps to accommodate the stretching caused by body movements and helps to resist tearing.

The dermis also contains a number of specialised structures including:

+ some **sensory receptors** that are sensitive to pain and others that receive information about touch, pressure or temperature

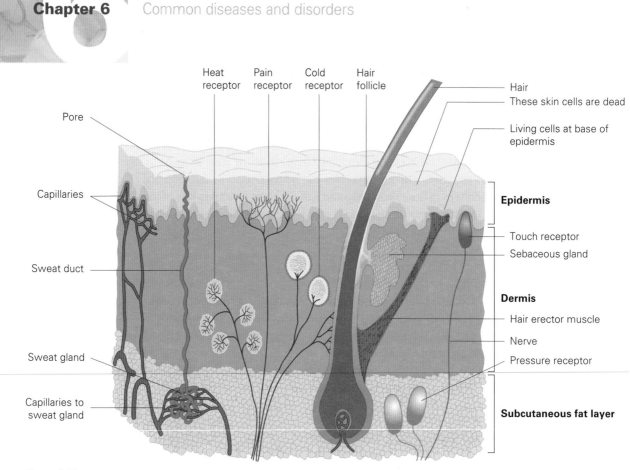

Heat receptor | Pain receptor | Cold receptor | Hair follicle

Hair
These skin cells are dead
Living cells at base of epidermis
Epidermis
Touch receptor
Sebaceous gland
Dermis
Hair erector muscle
Nerve
Pressure receptor
Subcutaneous fat layer

Pore
Capillaries
Sweat duct
Sweat gland
Capillaries to sweat gland

Figure 6.11
Structure of skin

+ **Langerhans cells**, which are part of the immune system. These detect foreign substances and play a role in skin allergy development.
+ **hair follicles**, which are the structures from which hairs grow. There are also tiny muscles that make the hair stand up (called hair erector muscles). Most of the skin surface produces short, fine hairs that serve little purpose. However, the longer hair on the scalp helps to prevent heat loss from the head. In cold conditions, the hair erector muscles contract, making the hairs stand up more. This increases the heat-insulating properties of hair on the scalp. Hairs inside the nose filter dust from the air we breathe.
+ **sebaceous glands**, which produce an oil (called sebum) that is released onto the shaft of each hair. Sebum spreads over the hair and skin. It helps to keep the skin moist yet waterproof and acts as a barrier against bacteria. It also produces body smells.
+ **sweat glands**, which secrete a salty, watery liquid that spreads over the skin and then evaporates, helping to keep the body cool

The bottom layer of the skin is called **subcutaneous tissue**. This contains connective tissue, fat (known as **adipose tissue**) and blood vessels. The fat serves as a heat insulator and the blood vessels supply the skin with oxygen and nutrients.

Table 6.4 summarises the components of skin and their roles.

Component	Main roles or functions
Epidermis	Protection against ultraviolet radiation
	Barrier protection against disease-causing organisms
	Protection against damage by abrasion
Dermis	Protection against tearing and piercing
	Receiving sensory information about pain, temperature, pressure and touch
	Immune protection against disease-causing organisms
	Temperature regulation (hair erection and sweating)
	Sebum production for waterproofing and bacterial protection
Subcutaneous tissue	Heat insulation
	Blood supply

Table 6.4
Skin components and their main roles

Disorders of the skin

Blackheads

Blackheads (also known as **comedos**) are a symptom of the skin condition **acne**. A blackhead forms when a skin pore at the opening of a hair follicle becomes blocked by a plug containing a mixture of sebum, bacteria and melanin. It is the melanin that makes the blackhead dark in colour (not dirt, as is commonly believed). The bacteria feed on sebum and produce an acidic waste that causes inflammation. Blackheads are most common when the skin is producing the largest amounts of sebum. This is during adolescence, when hormonal changes increase production. In teenaged girls, acne become worse about a week before a period.

Although difficult to prevent, washing with soap and water is a useful precaution. Completely removing make-up also reduces the risks. Face creams do not help to reduce acne because they tend to block pores in the same way that sebum does. Acne is not caused by diet.

Blisters

Blisters are round or oval bumps on the skin in which fluid has accumulated between the dermis and the epidermis. Blisters can be caused by burns or by chafing — for example, when using scissors for a long period or walking in new shoes. They can also be caused by some skin diseases and by viruses (e.g. cold sores and shingles). The fluid in a blister is blood serum, i.e. blood without the red corpuscles. This fluid helps the healing process.

Scabs

A **scab** is a hard crust that forms soon after a wound that pierces the skin and causes bleeding. It is made up of a mixture of **fibrin** (protein fibres that are the end-product of blood clotting), blood platelets and cells from the skin surface. The scab helps to prevent bacteria from entering a wound and infecting it. It also shields the wound from further damage, giving time for the skin to heal. The scab then dries up and falls off.

Rashes

A **rash** is an area of inflammation of the skin. Rashes are often itchy and may be accompanied by a high body temperature. There are different types of rash, including:

+ **localised rashes**, which are present on only small areas of the body, for example those caused by ringworm, candidiasis and scabies, and nappy rash in babies
+ **generalised rashes**, which cover a larger area and, rarely, the whole body. Examples of generalised rashes are those caused by measles and chicken pox.
+ **macular rashes**, which are flat spots (rather than raised spots) on the skin. These have a different colour or texture from the rest of the skin.
+ **raised rashes,** which are red bumps on the skin that are either **papules** or **nodules**. Papules are small bumps or raised spots on the skin, such as blackheads or other types of acne; nodules are larger skin lumps.

Headaches

The pain in a headache arises from the meninges and the scalp and its blood vessels and muscles. Usually, headaches are caused by minor problems. However, they can also occur in serious conditions, such as meningitis and brain tumours.

Causes of headache

Headaches can be triggered by a wide range of conditions including stress, dehydration, hangover, prolonged travel, eating certain foods and spending time in a stuffy atmosphere. Migraine is a severe type of headache.

Stress

Stress refers to a person's responses to demanding situations. Whether people experience stress depends partly on their personalities and partly on how demanding the situation is. People are more likely to experience stress when:

+ they have worries or responsibilities
+ they are in situations that do not allow them to have complete control
+ they are under time pressure

These sorts of conditions occur in some work situations — for example, among military personnel during wartime, and among teachers and hospital staff.

Some people experience little stress, even in the most demanding situations. At the opposite extreme, other people experience stress in relatively undemanding situations.

Stress causes headaches when the muscles of the face, scalp and neck become more tense. This is called a **tension headache**.

Dehydration

Dehydration is a condition in which the body does not contain enough fluid. It can be caused by not drinking enough water, particularly when taking vigorous exercise in hot weather and dry air conditions. It can also be caused by diarrhoea and by consuming drinks that are **diuretic**, such as alcohol. A diuretic increases the loss of water from the body by urination.

Hangover

People who drink an excessive amount of alcohol often wake up with a combination of headache and nausea, called a hangover. This results partly from the diuretic effect of alcohol, described above.

Travel

Prolonged travel can also lead to headaches. This is sometimes because of dehydration, especially during air travel.

Stuffy atmosphere

A stuffy atmosphere can be caused by a lack of ventilation, particularly in a centrally heated place where people are smoking.

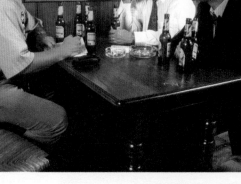

Alcohol and a stuffy atmosphere can both lead to headaches

Food and hunger

Some foods such as chocolate and cheese can trigger headaches in some people. However, a lack of food can have a similar effect.

Cluster headaches

Cluster headaches are a series of short headaches – sometimes several in one day – that occur over a period of a few days or weeks. They usually affect only one side of the head. Sometimes the eye on that side is painful too.

Migraine headaches

Migraines are painful, throbbing headaches that can last from several hours to 3 days. They usually start on one side of the head. Sometimes migraines are accompanied by visual effects, such as flashing lights or geometric patterns. Nausea, vomiting and diarrhoea are other common symptoms.

Women are more likely to suffer from migraine headaches than men. The cause also seems to be partly genetic, because the condition tends to occur in several members or generations in some families, but not in others. Migraines can be triggered by circumstances, such as menstruation and tiredness, or by certain foods, including red wine, peanuts, chocolate, strong cheese, aspartame (a food sweetener) and caffeine.

Food poisoning

Food poisoning can be caused by infections or by toxins ingested with food. The usual symptoms are stomach pain, vomiting and diarrhoea. It can occur as soon as 30 minutes after eating or up to 2 days later. In many cases, it is relatively harmless, although elderly people and young children can become seriously ill.

Infective food poisoning

This can result from infections by bacteria or viruses.

Bacterial food poisoning

Salmonella is one of the commonest causes of food poisoning. *Salmonella* is a bacterium that lives in chickens and their eggs. The risk of food poisoning from infected chicken is reduced by cooking at a high temperature and by not storing chicken at room temperature.

Another common bacterium that causes food poisoning is *Campylobacter*, which occurs in poultry, unpasteurised milk, red meat and untreated water.

Other types of food-poisoning bacteria — such as *Escherichia coli* (*E. coli*) — can be transferred to food by poor food handling and hygiene practices.

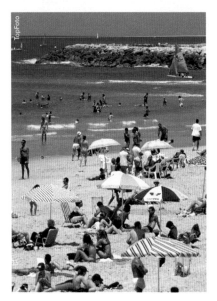

The Norwalk virus is common in sea water contaminated by raw sewage, as in some holiday resorts

Viral food poisoning

The most common type of viral food poisoning is caused by the Norwalk virus. This virus lives only in human cells. It is passed from person to person through faecal matter (sewage). The virus gets into food in several ways. For example:

+ on food that has been prepared by a person whose hands are contaminated with faecal matter. This is a problem with uncooked cold-served foods, such as salads and raw vegetables.
+ in seafood, such as shellfish, which have lived in waters contaminated by raw sewage. Sewage is pumped directly into the sea in many coastal areas.
+ in untreated drinking water and ice cubes made from untreated water. In the UK, tap water is very unlikely to contain the virus. Many other countries have water supplies that are much less clean.

Non-infective food poisoning

Non-infective food poisoning is caused by eating or drinking toxic substances.

Zinc

Although the metal zinc is needed in small quantities in the body, an excess is toxic. Zinc is sometimes used to coat iron to prevent it from rusting. However, zinc is easily dissolved by acids, so if fruit juice (which is acidic) is stored in a zinc container, some of the metal dissolves into the juice. Drinking this contaminated juice can produce food poisoning. Fruit juices should be stored only in glass or plastic containers.

Fungi

Fungi live on decaying vegetation in the soil. Their fruiting bodies (mushrooms and toadstools) are eaten by some people. Some fungi are poisonous and are occasionally eaten by mistake, either by curious children or by adults who mistake them for edible fungi, such as field mushrooms. Eating these species can cause a range of symptoms, from mild food poisoning to death.

Summary

The causes of food poisoning are summarised in Table 6.5.

Type of food poisoning	Agent	Example
Infective	Bacteria	*Salmonella, Campylobacter, E. coli*
	Viruses	Norwalk
Non-infective	Inorganic chemical	Zinc
	Biochemical food toxin	Poisonous mushrooms and toadstools

Table 6.5
Causes of food poisoning

Check your knowledge and understanding of the common diseases and disorders described in this chapter by considering these diagnosis exercises and then answering the questions that follow.

Try it out

Question 1

Matt has just started a course at university. He has enjoyed meeting new people and drinking with them in the Student Union bar. One morning, his friends have difficulty waking him. He complains of a headache and asks them to shut the curtains to keep out the bright light. His friends assume he has a hangover. Later, he gets up and is sick in the toilet. It hurts when he lowers his head. Is this a hangover or something more serious? Why has this happened to Matt just after starting at university?

Question 2

After having several different sexual partners in her teens, Melissa has now settled down with a partner and wants to have a baby. After trying for over a year, Melissa and her partner decide to see a GP to find out if anything is wrong. A specialist later finds scarring on Melissa's uterus and Fallopian tubes. What disease might have caused this scarring? Is it surprising that Melissa did not have any earlier symptoms?

Question 3

George is retired and spends most of his time sitting watching television. After getting a cold, he begins to feel much worse, with a wheezing cough and shortness of breath. What might be causing these symptoms?

Question 4

Miranda and Amir are in a restaurant overlooking the Mediterranean sea. Miranda orders pizza and beer. Amir orders a salad with shellfish and has some water with ice to drink. That afternoon Amir is very ill, with vomiting and diarrhoea. Name the disease-causing organism that is likely to have caused Amir's illness. Why was his choice of food and drink risky?

Question 5

Tom has just started at primary school. His parents notice that he is scratching his head a lot. When they look carefully, they find a round red patch behind his ear, mostly hidden by his hair. They also notice tiny hard blobs apparently attached to some of the hairs. What is the problem? Or could there be more than one problem?

Question 6

Tariq is trying to get to sleep when he notices a low humming sound. His wife wakes up and asks him what's wrong. He tells her about the sound, but she cannot hear it. He gets up and goes from room to room trying to find where the hum is coming from, but he cannot find a source. What might be causing the hum?

Try it out

Question 7

Martha took her tent to the rock festival. The weather was cold and she was lucky to be able to borrow a sleeping bag from some people in the tent next to hers. Two weeks later she noticed wiggly lines like pencil doodles on one of her ankles. On closer inspection she also found some small bumps on her skin. What caused these symptoms? What advice would you give to Martha to prevent this from happening again?

Question 8

Bruce, who lives in Australia, came to Wales for a holiday in August. He visited his grandmother who lives in a bungalow near farmland. The heating was on and Bruce found the house quite stuffy. A cat came and sat on his lap. The next day, Bruce's eyes were red and watering, his nose was running and he was sneezing a lot. Bruce's grandmother thought he had caught a cold. Think of another explanation for Bruce's symptoms and try to identify three possible causes of this in the description.

Question 9

Delyth is reading a book, when she happens to close one eye. She suddenly notices that the print on the lower left-hand corner of the page and the upper right-hand corner of the page is clear and sharp, but the print on the rest of the page is rather blurred. What is the problem with the eye she is using?

Question 10

Derek can see quite clearly and has never needed glasses to drive. Recently, he has found that in order to read a newspaper, he has to hold it as far away from his eyes as possible. Suggest two different eye dysfunctions that could be causing this.

The answers are given at the end of the chapter (see pp. 202–03).

The answers are given at the end of the chapter (see pp. 202–03).

Try it out

Summary tables

In the examination, you might be asked:

+ to apply your knowledge of common diseases and disorders by answering several different types of questions
+ to describe several diseases that have the same type of causal agent. For example, you might have to describe two different bacterial infections or two different types of allergy
+ to identify and describe diseases likely to affect one particular age group or diseases associated with lifestyle

The tables below should help you to prepare for these types of question.

Diseases and disorders common in babies and children	Diseases and disorders common in adolescents and young adults	Diseases and disorders common in elderly people
Meningitis	Gonorrhoea	Presbyopia
Head lice	Meningitis	Cataract
Ringworm	Scabies	Pneumonia
Common cold	Blackheads	Common cold
Scabies		Influenza
Glue ear		Progressive deafness

Table 6.6
Diseases and disorders associated with different age groups

Disease or disorder	Lifestyle
Gonorrhoea	Several different sexual partners
	Unprotected sex
Athlete's foot (*Tinea*)	Taking part in sport
	Swimming
Tapeworm	Eating infected undercooked meat and fish
Allergy to dander and feathers	Keeping pets
Tinnitus	Listening to amplified music
	Working with noisy machinery
Headache	Heavy intake of alcohol
	Prolonged travel

Table 6.7
Diseases and disorders associated with different lifestyles

Disease or disorder	Poor hygiene practice
Tapeworm	Infected person not washing hands after visiting the toilet
	Undercooking infected meat and fish
Dental caries Gingivitis	Not cleaning or flossing teeth regularly
Food poisoning	Storing food (e.g. raw chicken) at room temperature
	Not washing hands before preparing food

Table 6.8
Diseases and disorders associated with poor hygiene practices

Method of transmission	Examples
Coughs and sneezes	Meningitis, pneumonia, common cold, influenza
Sexual intercourse	gonorrhoea, thrush
Contact with infected people or surfaces	Athlete's foot, ringworm, head lice, scabies
Food	Tapeworm, food poisoning
Poor hygiene	Tapeworm, food poisoning

Table 6.9
Ways in which diseases can be transmitted, with examples

Sample examination questions with model answers

The answers given would score full marks. In some cases, alternative answers would be acceptable.

1 Certain groups of people are more likely than others to contract diseases.
   (a) Explain why children are more likely to catch colds than adults aged 30–40 years?   (2 marks)

   Children have not built up immunity to the viruses that cause colds. Adults will have been exposed to more viruses during their lives and will have developed immunity to them.

   (b) Explain why vegetarians are less likely than other people to suffer from tapeworms.   (2 marks)

   Tapeworms are found in meat and fish. Vegetarians do not eat these foods, so are less at risk.

   (c) Give two reasons to explain why people in hospital are more likely to become seriously ill with pneumonia than people not in hospital.   (4 marks)

   One reason is that people in hospital are ill and their immune systems are likely to have been weakened by their conditions. This makes it more likely that they will be unable to resist the effects of pneumonia.

Another reason is that most people in hospital spend most of their time lying in bed. This position makes it difficult for them to clear their lungs of the fluid that accumulates in pneumonia.

(d) Zeinab is 18 years old and keen on sports. On most days she goes for a run in the morning, then has a quick shower before going to school. After school she goes swimming. Suggest and describe one infectious disease that is commonly linked to a lifestyle such as Zeinab's. Refer to the description above in your answer. (7 marks)

Zeinab is at risk from athlete's foot. This is a fungal infection, also called *Tinea*. This fungus grows on the skin of the foot, mostly between the toes. The skin gets itchy, cracked and looks white. Infection is most likely to occur when the skin is warm and wet. When Zeinab goes running, her feet will get sweaty. When she has a 'quick shower' she might not dry her feet properly. Swimming will also keep her feet moist. She might pick up the infection by walking barefoot at the swimming pool.

Total: 15 marks

2 (a) Describe one function of the skin. (2 marks)

One function of the skin is to protect the body from infection. It does this by forming a barrier that helps to prevent disease-causing organisms from entering the body.

(b) Explain how a blackhead is caused. (4 marks)

Blackheads are a symptom of acne. A blackhead forms when a pore in the skin becomes blocked with sebum, bacteria and melanin. Sebum is produced in the sebaceous glands in the dermis, which is the middle layer of the skin. Melanin is a pigment. It makes blackheads appear black.

(c) People with normal vision can read print comfortably at a distance of 30–40 centimetres. They can also read car registration plates at a distance of 20 metres. Three people, A, B and C, all have different dysfunctions that affect their eyesight. Data in the table below show how their vision is affected when they are not wearing glasses or contact lenses.

Person	Comfortable distance for reading print	Able to read registration plate at 20 metres
A	10 cm	No
B	90 cm	Yes
C	90 cm	No

Referring to the data in the table, suggest and describe the dysfunction each person has. (9 marks)

Person A has myopia (short-sightedness). In myopia, the eyeballs are too long. People with myopia can focus on nearby objects but not on distant ones. That is why Person A has to be very close to read print and cannot read the registration plate, which will appear blurred.

Person B has hypermetropia (long-sightedness). In hypermetropia, the eyeballs are too short. People with hypermetropia can focus on distant objects but not on nearby ones. This is why Person B has to hold the print a long way away (90 cm) to be able to read it but can read the registration plate easily — and probably could if it was even further away.

Person C has presbyopia. In presbyopia, the lenses of the eyes become stiff and the focus cannot change. Person C's eyes probably focus in the middle distance. This is why Person C cannot focus much closer than 90 cm or as far away as 20 metres. Person C is probably elderly.

Total: 15 marks

Answers to 'Try it out' questions

Page 167

If the bacterial population doubles every half-hour, there will be over a million bacteria after 10 hours. The exact number is 1,048,576. However, in reality thousands of these would die. It is easy to see how infections (in people who do not have immunity) can become quite serious in only one day.

Pages 197–99

(1) There is a possibility that Matt has meningitis. By mixing with a lot of new friends, he might have picked up the disease from someone who carries it but who is now immune.

(2) Melissa might have contracted gonorrhoea from one of her sexual partners. About half of women with the disease show no symptoms.

(3) George might have pneumonia.

(4) Amir's disease could be caused by the Norwalk virus. This can be carried by shellfish, in water and ice polluted by human faeces and on uncooked food prepared by someone with unwashed hands.

(5) There is more than one problem. The round patch is probably ringworm. The blobs are the eggs of head lice.

(6) The hum is caused by tinnitus.

(7) Martha's symptoms are caused by scabies mites. To prevent this happening again, she should avoid sharing a sleeping bag, clothes or towels.

(8) Bruce could be affected by airborne allergens. His symptoms could have been caused by grass pollen (bungalow near farmland), animal dander (cat sat on his lap) and dust mites (stuffy, heated house).

(9)   Delyth is suffering from astigmatism.

(10) Derek could have long-sightedness (hypermetropia) or presbyopia.

Further reading

The British Medical Association (2004) *The British Medical Association A–Z Family Medical Encyclopedia*, Dorling Kindersley.
Komaroff, A. L. (ed.) (2003) *The Harvard Medical School Family Health Guide* (UK edn), Cassell.

Websites

Department of Health:
   www.dh.gov.uk
The Merck Manual of Medical Information:
   www.merck.com/mmhe/
The National Electronic Library for Health:
   www.nelh.nhs.uk
NHS Direct online medical information:
   www.nhsdirect.nhs.uk/
Patient UK:
   www.patient.co.uk

7 Needs and provision for elderly clients

This chapter contains background information for **Unit 7: Needs and provision for elderly clients.** It also includes guidance to help you with the coursework assessment for this unit.

The first four sections provide background material on health and social conditions and on service provision. The remainder of the chapter deals with planning your coursework, collecting data and writing your report.

Health conditions

The proportion of elderly people in the population has been rising for some time, and is expected to continue to rise for the next 20–30 years.

As people grow old they become increasingly likely to experience problems with their health. However, there is wide variation among individuals. For example, some 80-year-olds are fitter and healthier than some middle-aged people.

This section outlines the conditions most likely to affect people as they grow older.

Heart disease

Ischaemic heart disease

The most common heart disease is **ischaemic heart disease**. The heart acts as a pump that supplies blood to muscles throughout the body. The blood transports oxygen (absorbed into the blood in the lungs) and nutrients, especially blood sugar. Oxygen and blood sugar enable muscles to continue working. However, the heart itself is mainly composed of muscle. To function properly, the heart muscle must have its own supply of oxygenated, nutrient-rich blood.

The arteries that supply blood to heart muscle are called the **coronary arteries**. These arteries run round the outer wall of the heart in an irregular shape, rather like a thin coronet on someone's head. 'Coronary' means 'crown-like'.

Ischaemic heart disease is caused by **atherosclerosis**, which means hardening of the arteries. In atherosclerosis, the arteries become narrower because of deposits of cholesterol and other substances on the linings of the arteries. This means that they are less able to provide a strong supply of blood. On exertion (for example, by climbing stairs), the heart might not be able to supply the extra demand made by the muscles of the body. Atherosclerosis tends to occur in arteries all over the body. However, the condition is particularly serious when it affects the coronary arteries, which become less and less able to supply the blood the heart muscle needs to keep working. The pumping action of the heart becomes less effective and this in turn reduces the blood supply to the heart. The result might be a catastrophic event called a 'heart attack'. Regular exercise, not smoking and a diet low in saturated fat helps to prevent this kind of heart disease.

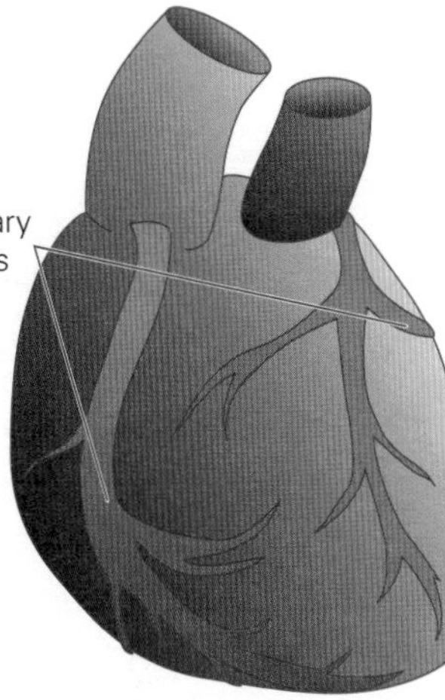

Coronary arteries

Figure 7.1
Coronary arteries supply the heart muscles with blood

Heart failure

Heart failure is the inability of the heart to meet the demands of the body for oxygenated, nutrient-rich blood. People with heart failure feel weak and tired and are unable to exert themselves. One cause is ischaemic heart disease (described above), but other causes include anaemia, hypertension (high blood pressure) and defects in the heart valves. One effect is **oedema**, which is a tendency for fluid to accumulate in the body tissues, for example in the legs, which appear swollen. Fluid also accumulates in the lungs. This is called pulmonary oedema.

Cerebrovascular accidents

Cerebrovascular accidents are commonly called **strokes**. They result from a problem with the blood supply in the brain.

A **thrombosis** is a blood clot that becomes lodged in an artery. When a blood clot blocks an artery, the blood supply is (sometimes temporarily) cut off to the tissues supplied by that artery. Blood clots can easily develop in the veins of the legs. These can become dislodged, pumped around the body and become stuck somewhere else. A blood clot in an artery to the brain can result in a stroke.

An **aneurysm** is an abnormal dilation of an artery. This can result in the artery splitting or bursting. If it happens to an artery supplying the brain, then blood leaks into the brain. This causes two problems:

+ Blood does not get to the brain tissue the artery normally supplies.
+ Blood can accumulate in the confined space inside the skull and put pressure on the brain, causing more damage. This is called a **haematoma**.

Nerve tissue (including the brain) is very sensitive to an interrupted blood supply and rapidly dies. Unlike tissue in other parts of the body (such as muscle, skin and bone), nerve tissue cannot regenerate itself. Cerebrovascular accidents can be fatal. However, more often they lead to temporary or permanent disability. The location of the stroke determines the effect on the body.

Cerebrovascular accidents are more likely to occur in people with **hypertension**. Smoking is a major risk factor.

Effects of a stroke

The most noticeable effects of a stroke are **paralysis** and loss of speech. Paralysis is the loss of the ability to move muscles in a part of the body. The parts of the brain that send nerve impulses to muscles are called the **motor areas**. There are two — one in each hemisphere. The motor area in the left cerebral hemisphere controls muscle movements of the right-hand side of the body; that in the right hemisphere controls movements of the left-hand side of the body.

Typically, a stroke affects only one hemisphere. A stroke affecting the motor area in the right hemisphere is likely to result in a paralysed left arm and leg. In addition, the muscles in the left-hand side of the face might lose 'tone', so that it seems to have sagged or collapsed. (Muscle tone is the normal tension that exists in muscles.)

Speech production is controlled by the left hemisphere — there are no speech areas in the right hemisphere. This means that a stroke affecting the left hemisphere is likely to result in impaired speech, whereas a stroke in the right hemisphere will not.

There are other effects of stroke that are less obvious to observers. These include effects on sensory abilities. A stroke affecting one of the somatosensory areas in the brain is likely to lead to numbness because the parts of the brain that received skin sensations have died. Vision can also be affected. For example, some stroke patients appear to lose awareness of anything on their right-hand side.

Sensory impairments

Hearing loss

Most people gradually lose hearing sensitivity as they grow older. This begins quite early in adulthood but is usually most noticeable in elderly people. The main cause of this hearing loss is progressive damage to, and deterioration of, the hair cells in the cochlea.

Hair cells can be damaged or killed by powerful vibrations transmitted from the middle ear. This type of hearing loss is much greater in people who listen to highly amplified music (via speakers or headphones). Working in a noisy environment, using machinery such as pneumatic drills, can also be a problem unless ear protection is worn.

In most people, the ability to hear the highest-pitched sounds is lost earliest. Some elderly people have hearing aids that occasionally make high-pitched whistling sounds. This is caused by feedback, in which the tiny microphone picks up sound from the loudspeaker built into the aid. You might think this would be very annoying for the wearers. However, they usually cannot hear these high-pitched whistles at all because of damage to the hair cells that vibrate to high-frequency sounds. Some older people find it easier to hear deep or mid-range voices than high-pitched voices.

This type of hearing loss cannot be reversed.

Visual impairments

The two conditions that most commonly affect vision in elderly people are presbyopia and cataract.

Presbyopia is a condition in which the shape of the lens becomes progressively more difficult to change. The result is that nearby objects are out of focus. Distance vision is less affected. Presbyopia occurs because as people grow older, the lens becomes stiffer, so its shape cannot change much. This is the reason why many older people have to use bifocal or reading glasses.

Cataract is a condition in which the lens of the eye becomes milky in appearance, preventing the person from seeing a sharp image. The older people are, the more likely it is that they will develop cataracts. In many people, the clouding does not affect vision seriously. However, in some cases, eye surgery is needed to restore vision. A simple surgical procedure is carried out to break up and remove the lens, which is then replaced by a plastic one.

Skeletal mobility problems

Two common disorders that affect mobility in elderly people are osteoarthritis and osteoporosis.

Osteoarthritis

Osteoarthritis affects the joints between bones, especially those joints that bear the weight of the body, such as the knees, hips, spine and neck. The fingers and wrists are also commonly affected. The main cause is the gradual loss of the smooth cartilage that covers the end surfaces of the bones at a joint. This smooth surface, together with lubricant synovial fluid, makes joints move smoothly. The cartilage tends to wear away with heavy use and as part of the ageing process. As it wears, small pieces sometimes break off and interfere with joint movement (see Figures 7.2 and 7.3). In addition, the ends of the bones are stimulated and grow small projections, which can limit joint movement. The result is joints that are swollen, restricted in movement and intensely painful. In some cases, the whole joint becomes distorted. This is most obvious when it affects the hands.

There is no cure for osteoarthritis, although regular exercise helps to keep muscles strong and these provide some support to the deteriorating joints, especially in the back. Exercise can also reduce the rate at which flexibility is lost.

People with relatively mild forms of the disorder often put up with the pain and inconvenience. Others regularly take analgesics (painkillers) and/or anti-inflammatory drugs.

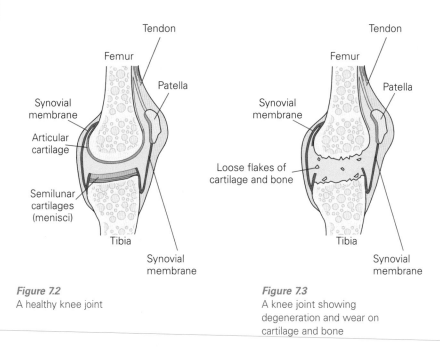

Figure 7.2
A healthy knee joint

Figure 7.3
A knee joint showing
degeneration and wear on
cartilage and bone

Osteoporosis

Osteoporosis is a condition in which the bones become less dense. Bone tissue becomes more porous and this reduces bone strength, increasing the risk of fractures. The gradual loss of bone tissue begins at around 50 years of age and is progressive. However, it does not create significant problems for everyone. Women are more at risk than men. This is because they tend to lose bone density more quickly than men, partly as a result of the reduction in oestrogen production after the menopause. Osteoporosis usually becomes apparent as a result of a fracture. Falls, which would not result in injury in younger people, often lead to fractures, especially of the wrist and hip.

Diabetes

There are different types of **diabetes**. The type that develops in elderly people is type 2 diabetes, in which the cells of the body become resistant to insulin. This leads to reduced blood sugar uptake by the cells from the blood. Therefore, there are high levels of sugar in the blood. This can lead to urinary infections, particularly in older people. It also increases the risk of other disorders, including atherosclerosis, hypertension and cataract. Problems can be reduced by regular exercise and a balanced diet.

Respiratory disorders

The function of the respiratory system is to enable oxygen to be absorbed by the blood and carbon dioxide to be removed. The system includes the airways (the trachea and the two bronchi) and the lungs.

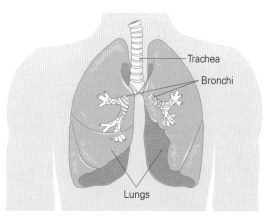

Figure 7.4
The airways and lungs

The most common respiratory disorders are viral infections, such as **influenza**, and bacterial infections, such as streptococcal **pneumonia**. Respiratory infections can occur at any time of life, but they tend to be most prolonged and have the most serious effects in people whose immune systems are weakened. This includes many elderly people. For this reason, an influenza virus, which might produce few symptoms in fit young or middle-aged people, could be fatal to elderly people. Retired people are normally offered a 'flu jab' every autumn to reduce this risk.

Pulmonary oedema (fluid in the lungs) is also more likely to occur among elderly people, especially those with heart failure.

Emphysema is a condition in which the tiny air sacs (alveoli) in the lungs are destroyed. It is caused by smoking or working in dusty conditions. However, as the damage is gradual and progressive, it does not become disabling until old age.

Bronchitis is a constriction or partial blockage of the bronchi, resulting in poor airflow into and out of the lungs. It can occur as a result of infection. It can also occur in cases of emphysema, in which case it is usually chronic (i.e. long-lasting).

Cancers

Cancers can affect people of any age. However, the longer people live, the more likely they are to develop cancer. Some cancers, particularly prostate cancer in men, develop very slowly over a long period and often become noticeable only in old age. People are living longer so the incidence of cancer in the elderly is expected to rise.

Incontinence

Incontinence is the loss of voluntary control over **urination** and **defaecation**.

In elderly people, urinary incontinence can be caused by a loss of control over the urethral sphincter muscle, which normally controls the opening and closing of the urethra. This loss of control may result from deterioration in the part of the brain and nerves that control this sphincter. Such deterioration can be caused by a stroke, a gradual loss of nerve tissue in the brain or by a neural degenerative disease such as Alzheimer's.

In older men, swelling of the prostate gland (sometimes, but not always, caused by cancer) restricts the flow of urine so that the bladder cannot be emptied completely. This leads to frequent dribbling of urine as the bladder overflows.

Faecal incontinence occurs less frequently. It can have a similar cause to urinary incontinence: loss of nerve tissue controlling sphincter muscles. However, it can also occur because of **constipation**, which is relatively common in elderly people. Constipation is more likely in people who take little exercise (such as an immobile elderly person), people who have little fibre in their diet and people whose pelvic muscles are weak and lack muscle tone.

Obesity

Obesity is now common in people of all age groups. Elderly people are sometimes at increased risk of becoming obese because other ill-health conditions prevent them from taking exercise.

Obesity increases the risk of some of the other conditions described above, including hypertension, diabetes and heart disease.

Confusion and dementia

Confusion

Confusion is a general term for a state of disorganisation of thoughts, disorientation and impairment of memory. Confused people might be unsure of where, or even who, they are. They might find it difficult to distinguish between reality and imagination. They might suppose themselves to be much younger than they actually are. They might fail to recognise familiar faces, including their own.

Confusion results from impaired brain function. It can be temporary – for example, as a result of a very high or very low body temperature or the effects of certain drugs. In older people, it is more often a chronic and progressive condition. An underlying problem is that from early adulthood onwards, there is a progressive loss of nerve cells in the brain. The effects of this are not usually noticeable until late in life, partly because as people get older, they find more 'short cuts' to handle information. For example, they might rely more often on stereotyped ways of thinking and understanding the world. Eventually, the accumulated effects become more noticeable, often in embarrassing ways – for example, someone mistaking her son for her husband.

Confusion in elderly people can be triggered by even minor infections, particularly urinary infections. Once the infection has cleared up, the confusion decreases.

Dementias

Dementias are progressive degenerative brain conditions that lead to confusion. They affect about 20% of people over the age of 80 years.

The usual cause is damage to nerve tissues. In some cases, this is caused by a series of mini-strokes, each causing small patches of localised damage. These mini-strokes often go undetected.

Another common cause of dementia is **Alzheimer's disease**, which causes a progressive loss of nerve tissue in the brain. Confusion gradually becomes more severe. Aphasias (language production difficulties) also occur. People with Alzheimer's can become disinhibited (i.e. lose their inhibitions) too, which can lead to behaviours such as aggressiveness, swearing and undressing in public. The condition is typically fatal about 10 years after onset.

Social conditions

A range of social conditions also tends to affect elderly people. However, there is wide variation in the extent to which these affect individuals. Some elderly people receive health and social care for many years, while others remain fit and independent until they die.

Isolation

Social isolation can occur for several reasons. Typically, older people lose social contact because a spouse dies, their children move to other parts of the country or long-term friends die. Reduced mobility means that some elderly people are less able to travel to visit other people.

Lack of occupation

Compared with other age groups, elderly people tend to lack occupation. Most elderly people do not work. Those who live alone have only themselves to look after. Ill health and reduced mobility can hinder people from taking part in a wide range of sport and leisure activities, as well as preventing them from carrying out some daily living tasks, such as cleaning and gardening. The result can be a lack of variety in their occupations, perhaps involving only watching television and reading. Lack of occupation can be harmful to people, partly because of psychological effects, such as boredom, depression and a lack of self-esteem, and partly because of the physiological effects of lack of exercise.

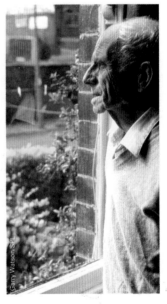

Elderly people are more likely to be socially isolated than other adults

Poverty

Poverty affects some older people. There are several reasons for this. Most elderly people do not work and, therefore, rely for income on state and company pensions, state welfare benefits and income from savings. A married woman who has not worked for most of her life will receive only the basic state pension. If her husband has died, she might not receive any of the occupational pension that he used to receive. Some occupational pension schemes pay a half-pension to the surviving spouse of a dead ex-employee, but others do not. Women who have worked for most of their adult lives are also likely to receive lower occupational pensions than men. This is mainly because women have tended to occupy lower-paid jobs. Generally, single elderly women have lower incomes than single elderly men.

If an elderly person lives alone in rented accommodation, the cost of rent and council tax is likely to be less affordable than for a couple living in the same house or flat. Elderly people are less able to carry out maintenance on buildings and gardens and so face additional expense to cover these tasks.

The poorest pensioners can receive a range of welfare benefits to prevent poverty. However, for various reasons, many do not claim what they are entitled to. These reasons include ignorance, a dislike of form filling, and objections to receiving benefits that they perceive as 'charity'.

Inadequate housing

Elderly people tend to be less able than others to maintain their homes. As a result, conditions can become cluttered, damp and insanitary. Some elderly people live in accommodation that has ceased to be appropriate to their needs — for example, a two-storey family house rather than a small bungalow or ground-floor flat. Poverty can make it difficult for them to find more suitable accommodation or to maintain their existing home.

Reduced independence

Some elderly people become progressively less able to do things for themselves. Impaired mobility due to medical conditions may prevent them from shopping or carrying out daily living tasks such as cooking, cleaning, bathing, dressing and undressing, and getting up in the morning.

Insecurity

Elderly people, particularly those living alone, often lack physical safety and psychological security. They might lack physical safety because frailty, combined with an unsuitable home environment, creates the potential for falls, scalds and burns. For example, the rooms in their homes might be cluttered with furniture and objects they could trip over. They might have stairs to climb. Physical safety is also at risk if they are taken ill suddenly, particularly if they are not then able to call for help.

Elderly people living alone might lack psychological security if they become anxious about the risks to their physical safety. The prospect of further declining health and increasing dependence might also cause people to feel anxious. Recently bereaved people might not have much experience of living alone and this could make them feel more anxious. As a result of misleading newspaper reports, some elderly people have an exaggerated fear of crime.

Cultural change

During the first 20 years of life, people acquire beliefs and attitudes from the culture they are growing up in. Usually, these beliefs and attitudes are acceptable and appropriate for the conditions in which people find themselves. During adulthood, these attitudes and beliefs are modified by experience, though not usually to a great extent. The beliefs and attitudes of elderly people are, therefore, similar to those they acquired during childhood and adolescence.

If there has been rapid cultural change during their lifetime, people's beliefs and attitudes, which were once appropriate, become increasingly irrelevant to the changed world they live in. The past century has been a time of very rapid change, which has affected many aspects of everyday life, including travel, education, health, work and leisure. To a young person growing up and adapting to life in Europe in the twenty-first century, the beliefs and attitudes of a 90-year-old can seem outdated. In turn, the beliefs and attitudes of the young person are likely to become increasingly outdated as they become older. This sort of cultural change can result in elderly people feeling uncomfortable and unhappy with what to other people are perfectly acceptable practices. For example, elderly Christians might be unhappy with a woman priest, because earlier in their lives all priests were men.

Low status/stereotypes

The elderly in Britain tend to be treated as people with relatively low status. They can be made to feel less important than younger adults — for example, when receiving services in shops. One reason is that elderly people have less power. For example, an elderly person might lack the confidence or the energy to complain about poor service, whereas a younger person would be more confident about making a fuss.

The behaviour of some people towards the elderly is influenced by stereotypes about elderly people, such as that they are slow-witted, intolerant and out of touch.

Service provision: health care

There is a range of services available to enable elderly people to cope with some of the problems outlined in the previous sections.

GP services

Everybody has the right to register with a general practitioner. It is particularly important for elderly people to be registered with a named GP, so that they can obtain access to a range of health services. A consultation with a GP is usually arranged by making an appointment. If their named GP is unavailable, patients will normally be offered an appointment with another GP working at the same practice or health centre.

Contact with a GP who knows the patient well is particularly useful for the elderly, who are likely to have chronic health conditions that need to be monitored.

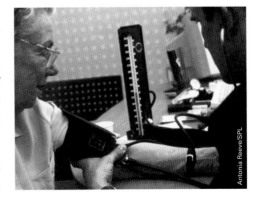

Contact with a GP allows chronic health conditions to be monitored

Antonia Reeve/SPL

In addition, the GP will be able to look out for the unwanted effects of medication prescribed to the patient on a long-term basis. For example, some of the drugs that are prescribed to reduce the risk of disease by lowering blood pressure can have harmful side-effects. It is sometimes necessary to try several combinations of these drugs in order to find the most suitable treatment. Careful monitoring of the patient by the GP is important during this process. A GP will also refer patients to other health services, including hospital services.

Elderly people living in the community are often encouraged to have a regular health check at their local GP surgery or health centre. Usually, this is carried out by a practice nurse, who will check blood pressure, ask about changes in health, request a urine sample, and take a blood sample for testing. This type of health check is designed to detect some of the medical conditions (such as hypertension, high cholesterol levels and diabetes) that are likely to affect elderly people. A practice nurse can also carry out immunisations, such as flu jabs.

Hospital services

Elderly people access hospital services in several ways, which are outlined below.

Accident and Emergency services

Following a stroke or heart attack, or an injury caused by a fall, patients are likely to be taken by ambulance to a hospital **Accident and Emergency department**, where they receive initial diagnosis and treatment. In some of these conditions, rapid treatment is important. For example, 'clot-busting' drugs administered soon after a stroke can dramatically reduce the resulting brain damage. After this initial treatment, elderly patients are likely to be transferred to a hospital ward for further treatment and/or observation. Many elderly people have impaired immune systems and poor physical fitness, so they tend to remain in hospital longer than other adults.

Outpatient treatment

Following a **GP referral**, a patient might be given a hospital outpatient appointment for a consultation with a specialist. This can lead to outpatient treatment, where the patient visits hospital several times (e.g. for physiotherapy), or to admission to a hospital ward for inpatient treatment.

Elective surgery

One type of inpatient treatment is **elective surgery**. Elective surgery refers to an operation that has been recommended by a hospital consultant, and agreed to by the patient, but which is not urgent.

An example is **orthopaedic surgery** to replace a hip. (Orthopaedic surgery means surgery to joints and bones.) **Hip replacement** operations are often used for patients who have great difficulty in walking because of osteoarthritis. The damaged top end of the femur is removed and a metal replacement is slotted into the end of the cut bone. A metal socket is embedded in the pelvic bone. The replacement has a smooth joint surface designed to fit into the pelvis and enable free and painless movement.

Another example of elective surgery is a **heart bypass** operation, used to treat atherosclerosis in the coronary arteries. The parts of the arteries that are most affected are bypassed using a section of healthy artery taken from elsewhere in the body or, alternatively, using a tube of synthetic material.

Because elective surgery is not urgent, planned operations are sometimes cancelled – for example, when the surgeon is required for an emergency operation following a heart attack or accident.

Audiology

People with hearing difficulties can be referred by their GP to a hospital **audiology** department. At an outpatient appointment, the hearing is tested. If a **hearing aid** is necessary, this will be supplied and fitted at another appointment.

Hearing aids do not restore hearing to normal. Until recently, they had the simple effect of amplifying all sound. This improved hearing in quiet conditions with only one source of sound – for example, listening to one other person talking. However, in conditions with a great deal of background noise (e.g. traffic, several people talking) people were often unable to pick out the sounds they wished to listen to. In addition, the amplified noise could be extremely annoying. This problem has been reduced in some public buildings by the **induction-loop** system, in which sound from microphones is transmitted and can be picked up by hearing aids, provided these are switched to induction-loop mode.

Recently, digital hearing aids have been introduced. These can be programmed to amplify more selectively, resulting in better hearing in some patients. They are available free under the NHS.

Some hearing aids hook over the ear, while others, which are bulkier but easier to adjust, have an earpiece connected to an amplifier worn in a pocket.

Some people (who are perhaps unaware of the free NHS service) purchase hearing aids from private providers. These are expensive. However, compared with aids that hook over the ear, some of these aids are very unobtrusive. The smallest aids slot entirely into the ear canal.

Optical services

Most eye surgery and treatments for eye disease (such as glaucoma and cataract) are provided by NHS **ophthalmology** departments. Other systems for correcting vision are provided by the private sector. These systems include contact lenses, glasses and laser corneal surgery.

A range of sight tests provided by opticians is free to people over the age of 60. (The optician is able to claim the cost from the NHS.) These tests are designed to detect short- and long-sightedness, astigmatism, presbyopia and glaucoma. Together with cataract, presbyopia and glaucoma are most likely to affect elderly people. More details of different eye conditions are given in Chapter 6.

Dental treatment

The teeth gradually deteriorate over time. This is because of dental caries and loss of gum tissue. The outcome is that elderly people sometimes need expensive treatment, such as bridgework. A dental bridge is a construction carrying one or more false teeth, which is secured to the remaining teeth and fills a gap left by loss of the natural teeth. In some elderly people, so many of the teeth are lost that a set of **dentures** (false teeth) is supplied, attached to a plastic false palate. Once people have lost all their teeth, they require little dental treatment, apart from the repair and modification of dentures.

Almost all elderly people have to pay for their dental treatment — one exception is people who are hospital inpatients. Although there are some NHS dentists, there are too few to meet demand at present. Most dentists are now private providers.

Chiropody

Elderly people sometimes have foot-care problems, partly because they lack mobility but also because they become less able to care for their own feet. Infections of the feet are more likely in people with diabetes and heart failure. Routine **chiropody** (also known as **podiatry**) is available, at a cost, from private providers.

NHS chiropodists tend to deal with more serious problems, such as toenail surgery and care of patients at risk from amputations (e.g. those with diabetes). NHS chiropodists can be based in a hospital department or clinic, or in a GP surgery or health centre.

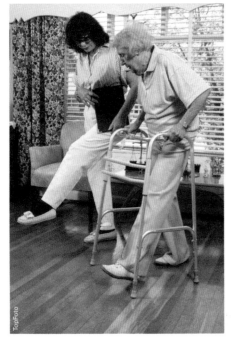

Physiotherapy helps elderly people to restore mobility after surgery or a stroke

Physiotherapy

Physiotherapy helps to restore muscle strength following surgery, to regain movement in stroke patients and to improve lung function.

Restoring muscle strength is important for people whose muscles have deteriorated. This could happen as a result of a long stay immobile in hospital or because of a long period of reduced mobility caused by arthritis. A hip replacement is likely to last longer in a person who develops strong muscles to support the joint.

Physiotherapy following a stroke aims to restore motor control, so that patients can walk again and manipulate objects. This is a long process because the control function lost because of dead brain tissue has to be taken over by neighbouring brain tissue. How successful this is, partly depends on the motivation and determination of the patient.

Some elderly patients will be treated by NHS physiotherapists in a hospital outpatient clinic; others might receive home visits.

Occupational therapy

NHS occupational therapists work with elderly people to maintain, improve or restore their ability to cope with everyday living tasks. A referral is made by a GP or, following hospital inpatient treatment, by a member of hospital staff for an occupational therapist to visit a patient at home. The therapist is likely to carry out a **needs assessment** that will take into account the ability of the patient to perform daily living tasks and the suitability of the home environment. Following this assessment, the occupational therapist can arrange for adaptations to be made to the home. For example, a downstairs room might be converted into a bathroom and/or suitable aids might be provided. The latter can range from mobility aids – such as walking frames and wheelchairs – to items designed for specific tasks, such as kettle tippers, bath hoists, extended tap handles or tap turners (Figure 7.5). Among elderly people, such aids are most commonly required to cope with problems arising from osteoarthritis.

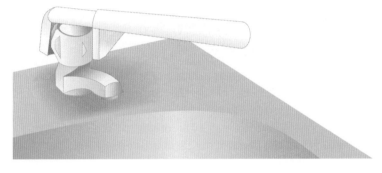

Figure 7.5
A tap turner clamped to an ordinary tap as an aid for an arthritic patient

Speech and language therapy

Speech and language therapists in the NHS often work with elderly people who have lost some of their language ability because of a stroke. They provide charts that patients can point to in order to indicate their needs. They also provide speech exercises to help people regain some language ability – for example, by encouraging them to say what they mean when they are unable to think of a particular word. In some stroke patients, language ability recovers quite soon after a stroke; in others, only partial recovery is possible.

Community health care

District (or community) nurses visit patients in their own homes to provide treatment (e.g. changing dressings), particularly for those recently discharged from hospital.

Diet

Dieticians give elderly people advice on diets that can help to reduce health problems, particularly in people with diabetes. Patients can get access to an NHS dietician via referral from a GP. Private dieticians are also available.

Elderly people in residential and nursing homes

Residential and nursing homes have some members of staff with nursing qualifications, who can change wound dressings, treat minor conditions and administer medication. The homes usually have an arrangement with a local GP surgery or health centre, so that a community nurse or GP can call on residents if necessary.

Service provision: social care

Social care tackles some of the problems that result from isolation, lack of occupation, poverty, inadequate housing, insecurity and reduced independence.

Needs assessment

For a client to gain access to social care provided by a local authority, a needs assessment has to be carried out. Typically, a social worker employed by the local authority visits the client at home and collects information to assess whether the local authority should provide services. The assessment is designed to find out whether the client is eligible to receive certain services, using a set of criteria.

Needs assessments consider the health of the clients, their ability to carry out daily living tasks, their level of risk (e.g. from falls or infections), the suitability of their accommodation and the amount of help they are currently receiving from informal carers.

Usually, each client is assigned to a category according to the level of need:

+ High category means that the needs of the client are critical – the client is at great risk of injury or illness.
+ Medium category means that the needs of the client are substantial – the current living conditions are unsuitable in a number of ways.
+ Low category means that the client could benefit from some provision, but is not at serious or immediate risk.

In the lowest category, the social worker will normally refer the client to other services but will not make local authority services available. Clients in the other categories will usually receive some form of care, depending on the availability of funds in the local authority social services budget.

Sheltered housing

Sheltered housing consists of (usually) rented flats or bungalows that are supervised in some way. Some units have a warden who lives in one of the flats, and a call system such as an alarm that can be triggered by a resident. This means that the elderly people feel safe and are less isolated. In an emergency, the warden is available to help or call for other services. Some units have a common room where residents can meet. This improves social contact. Sheltered housing provides security, while maintaining a level of independence. Each resident can feel 'at home' and has privacy.

Sheltered housing schemes are operated by a range of providers, including:
+ local authority housing departments
+ non-profit-making housing associations
+ charities
+ private, profit-making organisations

Each resident is liable to pay rent and maintenance charges to cover the cost of the accommodation, utility bills, maintenance, staffing and council tax. However, residents with low incomes are likely to be eligible for council tax rebates and, in some cases, rent rebates.

Residential and nursing home care

Residential homes

Elderly people who have become too frail to live independently can choose to live in a **residential home**.

Most residential homes are designed to cater for elderly people with only moderate health problems.

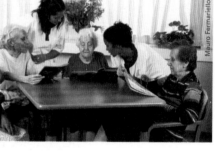

Staff in residential homes provide social contact

+ Each resident has a single room with a small bathroom and toilet attached.
+ Residents usually eat their meals in a communal dining room, although they can sometimes choose to eat in their own rooms.
+ Residents are usually allowed, or encouraged, to personalise their rooms.
+ Visitors are made welcome.
+ A communal sitting room enables residents to have social contact.
+ Various activities are provided, ranging from exercise sessions to crafts and singing.
+ Residential homes are equipped with specially designed bathrooms fitted with hoists.
+ Staff provide meals, activities, baths and social contact. They may help to get residents up and dressed and aid with toileting.
+ Additional services that are usually provided include visits to hairdressers and chiropodists, and occasional short outside trips.

Residential homes provide a higher level of supervision and security than sheltered housing, but residents have less independence.

Some residential homes are provided by local authorities, but most are run by private providers, some of which are profit-making organisations. Other homes are run by non-profit making charities and housing associations.

Residential care is funded in two ways. Local authority social services have a budget that they can use to fund places in residential care. Access to this funding is via a needs assessment and is means-tested. People with more than £20,500 in assets or savings do not receive local authority funding and have to pay the costs themselves. People who have assets less than this amount and who are in the greatest need of residential accommodation will receive funding.

In Scotland, the situation is different. Local authorities provide free residential care for all who are assessed as needing it, regardless of income.

In the remainder of the UK, the low level of funding for residential care has resulted in some privately run homes closing because they are no longer profitable. This has created a shortage of residential places.

Nursing homes

Nursing homes are similar to residential homes, although they tend to cater for people who have greater health needs — for example, those with Alzheimer's disease and terminal illnesses. They have a higher proportion of qualified nursing staff and their fees are higher.

Day care

Day care is provided in day-care centres or sometimes in residential homes. Elderly people living in the community visit the centre (perhaps twice a week) to spend the day. While there, they can socialise, take part in activities, have midday meals and perhaps take baths. Day care provides occupation and social contact for people who might otherwise be isolated. Day-care staff are in a position to notice changes in their clients so that if necessary they can be referred to other services.

Home care (domiciliary care)

Domiciliary care means practical help with daily living tasks, provided by a person who visits clients in their own homes. This care can include getting clients up in the morning, and helping with cleaning, bathing and cooking a meal. Domiciliary care enables clients to remain in their own homes, extending their independence.

Following a needs assessment, domiciliary care can be provided by a local authority social services department. The actual provision is sometimes carried out by local authority employees, but more often by private or voluntary agencies contracted and paid by the local authority. In some cases, clients are charged a fee for this service. Domiciliary care is also available from private providers, at full cost.

Meals on wheels

Local authorities usually have a 'meals-on-wheels' service that provides hot midday meals for elderly people on weekdays. Clients have to pay a small charge for this service.

Informal care

Many elderly people rely wholly or partly on friends, neighbours and relatives to provide care. This is called informal care. For example, an elderly relative might live with a son or daughter, who provides security, social contact and help with daily living tasks. Informal carers often visit elderly people in their own homes – for example, to provide social contact and do shopping and house maintenance.

More limited, informal care is provided by people who visit residents in residential and nursing homes.

Personal emergency response systems

These are systems to enable an elderly person to call for help in the event of an accident or sudden illness. The user wears a call-button on a cord around the neck. In an emergency, he/she presses the button. This signals an alarm call at a monitoring centre. Someone at the centre then telephones the caller to check whether or not the call was a false alarm. If the client confirms that help is required, the appropriate emergency service is alerted. If the client does not answer the telephone – he/she may be unconscious or have had a fall – an ambulance is sent as soon as possible.

This system provides security for elderly people living alone. It reduces the consequences of an accident or sudden illness, enabling them to continue to live independently.

Personal emergency response systems are provided by charities and profit-making organisations.

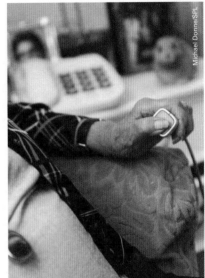

A personal emergency response system helps to improve safety and psychological security

Voluntary agencies

A number of local and national voluntary organisations help to provide some of the types of social care described above. For example, **Help the Aged** provides support for individuals to continue to live independently. This organisation also provides a telephone helpline, called SeniorLine, which gives advice on welfare benefits, together with information on health and social care provision.

Age Concern provides various services, including lunch clubs, day centres and home visiting. It also runs Aid-Call, a personal emergency response system (see above).

Welfare benefits

Some welfare benefits for elderly people are means-tested. This means that they are provided only for people below a certain level of income or wealth. Other benefits are not means-tested – they do not depend on income or wealth. The benefit figures given below were correct as of April 2005.

Means-tested benefits include:

+ **Pension Credit.** This is a benefit paid to people aged 60 years or over. Its purpose is to top up the income of poor people to a level of £109.45 per week for a single person or £167.05 for a couple.

+ a savings credit that can be claimed instead of, or in addition to, the basic pension credit. It rewards people who have low savings or a small occupational pension. This can be up to £16.44 for a single person and £21.51 for a couple. These two benefits can be claimed by filling in a form giving details and evidence of income.

+ **Cold Weather Payment.** This is automatically awarded to people who receive Pension Credit, but only if winter temperatures in their area fall below a certain level.

Non-means-tested benefits include:

+ **Attendance Allowance**. This is payable to people over 65 who, because of illness or disability, need help with personal care. The highest rate of £60.60 per week is for people who need care both day and night. The lower rate of £40.55 per week is for people who only need care either in the daytime or in the night-time. To receive this benefit, claimants have to fill in a form indicating their level of disability.

+ **Winter Fuel Payment**. This benefit is paid to people aged 60 years and over. The amount varies according to age. In the winter of 2004/5, a person aged over 80 and living with other people received a £200 payment.

Service provision for the elderly is summarised in Table 7.1.

Social condition	Relevant service provision
Social isolation	Day centres
	Domiciliary care
	Residential and nursing home care
Lack of occupation	Day centres
Poverty	Welfare benefits
Inadequate housing	Sheltered housing
	Adaptations
	Residential and nursing homes
Reduced independence	Domiciliary care
	Residential and nursing homes
Insecurity	Personal emergency response systems
	Sheltered housing
	Residential and nursing homes

Table 7.1
Service provision for the elderly is designed to cope with different social conditions

Planning your coursework

You need to produce a report based on what you have found out about one elderly person.

Finding an interviewee

+ Your interviewee should be at least 70 years old.
+ You will find producing your coursework much easier if you can find a suitable elderly person to interview. The ideal interviewee probably does not exist, but would be someone who:
    + is patient
    + is interested in taking part
    + is able to hear and speak quite well
    + has an interesting range of problems
    + is receiving several services

+ If the person you interview is very fit and well and does not need any services, you will not have much to write about.
+ It would be ideal if you and your interviewee already know each other quite well. Then, you will both be more relaxed in the interview situation.
+ If you know several elderly people, you could chat informally to them all. Then, on the basis of what you find out, decide which one to study in more detail.

Choosing an option

The unit assessment requires you to look at three topics. You must include a needs description and an account of service provision. For the third topic, you have a choice between 'comparison' or 'consequences'.

The 'comparison' topic involves comparing your interviewee's experience of growing up with your own experience. If you choose this option, you will have to ask your interviewee about aspects of their early life – up to the age of 25 years. In your report, you will also include an objective account of your own life up to the present (or up to 25 if you are older). You might need to check some of the information with a parent. This topic is likely to be quite interesting for your interviewee and for yourself, although it is also quite personal.

The 'consequences' topic looks at what it is like to grow old, from the perspective of your interviewee. The aim here is to enable you to explore the interviewee's own experience.

Clearly, the choice made between these two options will shape the questions you ask in your interview. You should think carefully before making your choice. One option might work quite well with some interviewees, but not with others. If you like, you could ask your interviewee to state a preference.

Collecting data

You should familiarise yourself with the background material given earlier in this chapter before designing your interview schedule.

Recording what you already know

Before interviewing your participant, you should record whatever you already know about him or her that might be relevant to your report. There is no point in asking questions to which you know the answer or to which the answer is obvious, such as 'Do you wear glasses?'

Interview planning

You will need to interview your participant in depth, making sure that you find out as much of the information you need as is possible.
+ You should first list all the topics you need to find information about.
+ Then you should structure these topics so that they follow logical themes – for example, a section about medical treatment being received, another section

about managing in the home – rather than jumping from one topic to another at random.

+ Your list of topics should be organised into an interview schedule, which lists the questions you want to ask and provides plenty of space for you to record replies.

The questions should aim to find out about the health and social conditions of the participant, the services received (at present and recently) and the opinions held about those services. You will also have to find out about any unmet needs.

The questions you ask will depend on what you already know about the person. If you have learned and understood relevant background material – such as that included in this chapter – you will be in a good position to know about services that could benefit your interviewee. Your participant might be unaware of some of these services, in which case your interview could be of practical use. For example, you might find that your interviewee is worried about being taken ill at home and not being able to let anyone know about it. You could then mention the availability of services such as Aid-Call.

However, you should not give the impression that you are an expert on health or social care. In particular, you should not attempt to diagnose illness or give advice. At most, you should give information that would enable the interviewee or an informal carer to contact a service provider.

You will have to decide how to find information for the optional topic 'comparison' or 'consequences'. A possible approach is to start the interview with one of these topics, because they might be easier for your interviewee to talk about than the compulsory subjects.

There will be a great deal of material to cover, so you might find it useful to conduct the interview over two or more meetings, rather than at one sitting. Advantages to this include the following:

+ It will be less tiring for interviewer and interviewee.
+ Both parties to the interview can refer to things that they forgot to mention or ask at a previous meeting.
+ Several shorter interviews enable a good working relationship to be built up.

Before carrying out your interview(s), you should discuss with your teacher what you are intending to do and ask. This should ensure that what you are doing is appropriate and ethical.

Interview technique

The interview is likely to be a strange experience for both you and your interviewee. It might help if you can make it an informal occasion. It will not work well if you sit and read out your questions like a market researcher or (worse) like a television reporter interviewing a politician. It would be better to adopt a more conversational style. The interview could consist of a mixture of everyday chat with some of your questions dropped in to stimulate conversation. This informal

Topic: hospital treatment

(1) Have you had to stay in hospital recently? (If no, go to item 19.)

    Yes ☐   No ☐

(2) What were you in hospital for?

(3) What was it like when you were in hospital?

(4) Did the treatment make you feel better afterwards? If so, in what ways? If not, how did it make you feel?

(5) How

Figure 7.6
Extract from an interview schedule

style of interviewing is likely to produce quite a lot of irrelevant material (which you will not need to record) but will help to establish a working relationship that will make the interview productive as well as enjoyable.

It is important to realise that the experience of being interviewed can be rewarding and enjoyable for the interviewee. For example, some elderly people enjoy talking about their early lives.

It is important to ask questions that are likely to elicit the information you need. For example, it would not be effective to ask 'What are your health needs?' because this is likely to be an unfamiliar phrase to most interviewees. Instead, it would be better to ask, 'Are you well?' or 'Is anything wrong with your health?' Similarly, it would not be effective to ask an interviewee about a 'needs assessment'. Instead you could ask 'Did anyone come to see you, to find out what you needed?'

You should understand that an interviewer should not disempower the respondent or act in a controlling or dominating manner, but should draw out, encourage, give choices and listen to the respondent.

More information about interviewing can be found in Chapter 9, pages 256–59.

Ethical precautions

It is very important to follow the ethical precautions described in the unit specifications available from AQA. If you do not have a copy of the specification for this unit, you can look it up on the AQA website (www.aqa.org.uk).

You should consider carrying out your interview in the presence of another responsible adult, such as a relative of the interviewee. This would have the advantage that the other adult could intervene if, for example, your questions were too intrusive or the interviewee wanted to withdraw. A relative might also be able to supply some of the information you need, although care should be taken to avoid the relative answering the questions, rather than the intended interviewee.

You should avoid asking direct questions that are potentially embarrassing or offensive to the interviewee. For example, you should not ask, 'Do you suffer from incontinence?' It is much better to ask a general question about health and let the interviewee disclose any further information.

The interview might reveal information of a very personal nature. You have to make a judgement about what to include in your report. In any case, it should *never* be possible for a reader to identify the interviewee. The name of the interviewee must not be given.

Trialling

You will find it helpful to do a trial run of part or all of your interview schedule with someone who can give useful feedback. This might be a fellow student, parent or teacher acting the part of an elderly person. Trialling will enable you to find out which questions work and help you to develop a quick and effective recording style. By enabling you to practise your interviewing technique, it might also give you confidence.

Writing the report

Detailed guidance on the contents of each section of the report is given in the unit specification.

Section A: Introduction

This should include a statement about what you have included in your report and a description of the elderly person.

Section B: Method

To score high marks, this section of the report should give an accurate description of when and how you collected information from, and about, your interviewee. It should also include a clear account of the ethical guidelines you followed. The evidence supporting this (including the original interview schedule or a photocopy) should be included in the Appendix.

Section C: Findings

To score high marks, this section of your report should include an accurate and detailed account of the interviewee's health and social conditions. For example, if the interviewee has diabetes, you should include some background information about this condition. It is quite likely that some aspects of the interviewee's health or social conditions are not covered in this chapter. You should consult additional sources for more information.

You should also describe what you have found out about the services your interviewee receives. It is not sufficient to rely on what your interviewee tells you. Find out some background about the services he or she mentions.

You should suggest any services that your interviewee is not currently receiving but from which they might benefit, either now or in the next 5 years. It is important not to miss out any services that your interview shows are obviously relevant.

Note that you should not include health and social conditions or services that are not relevant to your interviewee. For example, including information about deafness and surgery for prostate cancer when your interviewee is a woman with good hearing would be irrelevant.

You should evaluate the provision your interviewee currently receives, together with any others you suggest. This evaluation should be a description of any advantages or disadvantages of the provision for your particular interviewee. For example, with reference to residential care, you might refer to the advantages of security and social contact and the disadvantages of loss of some independence and privacy. As another example, you could refer to the health benefits resulting from medication to reduce hypertension and also the risks of specific side-effects.

Organisation

Your report should be well organised. It will contain a number of different topics, so you need to think carefully about the most logical order. The guidance given in the specification suggests how to divide the main sections into subsections.

You should also take care to organise the information so that there is a minimum of repetition. The report should be concise, not rambling. You will not gain more marks just by filling more pages.

Marks for interview technique

There are marks available for the design of the interview schedule and the use of interview technique. This will be partly evidenced by the completed copy of your schedules, included in the Appendix. You will be assessed on the appropriateness of the questions you asked (including how appropriate they were to the person you interviewed). Further evidence will come from the effectiveness of your recording method and from the quotes you obtained (and used in Section C).

Further reading

Information about services and needs assessment
Moore, S. (2002) *Social Welfare Alive!*, Nelson Thornes.

Information about services and health conditions
Komaroff, A. L. (ed.) (2003) *The Harvard Medical School Family Health Guide* (UK edn.), Cassell.

Information about health conditions

The British Medical Association (2004) *The British Medical Association A–Z Family Medical Encyclopedia*, Dorling Kindersley.

Websites

Useful general websites

Department of Health:
 www.dh.gov.uk

The Merck manual of Medical Information:
 www.merck.com/mmhe

The National Electronic Library for Health:
 www.nelh.nhs.uk

NHS direct:
 www.nhsdirect.nhs.uk/

Patient UK:
 www.patient.co.uk

Particular organisations

Age Concern:
 www.ageconcern.org.uk

Help the Aged:
 www.helptheaged.org.uk

Needs and provision for early-years clients

This chapter contains background information for **Unit 8: Needs and provision for early-years clients**. It also includes guidance to help you with the coursework assessment for this unit. The first two sections provide background material on the needs of early-years clients and on service provision. The last three sections deal with evaluating services, collecting data and writing your report. You should find the background material on child development in Chapter 4 useful.

Needs of early-years clients

There are different ways of describing human needs. The physical and psychological life-quality factors covered in Unit 1: Effective caring can be regarded as 'needs'. These life-quality factors apply to children just as much as to adults.

Physical needs or health needs

Physical and health needs include exercise, adequate nutrition, physical safety and hygiene, physical comfort and freedom from pain.

Exercise

The need for exercise is met by a combination of things including:

+ clean, uncluttered floor space
+ toys to assist walking

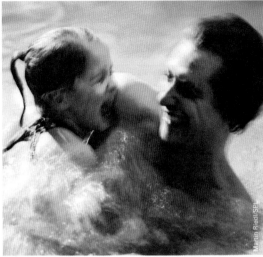

Meeting children's need for exercise includes giving them regular opportunities to swim

* ride-on toys
* safe outdoor space
* regular opportunities to run, swim and walk
* climbing frames, slides, swings and other large play apparatus

Adequate nutrition

The need for adequate nutrition is met by feeding a diet that is appropriate for the age of the child. The diet should enable physical growth but minimise the risks of developing health problems, such as obesity and dental caries.

Formal service providers are likely to follow nutritional guidelines when providing food for children.

Physical safety and hygiene

The need for physical safety is met partly by ensuring that the home environment is suitably adapted — for example, by keeping medicines and domestic cleaning fluids out of reach, fires guarded and upstairs windows secured. The need for physical safety is also met by systems and organisations designed to protect children from abuse or neglect.

The need for hygiene is met by bathing children, regularly cleaning and disinfecting surfaces that children come into contact with, and washing clothes and toys.

Formal service providers are likely to have a set of health and safety guidelines to follow.

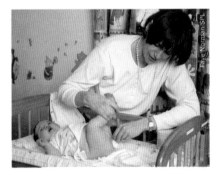

Prompt nappy changing helps to ensure an infant's physical comfort

Physical comfort and freedom from pain

These needs are met by procedures such as nappy changing, having a supply of clean clothes in the event of an incontinence accident and by seeking medical attention when a child has a painful rash, a high temperature or severe pain.

Social and emotional needs

Social and emotional needs include social contact, social support, approval and psychological security.

Social contact

From early infancy, children show an interest in other people. For the first 3 years of life, during which children are most strongly attached, the need for social contact is mainly restricted to contact with familiar people. After this, children become interested in contact with other children. Social contact also provides opportunities for learning.

Social support

The need for social support occurs most in potentially stressful situations. Children tend to seek increased social contact with familiar adults when they are ill, tired, in pain or afraid. Providing contact (often including physical contact, such as a cuddle) is an important way of minimising the distress caused to a child in such situations. For example, when receiving an immunisation injection or meeting new people for the first time, children benefit from the social support of a parent.

Formal service providers often recognise this need and make arrangements for the child to be accompanied by a familiar person.

Approval

Most people need to feel positive about themselves. They need to see themselves as worthwhile, with positive features and abilities. In other words, people benefit if their concept of self includes believing good things about themselves and having high self-esteem. When children are developing their self-concepts throughout most of the early-years period, they are very dependent on the opinions that others feed back to them.

Parents can show approval (positive regard) by:

+ listening to their child
+ appearing to be interested in some of the same things as the child
+ playing alongside
+ showing affection
+ praising

It is much better for the child if positive regard is shown only in response to **adaptive behaviours**. Adaptive behaviours are those behaviours that are likely to benefit the child in the long term. **Maladaptive behaviours** are those that are likely to harm the child in the long term. Maladaptive behaviours include anti-social behaviours, such as displays of aggression and violence, which lead other people to dislike the child. They also include behaviours that could directly harm the child, such as risk-taking activities. In young children, maladaptive behaviours can be reduced by not rewarding them with attention. In older children, they can be reduced by calm and reasoned persuasion.

Some adults adopt a different approach. They make a big fuss about maladaptive behaviours. For example, they might punish or criticise the child and use negative labels, such as calling the child 'bad'. They tend to ignore adaptive behaviours. This approach is likely to have the opposite effect to that intended.

Formal service providers usually employ staff (such as nursery nurses) who have been trained to develop adaptive behaviours in children.

Psychological security

Infants first begin to show signs of psychological insecurity when they form specific **attachments**, usually to their parents. This need can be met by ensuring that the child is not separated from a person to whom he or she is attached. Some psychologists believe that the quality of a child's attachment depends partly on the extent to which parents show **'sensitive responsiveness'** to the child. This means carefully observing the child and responding positively. A parent who shows sensitive responsiveness is likely to smile back at an infant who smiles, to respond to the child's vocalisation with speech and to notice quickly when a child is distressed.

In pre-school children, the need for psychological security can be met by:

+ removing the cause of the insecurity – for example, by explaining to the child that ghosts do not exist
+ providing social support – for example, if a child is very anxious about starting school, the parent can visit the school with the child beforehand so that the first day will not seem so strange or threatening

Educational or cognitive needs

These include occupation, stimulation, learning resources, choice and autonomy.

During the early-years period, children are effectively self-educated. A great deal of learning takes place, but most of it does not result from teaching. The child makes use of the resources around them (other people, toys and objects in the everyday environment) to gain knowledge, experience and understanding. For example, infants and toddlers use their parents as language resources, listening carefully to their utterances, engaging them in conversation and asking questions. They also learn about the physical environment by exploring the possibilities of toys in what is called **discovery play**. Adults can help by responding to the educational demands of the child, by providing access to stimulating play equipment and new environments (such as arranging visits to parks, castles and museums) and by setting challenges. Formal and informal service providers supply human and toy resources that give opportunities for occupation and stimulation.

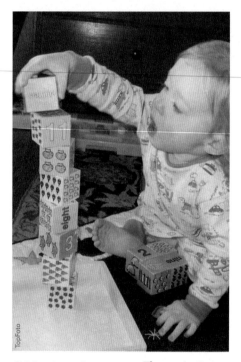

Children learn about their environment by discovery play

TopFoto

The curiosity young children show about all aspects of their world is probably to some extent maturational. In some people, this curiosity disappears later in childhood.

It is useful for children to be given choices from an age when they show an interest in choosing. It is a mistake to try to direct or control the play or learning of a young child. Older children can adapt to timetables for learning, but during the early years children learn most by following their interest at the time. Giving a child choices (for example, about food and birthday presents) can help to develop autonomy. It is important for children to achieve autonomy – to be self-controlling and self-directing — if they are to become independent adolescents and adults.

Cognitive developments include an understanding of the world and also language.

Needs of children of different age groups

For the unit assessment, you must choose one age group from the following:

+ infant — from birth to the second birthday
+ toddler — from the second birthday to the third
+ pre-school — from the third birthday to the fifth
+ school age — from the fifth birthday to the eighth

This unit does not include primary education, i.e. the schooling of children in the 5–8 year age group.

While children in all these age ranges have the same general needs, there are some quite significant differences at different ages, as the following examples show:

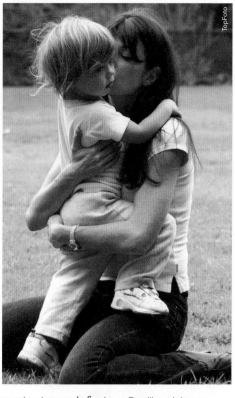

+ Resources for meeting exercise needs become more important once the child can walk. The needs change with developing gross motor skills.
+ Infants' nutritional needs are initially best met by breast-feeding. Later, infants adapt to a more varied diet.
+ Ways of ensuring physical safety also change with age. For example, an infant who is unable to roll over is more at risk of **sudden infant death syndrome** (cot death) if put down to sleep face downwards and if the parents smoke. When infants start to walk, different ways of ensuring physical safety become important, such as preventing unsupervised access to stairs.
+ Washing toys is particularly important for infants, who frequently suck them.
+ Physical comfort is particularly important for infants who wear nappies, because, unlike older children, they can do nothing to maintain their own comfort.

Familiar adults can provide psychological security to children who are attached to them.

+ Social contact with familiar carers becomes extremely important once infants begin to form specific attachments (from around 7 months). This continues until about age 3 and remains quite important throughout childhood. It means that a 1-year-old child who wakes fully during the night is quite likely to become distressed if not comforted by a familiar person.
+ Approval becomes particularly important once a child has begun to develop a self-concept (from around 8 months).
+ The need for psychological security arises at around the same time as the onset of specific attachment.

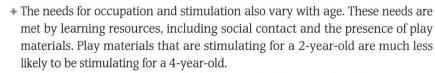

+ The needs for occupation and stimulation also vary with age. These needs are met by learning resources, including social contact and the presence of play materials. Play materials that are stimulating for a 2-year-old are much less likely to be stimulating for a 4-year-old.
+ Resources that are appropriate for language development also differ over time. For example, picture books for young infants are likely to be very short and possibly washable, while books for school-age children should be suitable for them to read. Parents often use a simplified form of speech when talking with infants (sometimes called 'motherese'), but more adult speech with pre-school and school-aged children.

Service provision

Some of the needs described above are provided by formal services, such as hospitals and nursery schools; others are provided by informal carers, such as parents and babysitters.

In any of the key age groups during the early-years period, a child is likely to receive care from both formal and informal providers, although most children experience a wider range of formal services as they grow older.

Some early-years services are mainly intended to provide basic childcare, i.e. to look after pre-school children while parents go out to work. The demand for this type of service has increased recently because of government policies designed to encourage more people to work full time. For example, the Childcare Tax Credit helps parents with the cost of childcare.

Formal provision

There are various formal services available to early-years clients.

Primary healthcare services

Primary healthcare services are based at the local GP surgery or health centre. They include GP consultations, developmental screening and assessments by a health visitor, and immunisation.

Secondary healthcare includes inpatient care in children's wards

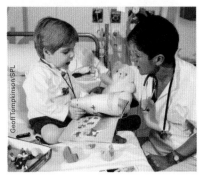

Secondary healthcare services

Secondary healthcare includes hospital services, such as:

+ screening by a paediatrician immediately after the child is born
+ tests for a range of disorders, including phenylketonuria (PKU) and developmental dysplasia of the hip
+ treatment for serious infections (such as meningitis) and after accidents
+ surgery
+ outpatient clinics to check and correct conditions such as glue ear and speech defects (speech and language therapy)

Child protection

The protection of children from neglect and abuse involves the police service, local authority social services departments and the NSPCC (the National Society for the Prevention of Cruelty to Children). Social services will work with families to try to help them provide better care for their children. If it is believed that significant harm is likely to come to the child, one of several legal orders can be imposed, which transfer the care of the child to social services.

In most areas, the NSPCC keeps a Child Protection Register, which records those children in that area believed to be at risk of harm.

Children who are judged to be in need of protection are supported by means of either a care order or a supervision order:

+ A **care order** takes the child into the care of the local authority social services department. The child is likely to be looked after in a foster home or a children's (residential) home.
+ A **supervision order** means that the child remains with the family, but social workers support the family in providing effective care for the child and supervise the child's treatment and progress.

When neglect or abuse is detected, or suspected, it is often necessary to act quickly to prevent further harm. Emergency protection can be arranged in three ways:

+ An **emergency protection order** can be applied for by any concerned adult (e.g. a teacher). A magistrate has the power to grant this order. The child is temporarily removed from home to a place of safety — normally with foster parents.
+ Under a **police protection order**, some police officers have the legal power to remove children from their homes for up to 72 hours, normally into the care of foster parents registered with the local social services department.
+ A **child assessment order** can be applied for by the NSPCC or the local authority. The child can be removed from the family for a maximum of 7 days, during which the child is assessed.

Police checks

Although most abuse happens in the child's own home, child protection measures exist to protect children from abuse in other situations. People who work with children must have a police check to find out whether they have a criminal record of child abuse.

Foster care

Foster care is usually provided within families. Parents volunteer to look after a child either for a short time or on a more permanent basis. Those who specialise in short-term care often take children who are judged to be at risk of harm at very short notice. Foster carers are registered with local authority social services departments and are paid.

Parents of children in foster care still have legal rights over their children, who can be returned to them by a court order.

Residential care

Some children who are in the care of the local authority on a long-term basis are accommodated in residential homes, called children's homes, although in most cases living in a family environment is regarded as better for children. Some children with learning disabilities also live in residential homes, especially those who attend a special school a long way from home.

Family centres

Family centres are run by local authorities. Staff at family centres provide support for families in which children might be at risk or who feel that they need help with parenting. They help to prevent poor treatment of children and to rehabilitate parents who have neglected or abused children in the past. They provide support groups, sessions to improve parenting skills and supervise contact visits, in which children in the care of the local authority have contact with their parents.

Child guidance service

Child guidance services are provided by local authorities. They are staffed by educational psychologists and social workers. They provide advice, support and counselling for families who have children with emotional or behavioural difficulties. For example, they support the families of children with autism or hyperactivity disorders.

SureStart

SureStart is a government programme targeted at children under 14 years of age who are likely to suffer deprivation. It is most likely to be provided in disadvantaged areas, where services for children are inadequate for the needs that exist. SureStart provides childcare, assists with health and emotional development, and helps parents to find work.

Pre-schools and playgroups

These cover a range of provisions. The most formal provision is called a **pre-school** and is provided by local authorities. Provision is typically two or three half-day sessions per week in a church hall or community centre. The main function is to provide social play facilities to (mainly) 3- and 4-year-old children, who otherwise would not have this opportunity (i.e. children who do not attend day nurseries or nursery schools). A small charge is made for each session.

Less formal playgroups are provided by voluntary groups — such as teams of parents — within the local community. Playgroups are staffed by volunteers, and parents are asked to contribute towards running costs.

Parent-and-toddler groups

Parent-and-toddler groups typically meet once a week in a church hall or community centre. They are usually run by volunteers and not for profit. In contrast to playgroups, the parents remain with their children. These groups provide parents with social contact and social support, as well as giving their children opportunities for interaction with other children. A parent who does not work and is otherwise socially isolated can benefit from this support and is also more likely to hear about other available services.

Day nurseries and crèches

Day nurseries take children from 0–4 years for up to 5 days per week. They provide play materials and activities appropriate to the ages of the children attending. The staff normally includes qualified nursery nurses and possibly a nursery teacher. Day nurseries enable parents to go out to work and leave their children at the nursery during working hours.

Some day nurseries are provided by local authority social services departments. Places here are available mostly for children believed to be disadvantaged and deprived.

Other day nurseries are run by voluntary organisations or by private, fee-charging providers.

Crèches are private day nurseries run by employers to provide day care for the children of employees. They have the advantage that parents are usually working nearby in case the child needs them.

The key function of day nurseries and crèches is to provide good-quality childcare to enable parents to work full time.

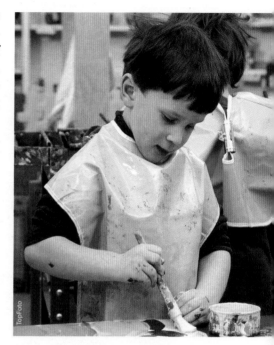

Nursery schools provide structured activities

Nursery schools and classes

Nursery schools are provided by local education authorities. They are staffed by qualified nursery schoolteachers and nursery nurses. They provide early-years education, mainly to 4-year-olds. This does not include formal teaching, but the activities are more structured and planned than in day nurseries or pre-schools. Learning is mainly play-based. Nursery education is intended to encourage social and cognitive development, and to help the child's transition into primary school.

Nursery education is also provided in primary schools, most of which now accept children from the age of 4 years. However, children do not start on the primary curriculum until around their fifth birthday.

The key function of nursery schools and classes is early-years education. They also enable parents to work full time.

After-school care

Some schools make arrangements for children to remain at school at the end of the school day, in order to fit in with the work patterns of their parents. After-school care is designed to create a homely, relaxed atmosphere.

Childminders

Childminders provide day care within their own homes. Usually, there is only one childminder, looking after a small number of children. Childminders can be officially registered and inspected by Ofsted (the organisation that inspects schools). In order to be registered, the childminder has to ensure that the premises are safe and appropriate for the number of children cared for. Childminders are not required to have any specific training or qualifications. Unregistered childminders are, in effect, informal carers.

The key function of childminding is to provide childcare while parents go out to work.

Toy libraries

Some childcare organisations, such as nursery schools and day nurseries, have collections of toys that children can borrow. Such collections are called **toy libraries**. They make available a range of toys for children of parents who otherwise might not be able to afford them or who usually buy toys that are of little educational value. For example, a model car is much less valuable educationally than a set of construction bricks, which a child can use to build a toy car and many other things.

Charities

The **National Society for the Prevention of Cruelty to Children** plays a major role in counteracting neglect and abuse. In most areas, the charity employs staff who work with the police and social services on child protection. The NSPCC also keeps a register of children thought to be at risk.

Gingerbread is a voluntary organisation that supports single-parent families.

Informal provision

Parents

Parents usually provide for a wide range of needs, from nutrition, basic healthcare and hygiene to social support and cognitive needs. However, parents often have to try to meet the needs of a child while having additional responsibilities, such as employment and the care of other children. In addition, most parents are not trained in understanding and meeting the needs of children, so their actions are not always the most appropriate. However, parents do have the advantage of knowing their child well. Their attachment to the child often motivates them to act in such a way as to meet the needs of the child.

Other family members, friends and neighbours

It can be an advantage for a child to have contact with different informal carers. It increases the human resources available to the child, because different people have a range of knowledge and experience. Children being reared by only one parent also benefit if they have opportunities to attach to other adults. This makes the consequences of separation from the parent much less severe. Neighbours and grandparents often act as informal carers while parents, for example, are at work or in hospital.

Babysitters

One of the commonest forms of temporary childcare is babysitting. A babysitter allows parents to have leisure time to themselves. The arrangement can work well if the babysitter is well known to the child (so that the child has some attachment and can be comforted by the babysitter). However, problems can arise if an attached child wakes up to find an unfamiliar person looking after them. Babysitters often lack the knowledge and experience to cope with difficult situations such as this.

Informal support groups

Parents with young children often belong to an informal network of friends, who meet in each other's houses. This can provide support for parenting skills (especially for inexperienced first-time parents), as well as social contact for the children.

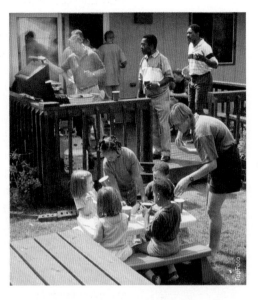

Parents with young children often belong to an informal network of friends

Evaluating services

There are several criteria you could use when evaluating early-years services.

Do services meet actual needs?

One important criterion is whether or not the services you have studied succeed in meeting the needs of children of the age range you have chosen. Services tend to have particular aims in mind. For example, they focus on child health or education. Their staff are often trained to meet one set of needs rather than a broad range of requirements. The result is that sometimes services succeed in meeting their stated aims but tend to neglect other needs that children have.

For example, think about children in hospital. The main focus of the staff might be on treating illness, with less attention paid to the child's needs for occupation and social support. If you decide to study provision for children in hospital, you might want to find out, for example, whether there are facilities for parents of 2-year-olds to stay in the same room as their children or whether there is a range of suitable play materials for 4-year-old inpatients.

In contrast, you might visit a day nursery that focuses on the social and cognitive needs of children and ask about their health and safety precautions. How often do staff at a toy library wash and disinfect the toys?

You might also consider to what extent services for children aged from 1 to 5 years take account of the attachment need of the child for contact with a familiar adult.

The ratio of staff to children can give an indirect measure of effectiveness. If the ratio is high (say, one member of staff to four children), the amount of individual care and attention given is likely to be greater than with a lower ratio of, say, 1:8.

Most formal service provision is covered by some form of inspection process and quality control. For example, registered childminders are inspected by Ofsted and the performance of hospital departments is measured according to national standards. As part of your evaluation of a service, you could ask to see the results of the most recent inspection or assessment.

How easy is it to access services?

Another important criterion is access to services. There might be some good-quality day-care provision in your area, but not enough of it to meet the needs of the community. If so, some of the children who could benefit from day care cannot access it. Alternatively, there might not be enough affordable provision for poorer families.

Access might also be limited by lack of awareness of the provision. When researching your local provision, you might have some difficulty in finding services. If so, parents are likely to find this equally difficult. This could be because of a lack of publicity for the service.

In other cases, access problems are caused by the location of service providers in relation to available transport. For example, a hospital might be outside a town, with a poor bus service and inadequate parking for those who travel by car.

Has the staff received appropriate training?

Formal service providers are usually staffed by people who have been trained (e.g. in speech and language therapy and nursing). Although training does not guarantee effectiveness, it increases the probability that staff will have the knowledge and expertise to recognise and meet the needs of children. Unpaid volunteers are less likely to have received formal training.

Have demographic changes led to an imbalance in provision?

Another criterion is the extent to which the existing provision matches the needs of the community. Demographic change refers to changes in size and structure of a population. Some communities experience rapid change, such as the building of new housing, which leads to an increase in population, or the arrival of a new group of immigrants. This might result in a mismatch between existing services and needs of the community.

Collecting data

You should use a variety of methods to collect data about local services for your report. You should first research printed and electronic sources. The reason for doing this first is to avoid wasting people's time asking questions to which the answers are readily available from such sources.

Sources

Printed sources

Sources such as Yellow Pages, local newspapers and directories of health and social services will help you discover some of the services that exist locally. You could also drop in to libraries and GP surgeries or health centres and collect leaflets advertising services.

Electronic sources

Local authorities, primary care trusts and hospital trusts have websites describing the services that they offer. These can also be sources of contact addresses and telephone numbers for more information. In addition, looking up the services using a search engine, such as Google, can provide useful information.

Formal service providers

Once you know something about the services available, you could select those that seem most relevant to the age group you have chosen and try to arrange a visit. Before a visit, you should think carefully about what you want to find out. Some information can be found simply by looking around (e.g. provision of play materials); other information can be found only by interviewing staff. When requesting a visit, you should explain the aim of the visit and outline what you want to find out. It is probably easiest to arrange a visit by telephone. You should then confirm in writing and keep a copy of your letter for inclusion in the research and analysis section of your report.

You will find it useful to draw up a form on which to record your findings during your visit. You should include the main questions you want to ask. Copies of this form can be used when visiting several different places. They will serve as interview schedules, reminding you of your questions and giving you space to record answers. More information on interviewing can be found in Chapter 9, pages 256–59.

Before requesting a visit, you should check with your teacher that the questions you intend to ask are appropriate and ethical. It is very important to avoid asking questions in a way that is likely to be offensive or insulting. For example, it would not a be a good idea to ask, 'Is hygiene up to scratch around here?' Rather, it would be better to say, 'What sort of hygiene precautions do you have to take in this centre?'

Informal service providers

A good way of finding authentic information about the availability, accessibility and quality of services is to ask parents of young children. They will probably have had experience of contacts with health visitors, paediatricians, hospital services, play facilities, childminders, babysitters and so on. You could find out their opinions about the services their children have used, and those they would have liked their children to have been able to use but which were unavailable or inaccessible.

You could also ask parents and other informal carers their views about meeting the needs of children. Informal providers are unlikely to have received relevant training, so do not be too surprised if their views are not the same as those of people who have been trained.

Scope of data collection

There is a risk that when researching for this unit assessment, you might collect a great deal of information, much of which is of insufficient depth to enable you to score good marks in your report. Rather than trying to find something out about the whole range of services listed in the specification, you should try to identify a selection that is most important for the age range you have decided to study. Your selection might also be influenced by the parents and children with whom you have contact. For example, if you know a child who has recently received hospital treatment, this will give you access to some useful information for evaluating that service. If you know a family with a 4-year-old who attends parent-and-child exercise sessions at a local leisure centre and nursery classes at a local primary school, you might decide to focus on this age group and include those services, among others. If you know a child with a learning disability, this might inspire you to research some of the services available for children with such needs.

You should make sure that the services you study allow you to cover most of the needs identified in the first section of this chapter.

Writing the report

Section A: The needs of children in the chosen age range

Section A should be a description of the needs of children in the age range you have chosen. To score high marks, this should show accurate understanding of those needs. One way to do this is to illustrate what you say with examples drawn from your research, from what you have been taught and from published sources. This section scores the most marks — over one-third of the marks for the whole unit — so you must provide plenty of detail. You could communicate the importance of each need by describing the negative consequences for the quality of life and development of the child if that need was not met.

Section B: How the needs are met locally

Section B should describe services that are available locally. It should also explain how the services you describe meet the needs described in Section A. This is really a matching exercise, based mainly on the aims and intentions of each service. For example, you could describe how immunisation helps to meet the health needs of a child or how the provision of play apparatus in public spaces meets the need for exercise.

Section C: Research and analysis of local provision

Section C should include evidence of the research you carried out in order to collect the information for this unit. It should not be simply a collection of documents.

The section should begin with a clear and logically structured description of how you collected the information. It should make reference (e.g. by referring to later page numbers in the report) to the evidence for this process. After this description, you should then include the most important documents in your research process. These are likely to include copies of request letters written by you and completed interview schedule forms. (These should be either the originals or photocopies.) You could also include leaflets and pages printed from website sources, although these should not be very extensive or bulky.

Section D: Evaluation of local provision

Section D should be a logically organised evaluation of the service provision you described in Section B. It is important that judgements you make about service effectiveness are supported with evidence and/or reasoned argument. One way of doing this is by referring to information you collected and reported in Section C. You should use a range of criteria, such as those included in the 'Evaluating services' section of this chapter. You should also refer to other criteria if these are relevant.

Use your judgement when making evaluations based on the responses of people you have interviewed. For example, if people have described a service as a 'waste of time', this should carry less weight than a more specific, better-informed, comment.

Further reading

Beith, K. et al. (2002) *Diploma in Child Care and Education: Student Book*, Heinemann.

Bruce, T. and Meggitt, C. (2002) *Child Care and Education*, Hodder Arnold.

Websites

Local authorities and health trusts will have their own websites.

Information about local childcare services:

www.childcarelink.gov.uk

Gingerbread:

www.gingerbread.org.uk

Birkbeck College runs a website dealing with evaluation of the SureStart programme at:

www.ness.bbk.ac.uk

The National Society for the Prevention of Cruelty to Children:

www.nspcc.org.uk

Ofsted (Office for Standards and Education):

www.ofsted.gov.uk

SureStart:

www.surestart.gov.uk

Complementary therapies

This chapter contains information you need for **Unit 9: Complementary therapies**. The first three sections provide background material and cover concepts that are important in understanding these therapies. The last three sections give detailed guidance on how to plan and write your report.

Key concepts

Holism

Holism refers to the belief that health and wellbeing are influenced by the physiological state of the body and by feelings and cognitions. Feelings often associated with ill health include sadness and anxiety. Cognitions often associated with ill health are negative beliefs, such as the perception of helplessness and low self-esteem.

People who think of their health in this broad way, i.e. including feelings and cognitions as well as the physical state of the body, are said to have a holistic concept of health. This is described in more detail in Chapter 3.

This belief in holism has given rise to an approach to therapy that takes account of all those influences and is called the holistic approach. A simpler, but less precise, way of describing the holistic approach to therapy is that it is any approach that takes account of both the body and the mind.

During the last century, some conventional medical practitioners tended to ignore the feelings and cognitions of patients. It is now well known that stress and depression can delay recovery from illnesses and that beliefs can affect people's health. For example, people who believe that they have some control over their own health and who believe they can get better are more likely to survive serious disorders such as heart disease and cancer.

Today, conventional medical training encourages a more holistic approach. Many practitioners of complementary and alternative therapies also adopt a holistic approach, although some tend to ignore the physical aspects of ill health.

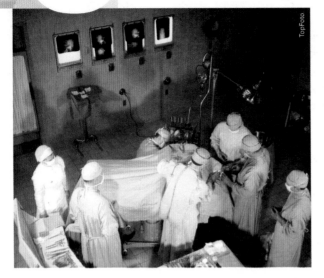

TopFoto

Conventional therapies

The term 'conventional therapy' is used to mean the range of therapies traditionally used by trained medical practitioners. This amounts to the therapies typically provided by NHS practitioners. It is based on the practice of looking for evidence of illness (disease symptoms, bacterial infection, tissue damage etc.) and selecting treatments, including medication and surgery, to eliminate or correct the cause of the illness.

A simpler way of defining conventional therapies is to say that it covers therapies other than complementary and alternative therapies.

Surgery is a conventional therapy

Evidence-based medicine

Conventional therapies have derived mainly from evidence-based medicine. Evidence-based medicine originated in Europe about 150 years ago, when scientific methods of research began to be used more systematically and effectively. For example, the discovery by Pasteur that infections were caused by 'germs', or microorganisms, led the way to more effective prevention of diseases such as pneumonia and tuberculosis. Before that time, such infections were attributed to other causes such as 'bad air'. Evidence-based medicine questioned traditional explanations of illness and replaced them with explanations that could be tested. The approach (common to sciences) is to test an explanation for an illness by observation and experiment. The results of such research led to a rapid increase in understanding of the causes of disease and of the functions and systems (e.g. the immune system) of the body.

A similar approach was applied to testing therapies. The effects of using particular therapies were observed and only those therapies that were successful were developed. Scientific testing of medicines involves 'clinical trials'.

Evidence-based medicine soon came to dominate healthcare provision in wealthy countries, and it continues to thrive. Diseases that until recently often proved fatal, such as cancer, heart disease, poliomyelitis and diabetes, were cured or treated effectively for the first time in human history. Infant mortality, which was high in Britain only a century ago, has been reduced to a very low level and life expectancy has been increased. This is partly due to medical progress but also to improvements in public health (such as clean water supplies and sewage disposal). More recently, treatments for newly emerging diseases, such as AIDS, have been rapidly developed.

Although modern evidence-based medicine originated in Europe, its use has spread rapidly to other parts of the world.

Clinical trials

When new treatments in conventional medicine (including drugs and surgical procedures) are being developed, they are usually first tested using non-human animals. Testing is necessary because there is a significant risk that the treatment or therapy could have harmful or unexpected side-effects. While such trials are likely to involve harming or killing the animals (e.g. to see the effects on internal organs), they are regarded as less unethical than carrying out the same trials with human participants.

Some people understandably object to potentially harmful medical experimentation being carried out on non-human animals and consequently may refuse to receive conventional medical treatments. Other people believe that the potential benefits for humans outweigh the ethical disadvantages.

If a treatment turns out to be beneficial in non-human animals, it then has to be trialled with human participants. This takes place in **clinical trials**. A clinical trial uses volunteers who have a particular medical condition and follows the experimental method — the most powerful approach in scientific research.

The best form of clinical trial is called the **randomised controlled trial** (RCT). The sample of participants is split randomly into (usually) three groups:

+ The first group receives the new treatment.
+ The second group receives a **placebo** (a treatment known to have no direct physiological effect).
+ The third group (the **control group**) receives no treatment.

In a **single-blind RCT**, the participants who received the treatment or the placebo do not know which they have received. In a **double-blind RCT**, the researcher who is to assess the effects on participants does not know to which group each belongs.

The single-blind procedure prevents the participants from being affected by the expectation that receiving the treatment will have a certain effect. The double-blind procedure avoids the risk that the person assessing the effects could be biased by knowing who has, and who has not, received the real treatment.

Placebo effect

It has been known for some time that giving a patient a treatment that can have no direct physiological effect can produce improvements in the patient's condition. For example, less pain might be felt and the patient might become more active. This is called the **placebo effect**. Simply believing that some treatment has been received can produce improvements.

This creates difficulties for clinical trials. The problem is that if, in a trial, a new treatment produces an improvement, this improvement might be due to:

+ the direct physiological effect of the treatment
+ the placebo effect
+ a combination of physiological effect and placebo effect

It is for this reason that one of the groups in a clinical trial is a placebo group. The effectiveness of the treatment is assessed by comparing the participants who received the real treatment with the placebo group, to see whether those who received the real treatment improved significantly more than those who received the placebo. If they did not (and particularly if they did not improve as much), the conclusion is that the treatment is not effective for humans. In drug trials, the placebo version of the drug is often made of sugar.

Acupuncture can be used to complement conventional treatments

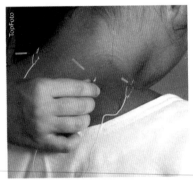

Complementary therapies

There are several different definitions of complementary therapy. A strict definition is that complementary therapies are those that are used alongside conventional medicines in order to provide a more holistic treatment. For example, acupuncture is sometimes used by NHS practitioners to assist in long-term pain control and several NHS hospitals make use of homeopathy. The role of complementary therapies can thus be seen to add to (or complement) conventional treatments. This definition distinguishes between complementary and alternative therapies.

Alternative therapies

Alternative therapies are defined as those intended to be used instead of conventional therapies. Their role is to replace conventional treatment with something different. For example, a person might take Chinese herbal remedies instead of medication prescribed by a GP.

Summary

Some complementary/alternative therapies and conventional therapies are listed in Table 9.1.

If the therapies had not already been categorised in Table 9.1, it would be quite difficult to guess whether some of the items were conventional or complementary/alternative therapies. One reason is that some complementary and alternative therapies are given names that sound scientific, i.e. ending with -opathy or -ology.

There is not always a very clear distinction between conventional and complementary therapies. For example, biofeedback is a technique based on principles of human physiology and scientific psychology.

Table 9.1
Selected therapies

Complementary/ alternative therapies	Conventional therapies
Acupuncture	Aversion therapy
Alexander technique	Cognitive-behaviour therapy
Aromatherapy	Dentistry
Ayurvedic medicine	Dialysis
Bach remedies	Diathermy
Biofeedback	Drug treatments/chemotherapy
Chiropractic	Electroconvulsive therapy
Crystal healing	Hormone therapy
Herbal medicine	Immunisation
Homeopathy	Occupational therapy
Hypnotherapy	Physiotherapy
Massage	Radiotherapy
Meditation	Speech and language therapy
Naturopathy	Surgery
Osteopathy	
Reflexology	
Shamanism	
Shiatsu	
Traditional Chinese medicine	
Unani medicine	
Yoga	

Criteria for assessing therapies

One of the problems that arise when trying to assess different therapies is that there is widespread prejudice about both conventional and complementary therapies. Some people, particularly those working in conventional medicine, tend to reject complementary therapies, regarding them as largely ineffective or as exploiting gullible clients for money. Other people are prejudiced against conventional treatments, believing that they often do more harm than good and worsen health.

Despite this apparent opposition between conventional and complementary therapies, they are not really in competition with each other. Conventional medical training now supports a more holistic approach to patient care than was the case in the last century. Those complementary therapies that are seen to be most effective are used alongside conventional treatment in the NHS. In addition, although there is some overlap, conventional and complementary therapies tend to tackle rather different problems. Conventional therapies treat more severe and acute conditions such as cancer, strokes and schizophrenia, whereas complementary therapies tend to focus on less severe chronic conditions, such as joint pain and stress.

Effectiveness of therapies

One of the most important questions to consider when assessing a therapy is its effectiveness.

How effectiveness is measured

Some complementary and alternative therapies have been assessed by clinical trials. However, a number of problems arise:

+ Clinical trials are expensive.
+ It is more difficult to get funding for research into complementary therapies than conventional therapies. As a result, relatively few trials have been conducted.
+ The practitioners of some complementary and alternative therapies do not accept the use of scientific methods of assessment.

Nevertheless, controlled trials have resulted in improvements in some therapies. For example, trials of herbal medicines have revealed which of these are effective for certain disorders. This enables ineffective or potentially dangerous treatments to be ruled out.

Another measure of effectiveness of treatment is to ask patients or clients how satisfied they are with their treatment and whether or not they feel better.

It is virtually impossible to assess the effectiveness of a therapy that is designed to promote general health rather than to treat specific symptoms.

Risks and benefits

Another important factor in assessing a therapy is the level of risk involved compared with the resulting benefits.

Some of the techniques used in conventional medicine are far more dangerous than most of those used in complementary and alternative therapies. For example, surgery that involves opening the chest is relatively dangerous. Any operation that requires a general anaesthetic also carries a small but significant risk of proving fatal. For these reasons, surgeons usually inform patients beforehand about the probability of harmful effects. In contrast, very few fatalities or serious injuries result from complementary and alternative therapies.

It would be easy to draw the conclusion that complementary and alternative medicines should always be preferred to conventional ones. Indeed, some alternative therapists believe this.

However, it is also important to consider the potential benefits of any therapy. A person who undergoes a major operation often does so because it is the only way of prolonging life. The benefit is continued survival. As a result, a patient might prefer an operation with a 30% probability that it will kill them, compared with a much higher probability that without the operation they will die soon. (Most conventional procedures carry a much lower risk than this example.)

Apart from the risks associated with particular therapies, there are also risks occurring from an inappropriate choice of therapy. For example, it would be risky to rely on an alternative therapy if a patient was suffering from a life-threatening condition.

Drug treatments often lead to unpleasant, sometimes dangerous, side-effects. This is true of both conventionally produced drugs and traditional herbal remedies. Drugs can also interact in unpredictable ways, so it is important not to combine taking a herbal remedy while, say, also taking medicine prescribed by a GP for hypertension.

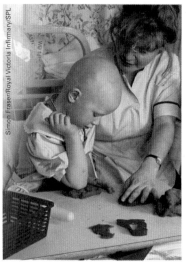

Anti-cancer drugs can cause hair loss

Did you know ❓

Herbal medicines work in very much the same way as drugs used in conventional medicine. In fact, many conventional drugs were originally obtained from plants. For example, aspirin was extracted from willow trees. As long as 2000 years ago, people used to chew willow twigs to cure headaches. Such drugs are now synthesised in pharmaceutical chemical plants, which can produce them cheaply and in a purer form than the plant derivative.

Invasiveness and unpleasant side-effects

Another criterion for assessing a therapy is to ask how **invasive** it is. The term 'invasive' refers to how much damage to body tissues a therapy causes.

The most invasive therapies involve surgery — for example, to open the skull or the abdomen. Slightly less invasive are surgical techniques using **endoscopy** (sometimes called keyhole surgery). Endoscopy involves smaller incisions or no incision, when inserted via a natural opening such as the mouth. Such therapies can be rather unpleasant. However, some minor surgical procedures, including the correction of heart arrhythmias and cataract removal, can be carried out using a local anaesthetic and with little or no discomfort.

Acupuncture is only minimally invasive (the needles are inserted into the skin, but not right through it).

Therapies that involve taking medicines (conventional and herbal) are much less invasive. However, they are sometimes extremely unpleasant.

For example, the most powerful conventional anti-cancer drugs produce nausea (a feeling of sickness), loss of hair and loss of appetite. Some herbal medicines taste very unpleasant.

Therapies that involve massage, exercise such as yoga and counselling are not at all invasive, although some involving vigorous manipulation (especially of the back) can be uncomfortable.

Homeopathic medicines, which mainly consist of water, are very unlikely to produce any harmful effects.

Is the therapeutic mechanism understood?

With some therapies, the reason for their effectiveness is quite well understood. For example, the way in which **vaccination** stimulates the immune system to produce antibodies against a particular disease-causing organism is well known.

With other therapies, the mechanism is not well understood. It might surprise you to know that there are conventional and complementary therapies that are used, even though we do not know how they work.

A classic example is the use of **electroconvulsive therapy** (ECT) in conventional psychiatry. This alarming procedure involves inducing an epileptic-like fit by the application of electric shocks to the skull of the patient. It can be very effective in treating people who have severe depression. How it produces its effect on the feelings of the patient is not known. However, it continues to be used because it is effective in cases where other treatments are ineffective.

The key point is that if a therapy is effective (and if the side-effects are tolerable), it should be used, even if the mechanism by which it produces its effect is not known.

A similar example is the use of **acupuncture**, which can help to relieve chronic pain. There is more than one possible explanation of how it works, so the mechanism is not yet fully understood.

Generally speaking, there has been more research into the actions of conventional treatments, so the actions of these treatments are better understood.

When therapies are effective, it is sometimes difficult to know whether this is because of a direct effect or a **placebo effect**. However, even if a therapy works only because of a placebo effect, rather than by some other process claimed by the therapist, it is still worth using.

The so-called '**caring effect**', which occurs in some therapies, can contribute to the overall placebo effect. When people receive a treatment from any practitioner, they become the focus of attention. For many people this is enjoyable and makes them feel better. This effect is probably at a minimum when the interaction between practitioner and patient is very brief or impersonal. For example, most patients only have brief consultations with their GPs. However, in consultations with practitioners in which the patient has to pay for treatment on the basis of time spent, the practitioner spends more time with the patient.

The caring effect is likely to be greater with complementary and alternative therapies than with conventional therapies. In the former, patients often have the

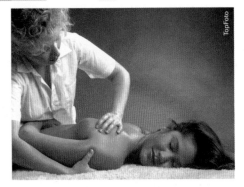

Techniques involving physical contact are likely to produce caring effects

chance to talk at length about their feelings to a practitioner who has time to listen carefully. The result is likely to be a noticeable caring effect.

Techniques involving physical contact, such as massage, are particularly likely to produce caring effects because many people enjoy being stroked or caressed.

How much the placebo effect contributes to the effectiveness of a therapy, and how much the effectiveness results from the intended effect of the procedure, can be found using clinical trials.

A coherent and credible knowledge base

Most therapies are based on a set of theories and assumptions about the functioning of the human body.

These theories vary in **coherence** and **credibility**. You must be the judge of this. If a theory seems to make sense to you and if you find it believable, then for you it is coherent and credible.

Take **homeopathy** as an example. Homeopathic medicines are made by taking a small quantity of a drug and diluting it repeatedly with water. Some homeopathic medicines are so dilute that they are, in effect, water. Only a few molecules of the original drug can possibly remain. You might find it difficult to understand how such a drug could have any effect, particularly as drugs used in conventional and herbal medicines are believed to be effective only in relatively high concentrations. The beliefs held by homeopathic practitioners about the effects of drug concentrations are at conflict with the beliefs of those who practise conventional and herbal medicine. This is an example of different therapies being based on conflicting beliefs.

Another example is different beliefs about **energy**. Conventional science-based dietetics and nutrition use the term 'energy' to refer to the chemical energy in food that can be converted into mechanical energy to produce work, such as moving muscles. The energy content of food can be observed and measured by burning the food in a calorimeter. This use of the word 'energy' is consistent with other sciences, such as physics and chemistry. In contrast, traditional Chinese medicine refers to 'life energy', known as 'qi'. This is quite different from the scientific use of the word. There is no evidence for the existence of this 'life energy' and it cannot be measured.

Therapeutic aims and procedures

Different therapies have different aims. They can be:

+ **remedial** — aiming to cure disease. These include homeopathy, and conventional treatments such as medication and surgery.
+ **preventative** — aiming to reduce the risk of an illness developing. These include reflexology, yoga and conventional immunisation.

✦ **palliative** — aiming to make symptoms tolerable. These include acupuncture and conventional analgesics to reduce pain.

Conventional therapies are used to prevent, cure and palliate a wide range of disorders, from skin diseases to schizophrenia.

Complementary and alternative therapies have been applied to a wide range of conditions. However, they tend not to be seen as the main treatment for acute (sudden) life-threatening diseases. They do not, for example, include surgery. If a person has cancer or pneumonia or has just had a stroke or heart attack, the usual treatment is conventional.

Complementary and alternative therapies tend to be used more for relatively minor disorders. They are also used in chronic (long-lasting) conditions that persist without being cured, such as some forms of back pain and arthritis.

Complementary therapies are sometimes used alongside conventional treatments in cases of cancer and heart disease.

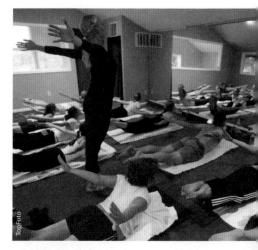

Therapies such as yoga aim to maintain health and prevent illness

Professional training, registration and quality control

Complementary and alternative therapies are mainly (but not entirely) provided by practitioners who do not have conventional medical training.

Several complementary and alternative therapies are not regulated by law. For example, anyone can start practising as a reflexologist without having any training. As a result, there is a risk that unregulated private providers with little skill or experience could give a poor service and exploit their clients — for example, by providing a series of expensive but unnecessary treatments. However, practitioners in various complementary and alternative therapies have joined together to provide some form of regulation and training. The governing bodies for each therapy can provide the names of qualified practitioners. Umbrella groups that aim to support practitioners of a wide range of complementary and alternative therapies have also been set up. These include the British Complementary Medicine Association (BCMA).

Some complementary and alternative therapies are controlled by law. These include chiropractic and osteopathy. In order to practise either of these therapies, a person has to register with the General Chiropractic Council or the General Osteopathic Council.

To reduce the risks associated with unqualified practitioners and unregulated procedures, it is important that practitioners attend accredited training courses and that practice is regulated by a professional body. This has been the case with most conventional therapies for many years. Increasingly, complementary and alternative therapy groups are organising training and accreditation systems, and setting up complaints and quality control procedures similar to those used in conventional medicine.

Availability and cost

All conventional therapies and some complementary therapies are available free from the NHS. Most complementary and alternative therapies are supplied by private practitioners and have to be paid for. Availability in your area can be found by using sources such as Yellow Pages. Listings are under 'alternative medicine/therapies', 'complementary therapies' and the name of the particular therapy.

Reasons for using complementary and alternative therapies

There are a number of reasons why increasing numbers of people use complementary and alternative therapies.

Dissatisfaction with conventional medicine

In some cases, patients become dissatisfied because they have medical conditions that cannot be cured, only palliated. For example, a person with osteoarthritis might receive prescribed medicines that reduce pain but do not cure the condition. This person might dislike the long-term use of painkillers (which can have negative side-effects) and so might look for some alternative.

Dissatisfaction can arise in cases where a GP diagnoses an illness, but either refuses to prescribe any medication or asks the patient to self-medicate, for example with non-prescription painkillers. Some patients who visit a GP expect to be provided with some form of treatment.

Dissatisfaction can also occur because of the unpleasant, painful and invasive diagnostic and treatment techniques that are sometimes used in conventional medicine. Some patients are repelled by the thought of having to undress and to undergo internal examinations.

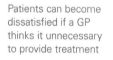

Patients can become dissatisfied if a GP thinks it unnecessary to provide treatment

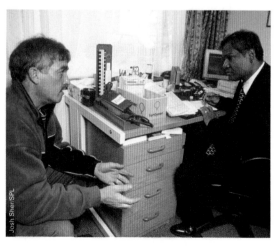

Refusal to treat

Because NHS services are mainly free of charge, practitioners try not to spend time and resources on patients who have no symptoms of illness. If a GP can find nothing wrong with a patient, no treatment will be given. Patients who are convinced that they are ill might not accept this and might visit complementary or alternative therapists, who are less likely to refuse to provide treatment. A therapist who has a holistic concept of health is more likely to accept a claim of illness, because according to this concept, if people do not feel well, they are ill.

Cultural background

People who have grown up in a culture in which alternative therapy is the norm are more likely to choose this therapy than conventional medicine. For example, people who have relied on traditional Chinese medicine for most of their lives are unlikely to change.

Appeal of exotic and different cultures

Alternative therapies appeal to some people because they are different. There is a romantic appeal in the idea that some ancient, preferably east Asian, philosophy has answers to problems that Western cultures do not. Some people are fired with enthusiasm by Hopi Indian ear candles as an exotic alternative to eardrops.

Prejudice against science and technology

Popular attitudes to science and technology change with time. Currently in Britain, there is widespread distrust of science and scientists, and resistance against emerging technologies, such as the production of genetically modified foods. Conventional therapies are technologies that have arisen out of medical science, and as such are also distrusted by some people.

This distrust is not universal. For example, in China, attitudes to science and technology are much more positive.

Ethical objections

Some people object to the exploitation of non-human animals for research into conventional medicine. One key objection is that this exploitation is morally wrong and that non-human animals have some of the same rights as humans. People who take this view are more likely to choose complementary and alternative therapies that have not been tested on these animals.

Religious objections

Followers of certain religions object to some conventional treatments. For example, Jehovah's Witnesses refuse to have blood transfusions. Members of the Christian Science sect (which is actually unconnected with science) object to conventional treatments such as chemotherapy for treating cancer. As a result, they are more likely to seek alternative treatments.

Choosing therapies and collecting background information

You are required to choose three different therapies and to write a guide about them. There are several different ways of approaching this task. You should think carefully and read background information before making your final choice of therapies.

One approach is to focus on a particular ill-health condition which your three chosen therapies can be used to treat. For example, you could choose a conventional treatment for cancer and two other therapies that can be used to complement this treatment. Another approach is to choose three contrasting therapies that are typically used for three different conditions.

Your choice of therapies might be influenced by your access to sources. For example, if you already know someone who is an alternative therapist, or someone who uses an alternative therapy as a client, you might choose this as one of your three therapies. Availability of practitioners in your local area might influence your choice too. You can choose a conventional therapy as one of your three choices, for comparative purposes, but no more than one.

You could choose three therapies from Table 9.1 on page 248, although you can also choose therapies not included in those lists. Your combination of three therapies should be unique for your centre. For example, you might choose osteopathy, herbal medicine and hypnotherapy; a fellow student could choose osteopathy, chiropractic and hypnotherapy.

The interview

The assessment for this unit requires you to interview at least one practitioner or client. This could be a conventional or alternative therapist, or a client of either. The person(s) you interview should have some connection with at least one of the therapies you have chosen to write about. For example, you might interview a physiotherapist about his or her own (conventional) treatment and ask for opinions of two complementary or alternative therapies that have similar therapeutic aims to physiotherapy.

Interview method

An interview is a research method in which the researcher asks questions of a single participant, and records the answers. Interviews carried out for research purposes can range from unstructured interviews to structured interviews. In either case, tape recording can be useful.

Unstructured interviews

An **unstructured interview** is one in which the questions and the sequence in which they are asked is not decided in advance. The interviewer simply asks the questions that occur at the time. However, the interviewer will normally have previously thought carefully about the aims of the interview, and the main topics to be covered will have been decided.

Advantages

+ The unstructured interview is flexible enough to enable the interviewer to follow up interesting statements from the interviewee. A chance remark by the interviewee could change the whole direction of the interview and lead to interesting information being revealed.

+ This type of interview can seem very informal, allowing the interviewee to relax and 'open up'.

Structured interviews

A structured interview is one in which the questions and question sequence are planned in advance. The interviewer usually produces a printed interview schedule, which includes the questions and spaces for recording the answers.

Advantages

+ Recording is easier than with the unstructured interview.
+ Less skill is required from the interviewer, so inexperienced researchers can use the method successfully.
+ Because different respondents are all asked the same questions, comparisons can be made between them.

Semi-structured interviews

A **semi-structured interview** combines the advantages of both approaches. In a semi-structured interview, a structured interview schedule is used and follow-up questions to explore 'side-issues' are added as the interview proceeds.

Writing interview questions

As with the questionnaire method (Chapter 2), interviews can include closed as well as open questions (see Figure 9.1).

(6) How long does a session with a client usually last?

(7) About how many sessions do clients usually need?
Least number ____ Typical number ____ Most ____

(8) How much do you charge per session? £ ____

(9) What does the treatment actually involve?

(10) Are there any risks or side-effects?

(11) Do you get clients to fill in a quality-control or satisfaction survey?
Yes ☐   No ☐   If yes, request a copy.

(12) Is there a system for making complaints?

Figure 9.1
An extract from an interview schedule

When asking a closed question, the interviewer might give the participant a range of possible responses. For example, 'Are you "very satisfied", "satisfied", "undecided", "dissatisfied" or "very dissatisfied" with the treatment you received?' Alternatively, the interviewer might ask the participant, 'On a scale of 1 to 5, how satisfied are you with your treatment (1 is very dissatisfied, 5 is very satisfied)?'.

Open questions often play a greater role in an interview, compared with a questionnaire. This is because the responses are recorded by the interviewer, so it is less demanding for the participant.

Recording answers to open questions is not easy. The participant might speak for several minutes in answer to a single question. A technique that can help in recording is to code the answers. For example, if you asked the question, 'Why did you decide to try osteopathy?', you could code part of the answer by using tick boxes on the interview schedule that include most of the common answers, such as, 'Recommendation by friend ☑'; 'Physiotherapy did not work ☑' and so on. Often it will be necessary to take brief notes to record the gist of the answer.

Trialling

Interviewing requires more skill than the questionnaire method, so it is very important to try out your interview schedule with someone who knows you before using the interview to collect data. The experience of running the interview, and the feedback from the other person, will tell you whether your schedule of questions and your recording methods are appropriate. It also gives you the opportunity to practise.

Ethical issues

As with other research methods, informed consent should be sought from participants. This should include an indication of how much time the interview is expected to take. Participants should be informed of the purpose of the interview and given anonymity. They should be told that they do not have to take part and that if they do, they have the right not to answer certain questions.

To remind yourself to follow the correct procedures, it is useful to include a statement of aims, anonymity, the right to withdraw and a request for consent at the start of the interview schedule. This can then be read out to the participant.

It is also important to avoid asking questions that are likely to upset, insult or embarrass a participant. For example, it would be tactless to ask a GP, 'Some people say that GPs often do more harm than good. Do you agree?' Equally, it would be wrong to ask an alternative therapist, 'Do you think you actually do any good, or is it all a big con?'

Useful question topics

Interviewing practitioners

To collect the information you need, consider including questions about:
+ how the therapy is believed to work
+ what procedures are involved

+ how long treatment takes (e.g. how many sessions and the length of each session)
+ the cost of each treatment session
+ what training the therapist has received
+ to which regulatory bodies the therapist belongs

It would also be useful to seek opinions about the other therapies you have chosen to describe.

Interviewing clients

You should consider asking why the participant decided to have the therapy in question and what the experience was like. For example, you could ask in what ways the therapy conformed to their expectations and in what ways was it different. You might also ask for their views on the effectiveness of the therapy. In addition, the bullet points above about procedures, treatment time and costs would be relevant.

Writing the guide

The recommended way to present your report for this unit is in the form of a guide. This could be in the form of a booklet intended for a person who is considering using complementary or alternative therapies. This means that the information should be well structured and appropriate for a reader, such as a teacher. It should be presented attractively and be interesting and informative to read. If you have a flair for design, you should use it to your advantage in this assessment. The guide should comprise the first three sections of the report as listed in the specification, i.e. an introduction, a section describing each therapy and a section of advice about each therapy. A suitable title for a guide (depending on the choice of therapies you make) could be something like, 'Back pain: three alternative treatments explained'.

The fourth section of the report is an appendix, which should not form part of the guide but which should accompany it.

Section A: Introduction

This section should be a brief general introduction to complementary therapies.

Section B: Describing therapies

To score high marks, you should describe your three chosen therapies accurately and in detail. The description should include the aims of each therapy and the procedures involved. You might also want to include a brief account of any beliefs or theory underlying each therapy. This will be useful when you evaluate the therapies. To help you to decide what to include, you should think about what questions the reader would want answers to.

Section C: Evaluating therapies

To score high marks, your advice in this section should be supported by reasoned argument and/or reference to your sources. You will probably find it useful to include quotations from your written sources and interviewees. All the criteria mentioned in the specification should be referred to for each of the three therapies, so as to give a realistic view of the advantages and disadvantages of each. If you have chosen three therapies that are intended to treat similar conditions, you can also compare these.

Section D: Appendix

The appendix is an important section of this report. It should not be merely a list of sources.

You should include references to books, articles and websites you have used to produce your guide. You should not rely on only one source for your information.

You should also include completed interview schedules for all the interviews you carried out. These should be the originals or photocopies of the originals. Inevitably, these will be quite untidy, with scribbled responses, notes in the margin and so on. It is much better to include these rather than a neater version copied out later, which will not look so authentic. However, if some of the answers you recorded are likely to be illegible to another reader (e.g. because you used shorthand), it is worth transcribing these more legibly onto a separate page.

You should include a summary of what emerged from the interview(s) you conducted. Since you are unlikely to interview more than one or two people, there is no point in processing data statistically. Rather, you should refer to relevant answers to selected questions to support your evaluations.

You are also required to provide 'commentaries' on your sources. This means that you should assess the quality of data you obtained. The main reason is because of the risk of bias attached to this topic. If, for example, a book or website appeared to be prejudiced in favour of, or against, a particular type of therapy, you should state this, supporting your statement with reasons and preferably including a quotation.

You should also do this for the person(s) you interviewed. You are making a judgement about a person you have interviewed, so it is particularly important that the source is neither identified by name, nor identifiable by position (e.g. 'my GP in Broughton Moor').

Further reading

The general textbooks listed below provide reasonably balanced, unbiased information. Books designed to promote one specific therapy are likely to be more one-sided.

Barnett, H. (2002) *The Which? Guide to Complementary Therapies*, Which? Books.
Thomas, P. (2002) *What Works, What Doesn't: The Guide to Alternative Healthcare*, Newleaf.

Numerous books relating to specific therapies are widely available in bookshops and public libraries.

Websites

The British Complementary Medical Association is an umbrella organisation for a wide range of complementary and alternative therapies:
www.bcma.co.uk

The British Medical Association website has extensive information and links to websites for specific complementary and alternative therapies:
www.bma.org.uk

Psychological perspectives

This chapter contains the information you need for **Unit 10: Psychological perspectives**. Each perspective is described, illustrated by examples (including applications) and evaluated. The applications included here are only examples; others are possible. This chapter also contains detailed guidance on how to plan and carry out your coursework.

What is psychology?

Some people think that psychology is just 'common sense' applied to people in everyday life; others think that it just refers to techniques designed to manipulate people. Another popular view is that psychology is the study of abnormal individuals or a type of 'new age' therapy. These are all inaccurate views.

Psychology is a science. The subject matter of psychology is how people act, feel and understand the world. Many psychologists carry out research on groups of people who are not special or different in any way. They do this to find out how people normally function. Only rarely do psychologists study single individuals who are special or different in some way. Some psychologists study non-human animals, usually as a way of understanding human behaviour and experience. Whenever possible, psychologists use scientific methods of research, such as experiment and observation.

Research psychologists are skilled at collecting and processing data statistically. They also follow a strict code of ethics, which leads them to treat people much better than, say, journalists or stage hypnotists sometimes do.

Psychology is very different from a common-sense unscientific approach to understanding people.

Some psychologists apply psychological knowledge to everyday problems:

+ **educational psychologists** apply psychology to assess and design learning programmes for children with learning difficulties
+ **clinical psychologists** apply psychology to help people who have mental disorders

+ **occupational psychologists** apply psychology to improve the workplace and worker productivity

Why study psychological perspectives?

The different perspectives described in this chapter can be seen as tools for understanding people. Such tools can be very useful when working with people, especially in early-years health and social care. Psychology is interesting because it is about humans and our everyday experiences. It can also help us understand ourselves.

Behaviourist perspective

The behaviourist perspective was most influential during the first half of the twentieth century, and includes the work of Skinner and Pavlov. Their theories are still relevant today.

Learning theory/operant conditioning

Learning theory is a misleading name. Most people think of learning as a process that involves a lot of cognitive work — thinking. The behaviourists believed that thought processes could not be studied scientifically, so psychologists should only study what could be directly and publicly observed, i.e. behaviour. When behaviourists talked about learning, they defined it as a relatively permanent change in behaviour. To the behaviourists, learning meant producing new or different behaviour.

Skinner described and refined learning theory, and explored the principles of **operant conditioning**. Operant conditioning is a procedure for bringing about changes in behaviour (i.e. learning). The principles are as follows:
+ Individuals are observed.
+ As soon as they produce the desired behaviour they are immediately rewarded.
+ Unwanted behaviour is ignored.

The behaviourists did most of their research using non-human animals, partly because it was much easier to control their environment and carry out well-controlled experiments.

Skinner devised a specially equipped type of cage to make experimentation easy. This was called a 'Skinner box'. Different boxes were designed for rats and pigeons, which were Skinner's preferred experimental animals.

A Skinner box can be used to demonstrate operant conditioning in rats. The box is equipped with a lever that a rat can press. This lever is linked to a supply of food and is arranged so that when the lever is pressed, a piece of food drops down into the cage. At the same time, the lever pressing is automatically recorded, so that the observation of the lever-pressing behaviour can be done without anyone actually having to watch.

Skinner's experiment is summarised below:

+ A fairly hungry rat is put into the box for the first time. The rat explores the cage and, by accident, treads on the lever. A pellet of food drops down and the rat eats it.

+ The rat continues to explore, tripping the lever several more times. By now, the rat is spending more time near the lever. Pressing the lever is being rewarded immediately with food.

+ The automatic recording shows that pressing the lever becomes more and more frequent, until the rat is full.

+ The rat is taken out of the cage and then returned to it next day. Straight away the rat runs to the lever, presses it and heads for the food tray for a reward.

Figure 10.1
A rat in a Skinner box

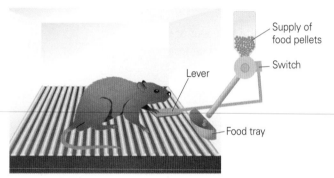

Supply of food pellets

Switch

Lever

Food tray

This simple procedure demonstrates that rewarding the (initially accidental) lever pressing has made this behaviour much more likely. The rat has learned to press the lever. The instant rewarding of behaviour like this is sometimes called **reinforcement** because it makes the behaviour more likely.

The **key feature of learning theory/ operant conditioning** is that behaviour that is immediately rewarded is likely to be repeated.

Applications

You might think that this simple procedure has little value apart from training animals to do circus tricks. In fact, it has important applications to humans too.

Biofeedback

Biofeedback is a system that people can use to learn to control stress. A sensor on the skin measures how moist the skin is and converts this measure into a musical tone. The wetter the skin is, the higher the note. People's skin becomes moist when they sweat and they sweat more when angry or under stress. By listening to the tone, people can gradually gain control over it and make it go lower. At the same time (without knowing quite how they are doing it), they are gaining control over their responses to stress and are staying calmer. Eventually, they can do this without the biofeedback machine.

In biofeedback, the reduction in tone from a high-pitched whine to a more pleasant hum is the reward. As soon as the person calms down, the tone changes, so the reward is immediate.

Other forms of biofeedback measure heart rate and electrical activity in the scalp.

Behaviour modification

Behaviour modification can be used to encourage people to act in more adaptive ways. It has been used with young offenders and with adults with mental illnesses or learning disabilities. The operant conditioning principle is used. A behavioural target is set and on achieving it, the person is immediately rewarded. For example, a violent offender might be given a token if he cooperates with others on a task for 10 minutes, without being aggressive. When he collects enough tokens, he wins a weekend's home leave. This use of valued tokens as rewards is sometimes called the 'token economy'. If the offender becomes violent, he is not usually punished, but he is temporarily removed from the situation and left alone, so that he cannot receive any rewards. This is called 'time out'. It is the nearest practical equivalent to ignoring the unwanted behaviour.

If the behaviour modification works, the offender becomes more able to control his violent behaviour and, therefore, becomes less likely to offend again.

Everyday examples

Parents often use behaviour modification techniques with their children without realising it. For example, when an infant says something interesting, they reward the infant with their attention.

Sometimes parents unintentionally reward unwanted behaviour.

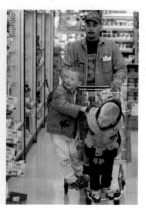
Parents sometimes reward unwanted behaviour

A toddler goes to the supermarket with her father. The toddler is very bored and starts taking items from shelves. The father notices and tells the toddler off. The toddler continues to create this kind of diversion; other shoppers stop and stare, and the father becomes embarrassed and angry. This is very entertaining for the toddler. The toddler is being rewarded with attention for unwanted behaviour. Eventually the father gives the toddler a chocolate bar, 'to keep you quiet'. This is another reward, and ensures that the toddler will 'make trouble' on future visits to the supermarket. Notice that the father in this example is applying the principle of operant conditioning without knowing it.

For children who get very little attention, even hostile attention, such as punishment, can be rewarding.

Try it out

Think of an alternative way the father could have behaved to the toddler in the supermarket.

What behaviours should he be rewarding?

Evaluation

Operant conditioning can be used to shape behaviour even if people do not wish to cooperate. In other words, it does not increase a person's autonomy. For this reason, some people object on ethical grounds to its application to humans. They argue that if a person's behaviour is to change, that person should make the decision to change. This happens in biofeedback, but not in behaviour modification. On the other hand, if behaviour modification helps people to become less violent or helps mentally ill people to behave in ways that make them more acceptable to society, this advantage might be seen to outweigh the ethical issue.

A general problem with the behaviourist perspective is that it ignores the influence of cognitions, i.e. what people think and believe about their situation. Yet, cognitive factors also influence behaviour and experience.

Figure 10.2
Pavlov's classical conditioning experiment

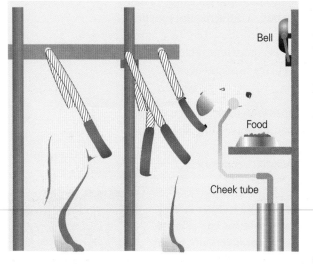

Classical conditioning

Classical conditioning was described by Pavlov, who discovered the effect while studying the salivation reflex in dogs. He inserted a tube into each dog's cheek to divert the saliva into a measuring tube. His plan was to measure salivation when the dogs were fed. Unfortunately the dogs could hear the sound of food bowls being prepared and began to salivate before the food was presented to them. Pavlov realised that this was a very simple form of learning.

The dogs had learned to link the sound of the food bowls with food. Pavlov then tried ringing a bell at the same time as giving the dogs their food. After a few repetitions of this pairing, the dogs would salivate when they heard the bell, even if no food was presented. The dogs had learned to produce the same reflex response to a new stimulus – the bell.

Pavlov used a harness to hold the dog still, and measured the volume of saliva produced before, during and after conditioning (see Figure 10.2).

Pavlov's procedure is usually set out as shown in Figure 10.3. It can be used with a variety of different stimuli and reflex responses.

Notice that what happens is that a new stimulus (such as a sound or a light) becomes linked to an existing reflex response.

The **key feature of classical conditioning** is the assumption that the pairing of a new stimulus with an existing unconditioned stimulus that produces a reflex response will lead to the new stimulus itself eliciting the reflex response.

Figure 10.3
Pavlov's conditioning procedure

(1) Before conditioning

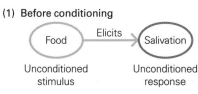

(2) During conditioning

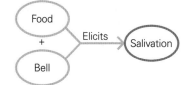

This pairing is repeated on several occasions

(3) Result of conditioning

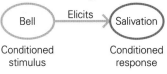

Applications

You might think there would be few uses for a conditioning procedure that only results in reflex responses. However, psychologists have found several ways of using this procedure to benefit people.

Aversion therapy

Aversion therapy is a technique designed to cure addictions, for example to alcohol. It relies on the vomiting reflex. The procedure is to invite the alcoholic to drink some alcohol that has had an emetic drug added to it. Emetics make people feel sick and in sufficient quantities cause vomiting. Usually, the amount of emetic is designed not to cause vomiting but to cause the unpleasant feeling people have before they vomit (nausea). The more that is drunk, the worse the person feels. The repeated pairing of different alcoholic drinks with the emetic leads to conditioning, so that eventually the smell and taste of an alcoholic drink, even without the emetic, makes the person feel sick.

This can be shown in a similar way to Pavlov's procedure (Figure 10.4).

Understanding phobias

Another application of classical conditioning is in the understanding of **phobias**. A phobia is an irrational, but intense, fear of some object or situation. Being frightened of poisonous snakes is not a phobia, because this fear is rational — such snakes can kill. However, being frightened of air travel is irrational (especially for people who travel in cars or who smoke). The latter activities are much more likely than air travel to result in death.

The idea is that in some (but not all) cases, phobias might have resulted from conditioning. Imagine that a child was painfully injured in a car crash. The kind of reflexes that occur when we are in danger — such as a dry mouth, sweating, increased heart rate — have, in this case, been paired (although only once) with the experience of being in a car. This 'one-trial conditioning' could result in a phobia. The next time the child is in a car, he or she might experience all those pain and fear reflexes and feel panicky. The child might know that this is irrational, but cannot stop the feelings.

Systematic desensitisation

Assuming that the above explanation of a car phobia is true, classical conditioning theory offers a clue to a cure. Pavlov found that if the conditioned stimulus (the sound of a bell) was repeatedly presented to a dog but never again paired with food, the conditioned salivation reflex began to decline. The principle here is to present the conditioned stimulus repeatedly without the unconditioned stimulus.

Applying this to the child with car phobia, you would have to expose the child repeatedly to cars while trying to avoid the pain and fear reflexes being triggered.

(1) Before conditioning

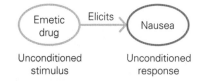

(2) Aversion therapy procedure

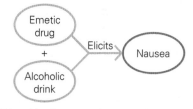

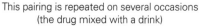

This pairing is repeated on several occasions (the drug mixed with a drink)

(3) Result of therapy

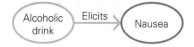

Figure 10.4
An aversion therapy designed to cure addiction to alcohol

This is not easy. **Systematic desensitisation** does this by exposing the child to representations of cars. For example, to start with the child is asked to look at a picture of a pleasant scene in which a car is shown in the distance. Meanwhile, the child is kept as calm as possible. Next, a picture in which a car is more prominent is presented, for as long as the child feels comfortable with it. At a later session, the child is shown some toy cars and invited to play with one of them. Later still, the child is asked to walk past and then sit in a stationary car. So long as the child does not become upset, this procedure gradually desensitises the child to the conditioned stimulus. Eventually, the child will happily ride in a car again.

This procedure can be used with a variety of phobias, such as **agoraphobia**, in which the person has an irrational fear of open spaces, such as streets and supermarkets. However, the technique does not always work, particularly if the cause of the phobia was not accidental classical conditioning.

Evaluation

As with operant conditioning, classical conditioning is a procedure that does not rely on the cooperation of people. Its use in the past has sometimes been unethical – for example, when electric shocks were administered to male homosexuals while they were looking at photographs of attractive men. This use of aversion therapy happened at a time when homosexual behaviour between adults was illegal and homosexuality was regarded as a disorder.

Classical conditioning is a very simple type of learning. However, humans also learn in much more sophisticated ways. The behaviourist perspective tends to ignore the influence of cognitions on behaviour and experience. A shocking, fictional portrayal of an unethical use of aversion therapy occurs in the film *A Clockwork Orange*.

Cognitive perspective

The words **'cognition'** and **'cognitive'** refer to ideas, thoughts, knowledge and beliefs that people have. Cognitive processes are concerned with thinking, memory, understanding language, and perceiving and solving problems. Social cognition is a person's understanding of what other people are thinking and feeling.

Humans have a strong tendency to try to make sense of the world around them. Early in childhood, people look for rules and patterns in life. For example, toddlers soon pick up the grammatical rule that words can be made plural by adding a letter 's'. When they come across words such as 'sheep' – which do not obey this rule – they are likely, on seeing several sheep, to make the mistake of saying 'sheeps'. This mistake illustrates the tendency to look for rules. However, the child's search for patterns and rules is usually successful.

The ideas, beliefs, patterns and rules we construct when making sense of the world are called **schemas**. Our set of schemas amounts to a description of how things work in our world. It is as if we have an internal model of the real world. We use this to guide our behaviour. This works quite well if the model is accurate

— for example, if our beliefs match reality. Inevitably, however, all of us have some inaccuracies in the way we perceive the people around us and other features of our world. Different individuals and cultures have different ways of thinking about the world. These inaccuracies and differences sometimes lead to misunderstandings.

Stereotypes are examples of schemas about groups of people. They are over-simplifications that, while sometimes inaccurate, help us to understand and predict the behaviour of other people. For example, a man might have a particular gender stereotype about men. He might believe that 'men don't show their feelings'. If so, he might assume that a male friend of his who has been bereaved, but shows little emotion, is actually very upset, but hiding it.

The cognitive perspective assumes that the behaviour and experience of people are influenced by what they believe and know.

Manuel believes that the people he works with dislike him. This might be true, but Manuel might believe this even if it were untrue. This belief could affect Manuel's experience — he might not enjoy going to work as a result. It could also affect Manuel's behaviour — he might show hostility to his work colleagues.

One effect of our tendency to build schemas is that we become susceptible to 'self-fulfilling prophecies'. A **self-fulfilling prophecy** is a belief that someone has, which influences their behaviour in such a way that the belief becomes true.

Manuel believes his colleagues do not like him. As a result, he shows hostility towards them. Even if they liked him to start with, they are now going to start to dislike him — so his belief comes true.

Another example is a common self-fulfilling prophecy about examinations. Some students believe they are 'no good at exams'. As a result, they do not do much revision, because if they are no good at exams, they believe that revision will not help them much. As a result of lack of revision, they perform poorly. This confirms their belief. However, if they did adequate revision, the same students might be quite good at examinations.

The **key feature of the cognitive perspective** is that our (sometimes inaccurate) perceptions and beliefs about the world can influence our behaviour and experience.

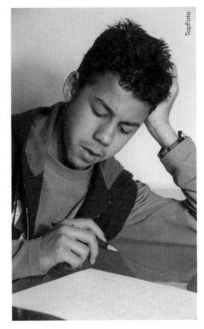

A self-fulfilling prophecy might affect this student's examination performance

Applications

The cognitive perspective is very useful in understanding people who have psychological problems. These often result from inaccurate perceptions that can make people miserable and make them act in ways that are maladaptive.

One example is **obsessive-compulsive disorder**. Some people have a compulsion to clean themselves and objects around them repeatedly. Compulsive hand-washing can occupy many hours of the day, making it impossible for the person to keep a job and interfering with relationships. For some of these people, the compulsion seems to stem from a belief that all microorganisms are extremely dangerous. This is an exaggeration of the actual risk.

The cognitive explanation also gives rise to a type of counselling in which the person's beliefs are examined and shown to be inaccurate.

Another example is behind one of the explanations for **anorexia**. Some people have very inaccurate perceptions of their own body size. Some anorexics continue to starve themselves because they believe themselves to be overweight.

Some therapies combine the cognitive perspective with a behaviourist approach, in what is called '**cognitive-behaviour therapy**'.

Evaluation

The cognitive perspective has the advantage of recognising that humans, more than any other species, are self-aware and are strongly influenced by beliefs and knowledge.

However, the cognitive perspective does not provide a full explanation. Biological factors, for example, also influence behaviour and experience.

Social influence

Humans, like some other species, are social, i.e. they tend to seek contact with other humans. Living in groups (and in larger structures such as cities) has certain consequences for behaviour. One consequence is the pressure to conform to group and societal norms.

A **group norm** is a behaviour or belief that is shared by most or all members of a group. For example, in a group of school-friends it might be the norm for each member to share sweets with the other group members. If a member of this group has some sweets, but eats them without sharing, the other members of the group are likely to disapprove. Behaviour that does not conform with group norms is called **deviance**. Deviance tends to lead to other group members exerting **group pressure** on the deviant individual. This can take the form of critical comments, or ignoring or even bullying the person. The effect of group pressure is to make the deviant member conform. It could be said that **conformity** is the price of group membership.

Societal (cultural) norms are behaviours, attitudes and beliefs that tend to be common to a whole society, culture or subculture. For example, some societies or cultures have norms such as being kind to animals or always wearing a hat or head covering when outdoors.

The process of learning to adapt one's behaviour and attitudes to that of the group is called **socialisation**.

Social influence can have such a strong effect on behaviour that people lack autonomy as a result. They feel that they cannot choose to do just what they want, but have to behave as others wish. This tends to reduce conflict within groups and societies.

Social influence is likely to be at its strongest when people are most dependent on the approval of their groups. For example, a young child is very dependent on his or her parents and is, therefore, likely to adopt their behaviours and attitudes. As children grow older, they come to depend more on their peers, such as school-friends. If the norms of their friendship group are different from the norms of the family group (and this is often the case), some conflict can occur when the individual acts according to the norms of the group they are not with at the time. For example, if a young person's family group uses a lot of swear words, but people in her friendship group do not, this can create conflict. If she swears a lot when with her friendship group, they might disapprove and like her less. If she does not swear with her family group, they might regard her as 'stuck up'.

Perhaps you did not find the swearing example very convincing. Think of an example of some other behaviour that is normal in your friendship group, but would be regarded as deviant if shown in your family group. Then think of an example of a behaviour that is normal within your family but would be deviant within your friendship group.

Try it out

As people reach adulthood, they come into contact with a wider range of social groups — for example, at work. They also tend to become more confident and less dependent on the approval of groups to which they belong. This enables them to become more autonomous and less influenced by other people. The ability to resist social influence is important in achieving autonomy.

The **key feature of social influence** is that it affects our behaviour, attitudes and beliefs, because we tend to conform to our group or society in order to gain acceptance.

Applications

We have already come across social influence as an explanation for conflict — for example, between children and parents.

Social influence also relates directly to other aspects of health and social care. If a group norm involves maladaptive behaviour, this is likely to have a negative effect on a person's health or wellbeing.

A classic example is the onset of smoking among young people. Young people who live in families where parents smoke, or who are members of friendship groups where smoking is a norm, are much more likely to start smoking themselves.

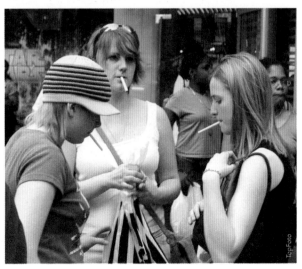

Social influence can lead people to take up smoking

Indirectly, this perspective can also be used to explain extreme antisocial behaviour. A person who is not at all dependent on others for approval (perhaps someone who experienced abuse and separation in infancy) is more likely to act in ways that infringe societal norms.

Evaluation

Social influence is useful for explaining some behaviours, but it is not applicable to all. An understanding of the perspective can help a person to become less socially dependent, and therefore more autonomous.

Biological perspective

The **biological perspective** assumes that behaviour and personality are strongly influenced by biological factors such as genotype and hormones.

Genes have a major influence on body structure and development. Maturation is a genetically programmed process of development that influences the onset of different abilities at different ages. For example, the patterns of development of language and of attachment seem to be maturational. More information on factors influencing development can be found in Chapter 4.

The similarities that occur between individuals (such as in the timing and sequence of language development) are to a large extent caused by the genetic similarity between humans. However, while genetically similar, no two people (apart from identical twins) are genetically identical. The genetic variation among us is partly responsible for differences in personality and behaviour.

For example, it is often noticeable from an early age that two children born of the same parents are quite different in temperament. Temperament refers to how active or calm or irritable an individual is. Two siblings can differ in temperament, for example, by one being tolerant of change and having regular sleeping patterns while the other is easily upset and frequently restless. Such temperamental differences usually persist right throughout life.

The hormone adrenaline can influence a driver's feelings and behaviour

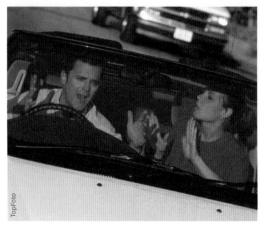

The feelings a person has involve brain processes and, to some extent, can be said to be the result of those processes. For example, damage to part of the brain (the frontal lobe) can lead to a change in personality. The presence or lack of biochemicals such as **hormones** and **neurotransmitters** can influence mood. Hormones are chemicals made by the body in endocrine glands. Hormones are released into the bloodstream and produce various effects, some of which influence behaviour.

For example, when a person is shocked, angered or alarmed by an event that has just happened, adrenaline is secreted into the bloodstream by the adrenal glands above the kidneys. Adrenaline is carried around the body by the blood and tends to keep the person aroused for some time afterwards. This arousal increases the probability that the person will take vigorous action, such as fighting or running away. It therefore indirectly influences behaviour as well as feelings. For example, it probably contributes to aggression and driver error following a conflict or 'near miss' between two car drivers.

Neurotransmitters are chemicals produced at the ends of nerve cells — at the point where they almost make contact with other nerve cells. They help to transmit nerve impulses from one nerve cell to the next. The presence or lack of neurotransmitters can also influence feelings. For example, there is some evidence that neurotransmitters called **enkephalins** and **endorphins** are released during vigorous exercise. These neurotransmitters are sometimes called 'natural opiates' because they seem to affect nerve receptors in the same way as opiate drugs, such as heroin. Two effects are noticeable:

+ Immediately following an injury, people often do not feel pain. The endorphins released seem to act as immediate anaesthetics.
+ After strenuous exercise, people often have a feeling of wellbeing. This is probably the result of endorphin release.

This neurotransmitter release is an important factor influencing wellbeing. It could also help to explain the placebo effect, in which an individual is given some drug or other therapy that is ineffective in itself. If people receiving the placebo or ineffective therapy believe it to be effective, they report feeling better. This suggests that the knowledge that they have received a treatment could itself trigger the release of endorphins.

Applications

Genetic similarity and variation can be used to explain a range of behaviours and health conditions. These include schizophrenia and autism, although genetic influence is unlikely to be the whole explanation.

The biological approach has given rise to a range of treatments. The most familiar example is the use of drugs to modify the chemical environment in the brain and so reduce the symptoms of mental disorders, such as depression.

The biological approach also helps us to understand the links between exercise and wellbeing.

Evaluation

The biological approach is important in understanding health and development. However, humans — more than other species — are also influenced by their ability to learn and by their cognitions.

A purely biological approach to understanding human behaviour, illness and health runs the risk of ignoring these other influences by simply treating the individual as a body rather than as a person.

Evaluating perspectives

In the 'discussion' section of your report you will have to evaluate the perspectives to which you have referred. Although some evaluation has been included in the descriptions above, you should also make judgements about how well each chosen perspective applies to your topic.

Overlap between perspectives

It might have occurred to you that the different perspectives described overlap or interact to some extent. For example, while the biological approach can explain why exercise leads to feelings of wellbeing, the learning theory perspective can help us to understand why it is that people can become 'addicted' to exercise. The immediate release of endorphins following exercise is pleasant, therefore rewarding, and reinforces the taking of frequent exercise.

Research methods, techniques and ethics

Research methods

Psychologists use a range of research methods, including experiment, correlations, observation, questionnaire survey and structured interview.

Experiment

The experiment is the most important scientific method used in psychology. Its great advantage over other methods is that it is the only one that comes close to answering the most important question in psychology: what causes a person to behave in a certain way?

Human behaviour is influenced by many factors, so there is never just one cause of a person's behaviour — there are many contributing factors. An experiment allows the investigator to select one factor, vary it, and see whether this variation has any effect on behaviour.

The easiest way to understand experiments in psychology is by comparison with an experiment often carried out by biology students.

The biology experiment aims to find out about factors affecting the growth of beans. You suspect that several factors (variables) influence how tall beans will become in a certain time. These factors include:

+ the amount of light they receive
+ the amount of water they receive
+ the temperature
+ the type of soil

You plant two trays with the same number of beans, equal distances apart. For a proper comparison about factors affecting growth, there should only be one variable that differs between the two trays. It could be any of the four variables listed above. Suppose you choose light — this is then the **independent variable**. You place both trays in a plant incubator on a windowsill, with a piece of paper shading one of the trays. This tray will, therefore, receive less light. The soil type and the temperature of both trays are the same and you give them the same amount of water. After 3 weeks, you measure the heights of the bean plants. Height is the **dependent variable**. The heights of the bean plants indicate whether or not light is an influencing factor in the growth of beans. It does not indicate that light is the *only* influencing variable. You would have to test each variable in turn to find out. Notice that if you had two variables (e.g. light and water), it would not be possible to draw a conclusion. Any difference in height could be due to either light or water, or both.

Psychology experiments are similar. Typically, a psychologist chooses a likely influencing variable, then takes two groups of similar people and makes sure that only one variable differs between them.

For example, in a famous experiment, Festinger and Carlsmith asked two groups of students to do the same boring task (turning pegs in holes). The only difference between the two groups was that students in one group were paid 1 dollar for doing this and students in the other group were paid 20 dollars. Afterwards, the students were asked to rate how interesting the task was in itself — to see if the amount of the reward made a difference. It did, but not in the way you might expect. The students paid 1 dollar rated the task as more interesting than those who were paid 20 dollars.

In this study, the independent variable was the amount of the reward. The dependent variable was the rating of how worthwhile the task was.

To sum up, an experiment is a study in which:

✦ the experimenter intentionally varies one factor (the independent variable) and observes the effect of this on another factor (the dependent variable)
✦ other possible influencing variables are controlled (kept the same)

Advantages and disadvantages

The main advantage of the experiment in psychology is that it gives the clearest evidence of what factors cause or influence behaviour.

A disadvantage is that in setting up the controlled conditions needed, the situation can sometimes become artificial and not enough like real life to find out anything useful. The term **ecological validity** is used to refer to how 'true to life' a study is. Some experiments, but not all, are rather low in ecological validity.

Correlation study

A **correlation study** is a scientific method in which two variables are measured to find out whether they are connected. Unlike the experiment, neither variable is manipulated or controlled by the researcher.

An example would be a study to see if there is a link between obesity and inactivity. For example:

+ randomly select 200 adult males
+ weigh each participant
+ supply each participant with a pedometer (a device that records the amount of walking movement)
+ record the pedometer readings after a fixed time period, e.g. 1 week

After collecting the data, it should be possible to determine whether there is any link between body weight and activity. The data might show that heavier people walked less. This would be a **positive correlation**.

Notice that, unlike the experiment, a correlation study does not indicate which variable influences the other variable. It could be that the amount of walking influences weight – so the people who exercise least end up weighing the most. Alternatively, it could be that weight which influences how much people walk. The heaviest people walk least because they find it more difficult.

Advantages and disadvantages

An advantage is that correlation studies are easy to carry out and they can reveal links between variables.

A disadvantage is that they do not indicate the causal nature of the link (i.e. which variable influenced the other).

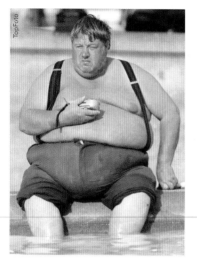

There could be a correlation between people's weight and the amount of exercise they take — but which factor causes which?

Observation

Observation is an important method of study in several sciences and the main method in astronomy. In psychology, observation means watching the behaviour of an individual or group and recording instances of specific behaviours. To be scientific, observation should be systematic – not just casual watching. The observer plans in advance which behaviours are to be recorded and uses a grid or tally chart to record the behaviours easily. The observer might use an electronic event recorder to register different behaviours simply by pressing a range of buttons. The number of times that each behaviour occurs is automatically totalled.

For example, Ainsworth et al. (1978) observed and recorded the behaviours of attached infants:

+ while they were with their mothers
+ with a stranger
+ when briefly separated from their mothers
+ when reunited with their mothers

They recorded behaviours such as crying, exploring and distance between mother and infant. This has become known as the **strange situation study**.

Advantages and disadvantages

A key advantage of observation is that what is recorded is the actual behaviour shown (typically) in a real-life situation. This means that observations are likely to have fairly high ecological validity.

One disadvantage is that the behaviour observed is likely to be influenced by the presence of the observer. If, on the other hand, a person were observed without being aware of it, this would be an ethical problem – invasion of privacy. Also, the method is rather time-consuming. It is difficult to collect accurate data about more than one person at a time.

Unlike an experiment, observation does not reveal cause–effect links.

Questionnaire survey

Rather than measuring or observing the behaviour of people, the questionnaire method involves asking them to report on their own behaviour and experience. For that reason, it is not as scientific or as rigorous as the methods described above.

The method relies on **self-report** – people telling what they do, think or feel. Each respondent has to read and fill in answers to the items on the questionnaire, before returning it to the researcher. People tend not to be very good observers of their own behaviour – they are naturally biased.

However, one way in which self-report methods are of value is that they enable researchers to collect information about beliefs and feelings, which cannot be collected by observation.

The questionnaire method is inferior to experiment and observation in studying actual behaviour. However, it is useful in studying attitudes.

Advantages and disadvantages

One advantage of the questionnaire survey is that it enables beliefs, feelings and attitudes to be studied. Another advantage is that it can be used to study a very large sample of respondents.

One disadvantage is that self-report is subject to bias. Unlike an experiment, this method does not reveal cause–effect links.

Interview

The interview is a self-report method. In a structured interview, the questions are planned in advance by the interviewer and printed out on a series of sheets, making up an interview schedule. The researcher asks each participant the questions and records the replies. A semi-structured interview, unlike the questionnaire, enables the researcher to ask supplementary questions, depending on the replies given.

The interviewer can also gauge how accurate the data are – for example, by seeing whether or not the interviewee is taking the interview seriously.

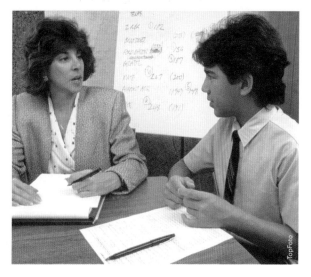

The interview allows the researcher to ask supplementary questions

Advantages and disadvantages

Advantages of the interview are that supplementary questions can be asked, and the interviewer can judge the accuracy of responses.

One disadvantage is that self-report is subject to bias. Another disadvantage is that the method is very time-consuming, because each respondent has to be interviewed separately. This means that it is difficult to study a large sample. Unlike an experiment, an interview does not reveal cause–effect links.

Case studies

Many case studies report on just one or two participants, when these are of special interest. Some of these are individual cases in which a particular therapy (such as systematic desensitisation) has been applied. The case study is not a method as such. In a case study, the method used is often a combination of observation and interview.

Advantages and disadvantages

The case study has no particular advantage. It is used mainly because a group of similar cases is not available for study. The study of one participant is better than none.

There are several disadvantages. For example:

+ the findings of a case study cannot be generalised to a population because the sample is too small to be representative
+ a case study cannot provide information about cause and effect or links between variables

Note that a piece of research using any of these methods is called a 'study'. Some people make the mistake of calling all studies 'experiments', when most of them clearly are not.

Sampling

The process of selecting people to take part in a study is called **sampling**. The group of individuals who participate in a particular piece of research is called a **sample**.

For a study to find out something useful about people, the sample studied should be representative of their population. This means that the data collected from a sample of, say, 100 members of that population should be typical of the population as a whole. Clearly, if the population to be studied was 7-year-old boys and girls in Britain and only one boy and one girl were studied, this tiny sample would not be representative.

Two factors together influence whether or not a sample is reasonably representative:

+ **Sample size** — to be representative, a sample should be as large as possible. If the population to be studied is quite small (e.g. people who received heart bypass surgery at West Cumberland Hospital in 2004), then all the cases could be studied.

+ **Sampling method** – a sample is most likely to be representative if it is randomly selected, so that every member of the population has an equal chance of being selected. Random sampling is quite difficult. First, a database listing the whole population (e.g. 7-year-old children in Leeds) has to be obtained. Then, a randomising function has to be used to select 200 of them.

In practice, sampling methods in psychology often fall short of this ideal. Typically, an **opportunity sample** is used. This could be people who happen to be available, picked in a haphazard way. If you carry out a study, you will probably have to use this method. The result is that many studies in psychology have been performed using university students as participants. University students are unlikely to be representative of many populations (apart from the population of university students).

In some studies, the sample used is self-selected, i.e. decided by the people who choose whether or not to take part. This happens in studies where volunteers are sought. It also happens in postal questionnaire studies where, typically, only a minority of people fill in and return the questionnaire. These people have there-fore selected themselves. Self-selected samples are no more likely to be represen-tative of their populations than opportunity samples.

Ethical treatment of participants

Participants should be treated well by researchers. **Ethical issues** include main-taining confidentiality, seeking informed consent, avoiding deception and distress, and giving participants the right to withdraw and debriefing.

Confidentiality

When data are collected from participants, and reported, this is usually done in such a way that readers cannot discover the identity of the participant. For example, questionnaires are usually anonymous. Participants may be named only if they freely agree to this.

Seeking informed consent

Participants should be asked whether or not they are willing to take part in a study. When seeking consent, the researcher should explain to the participant what is involved in the research. In some cases, this can be a problem. For example, if the researcher wishes to study very young children, the participants might not be able to understand what is said to them, so they cannot give informed consent. In such instances, parental consent is usually acceptable.

Another problem is that some research can succeed only if the participant is *not* fully aware of the aim of the study. For example, in a clinical trial of a new drug, some participants will receive the drug, some will receive no drug and some will receive a placebo (an inactive substance). The trial will work only if the partici-pants receiving the drug or the placebo are unaware which it is. However, the reasons for this can be explained to participants beforehand.

Avoiding harm and distress

A research procedure should be designed so as not to harm or upset participants. Distress can easily be caused. For example, a simple word-list memory experiment could be designed so that no participant is likely to recall all the words. You ask an adult male friend to take part, explaining that it is a 'memory test'. This friend has an inaccurate view of psychology and assumes that you are interested in studying him as an individual 'case'. When he remembers few of the words on the list, he assumes wrongly that this shows he has low intelligence. This leads to distress, which could have been avoided if the purpose of the study had been better explained.

Avoiding deception

Participants should not be given false information, unless this is strictly necessary for the study. Any deception used should be unlikely to cause harm or distress and the participants should be fully debriefed afterwards.

The right to withdraw

Participants sometimes change their minds about taking part once a procedure has begun. They should be told in advance that they have the right to stop taking part at any time. They should not be made to feel that they are under an obligation to the researcher to continue.

Debriefing

Debriefing happens after the data have been collected. It is a further — and probably fuller — explanation of the purpose of the study, what results are expected and what will happen to the data. It is also a chance to thank participants, reassure them that their results are similar to those of other people and to answer any questions.

Note: You might read about several famous studies carried out many years ago, which clearly breach these ethical guidelines. One reason is that such guidelines were not then in place.

Evaluating studies

Important factors for evaluating a study

On evaluating a study, there are several factors that should be taken into account.

Methodological factors

What method of study was used? For example, if a study used the correlation method, it can be evaluated by pointing out the advantages and disadvantages of this method, as applied to that particular study.

Sampling

You can make a judgment as to how representative the sample was of the intended population. For example, if the sample was large and randomly selected, it would be very representative. Note that if the description you have of the study does not include this information, you will not be able to evaluate this.

Ecological validity

You should make a judgement about whether you think the study was particularly high or low in ecological validity. You must be able to back up this judgement with reasons.

Some students seem to think that any experiment must have low ecological validity 'because it was done in a lab'. This is a mistake. Ecological validity is about whether the behaviour studied and the situation were sufficiently true to life.

For example, if a researcher is observing elderly people in the residential home where they live, this is likely to have high ecological validity. If the researcher is measuring how many words students can learn in a noisy classroom compared with a quiet classroom, this is also likely to have high ecological validity. However, if the researcher visits people in their own homes and asks them how they would feel if they were in hospital, this would have low ecological validity – the respondents are unlikely to be able to imagine how they would feel in this unfamiliar situation.

Ethics

You should make a judgement about the ethical issues raised by a study. Once again the evaluations should be supported with reasoned argument. If you think a procedure is likely to lead to distress, you should explain how. If you cannot find information about seeking informed consent, or debriefing, you will not be able to comment on these.

Likely benefits

You should assess any likely benefits that could follow from doing the study, such as improvements in care practice.

Example evaluation

This example is based on a fictitious study. You must not present it as a real study in your report.

Fictitious study: description

The aim of this study was to find out whether environmental factors could influence the perceptions people have of their own illnesses. The participants were patients at a health centre, which they attended for GP appointments. The study took place over two consecutive weekdays. All the adults who visited the health centre for appointments on those two days were studied. On one day there were 153 participants; on the next day, 127 participants.

On the first day, a series of posters was placed on the walls of the waiting area. The posters showed pictures of very ill people and close-ups of diseased tissues, together with warnings of the effects of smoking and lack of exercise. There were no magazines to read — only leaflets containing advice on topics such as living with AIDS and making a will.

On the second day, a different set of posters was placed on the walls of the waiting area, showing pictures of healthy children and adults taking exercise, cleaning their teeth and eating fruit. The leaflets were replaced with magazines about sport, healthy eating, wildlife and gardening.

Shortly before being called to the GP, each patient was asked anonymously to rate how ill or well he or she felt on a seven-point scale with 1 scoring as 'very ill' and 7 scoring as 'quite well'. Only one participant refused to give a rating.

Two days later, each participant received a letter from the researcher explaining the purpose of the study in detail, thanking them and inviting them to contact the researcher for further information.

The researcher found that the median rating for the first group was 3.5 and the median rating for the second group was 4.5. The researcher concluded that the posters and magazines in the waiting-area environment significantly affected the perceptions patients had of their illnesses.

Fictitious study: evaluation

Methodology

The study was an experiment. The independent variable was the waiting-area environment and the dependent variable was the rating of how ill each participant felt. One advantage of this method is that it showed evidence of cause and effect. The posters and leaflets were the only things different on the two days. Although self-report was used to find out how ill people felt, there was no alternative to this method in this case.

The sample was quite large and (although not randomly selected) reasonably likely to be representative of the people visiting their GPs in that area. It is unlikely that there would be any systematic differences between the samples on two consecutive days.

The study is likely to be high in ecological validity, because the participants were genuinely visiting their GPs. To the participants, this was a 'real-life situation' and they were probably unaware that the study was even taking place.

Ethics

The study can be criticised on ethical grounds. First, it is clear that participants did not have the opportunity to give informed consent. However, to do this would probably have made the experiment ineffective. If the participants had been told that the posters and leaflets were selected to influence their perceptions, they would probably not have been influenced in the intended way.

On the first day, the study might have caused distress to some of the participants. People sometimes read magazines in GP waiting rooms to calm themselves down or take their minds off their conditions. On the first day, everything available would have made them more likely to be worried and upset, so it was probably unethical to do this.

The researcher did attempt to debrief participants (by letter), but this method is far less effective than making personal contact with the participants.

The study could lead to some benefits, such as leading health centres to avoid presenting upsetting images of ill health in waiting areas.

The report

Deciding on a topic

In order to score high marks, your topic should be different from those of other students in your group.

The most important consideration is to choose a topic to which at least two of the four perspectives described above can be related. A topic that can only be connected to social influence, for example, would make it more difficult for you to score marks for application.

Your topic must relate to one of the following: health, illness, medical treatment, social wellbeing (including factors such as exercise), social-care practice and human development. Some examples of possible topics are given below.

Another consideration is to choose a topic in which you are interested. For example, you might be interested in mental disorder or in cognitive development.

Your choice of topic will also be influenced by the availability of information and on whether or not you intend to carry out a study of your own.

Suggested topics

Some topics make it easier to meet the requirements of this unit than do others. For example, the causes and treatment of mental disorders link up well with biological, behaviourist and cognitive perspectives. Some aspects of child development also work quite well, such as the development of aggressive or hyperactive behaviour.

The following topic suggestions show the range of topics available to you. You are not restricted to these.

+ **Psychological perspectives on autism** – there are several different explanations of autism and, therefore, this would enable you to refer to more than one perspective. You might be interested in this topic if you know someone who is autistic. However, for ethical reasons, you should not carry out your own research on autistic people.

+ **Psychological perspectives on individual differences** – individual differences are differences between any two people. An interesting version of this topic is to explain why two children from the same family (two siblings) are different in some ways (such as temperament and personality) but not others. This allows you to consider biological as well as learning-theory explanations. You might expect two children reared by the same parents to be very similar, but are they? This is really a child development topic. For ethical reasons, you should not study children, but you could find out about them by interviewing their parents.

+ **Psychological perspectives on smoking in adolescents** — why do some young people start smoking, while others do not? Explanations could include social influence, learning theory and perhaps even the biology of addiction. If you wanted to carry out your own study, you could look for differences between groups of people you know who smoke and who do not smoke. You could also, or alternatively, try to apply your knowledge of perspectives to ideas for helping people give up smoking.

+ **Psychological perspectives on anxiety about dental treatment** — why do people become anxious about going to the dentist, and how could this anxiety be reduced?

+ **Psychological perspectives on phobias** — you could study explanations and treatments based on different perspectives.

Finding information

Once you have chosen your topic, you will need to read plenty of background material in order to have a good chance of understanding how the different perspectives might apply.

+ To score high marks, you will have to spend time finding really appropriate studies.

+ To score in the top mark bands, you need to describe a minimum of two studies, one of which could be a study you have carried out yourself.

+ To be useful, a study must relate to the topic you have chosen and also illustrate one of the perspectives relevant to that topic.

Be prepared to look at a lot of websites and a range of psychology textbooks to find just what you want. If your school or college library takes magazines such as *New Scientist*, or if you can get hold of copies of the *Nursing Times*, you might find some useful studies there.

You should be careful to discriminate between articles that actually describe studies and general articles giving news or information about a topic. In itself, a magazine article is not a study, although it might give you useful background information. It might also refer to studies that you can then try to track down. Information from websites is most likely to relate to scientific psychology if you use the *Resource Discovery Network* for your searches. The address is given at the end of this chapter.

Summary descriptions in textbooks and magazines often do not give enough information to evaluate a study properly, so to produce a really good report, you may need to look at a copy of the original publication. For example, if your topic focuses on explanations for, and treatments of, autism, you might want to look at one of Simon Baron-Cohen's studies of cognitions in autistic children. Once you have tracked down a reference to the original article, which might have been published in a journal such as *Cognition* or the *British Journal of Psychiatry*, you would then ask the library to send for a photocopy of the article. You will probably have to pay for this service.

You might need to get hold of a book that is no longer in print. For example, to obtain more information about aversion therapy studies, you might want to look at Meyer and Chesser's (1970) *Behaviour Therapy in Clinical Psychology*. To obtain this, you would have to ask your school/college or local library to arrange an interlibrary loan.

Examples of suitable studies

Example 1: Social cognition in autistic children

Baron-Cohen et al. (1985) carried out a study in which they compared autistic children, children with Down's syndrome and unaffected children on the ability to guess or understand what other people are thinking. The child is told a story about Sally, Anne and a marble. Two dolls (Sally and Anne) are used to help the children understand the story (see Figure 10.5).

Sally has a basket in front of her and Anne has a box. Sally puts a marble in her basket; Anne's box is empty. Sally goes out, leaving her basket. (Here, the researcher removes the doll.) Anne moves the marble from Sally's basket to her box. Sally comes back. The researcher asks the child, who has been watching this, 'Where will Sally look for her marble?'

The researchers found that most of the normal and Down's syndrome children answered that Sally would look in her basket. However, most of the autistic children answered that Sally would look in Anne's box.

This study could be used to illustrate the cognitive perspective — showing that autistic children are less able than others to form accurate cognitions about what other people are thinking.

The reference

The words 'et al.' mean 'and others'. The full reference for this study is:

Baron-Cohen, S., Leslie, A. M. and Frith, U. (1985) 'Does the autistic child have a theory of mind?', *Cognition*, Vol. 21, pp. 37–46.

This reference names the three people involved in carrying out and reporting the study, the date when it was published, the title of the article and the title of the journal in which it was

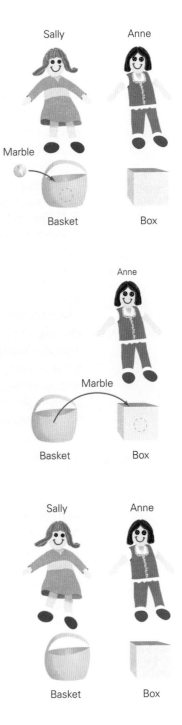

Figure 10.5
Dolls being used to help children understand the story about Sally, Anne and the marble

published (*Cognition*). It also tells you that this was the twenty-first volume of the journal and that the article can be found on pages 37 to 46.

Example 2: Body image of anorexic participants

In 1976, Garner et al. reported a study in which they asked participants, some of whom were anorexic, to look at photographs of themselves and adjust a lens (which could make the images look fatter or thinner) until the images looked exactly like themselves. The researchers found that most of the anorexic participants overestimated their body size (i.e. made the photographs look fatter than they really were), while most of the non-anorexic participants underestimated their body size (i.e. made the photographs look thinner than they really were).

This study could be used to illustrate the cognitive perspective – to show that inaccurate belief (an overestimation of body size) was linked to anorexia.

The full reference is: Garner, D. M., Garfinkel, P. E., Stancer, H. C. and Moldovsky, H. (1976) 'Body image disturbances in anorexia nervosa and obesity', *Psychosomatic Medicine*, Vol. 38, pp. 327–336.

Example 3: Does schizophrenia run in families?

Gottesman (1991) reported the results of a number of studies investigating schizophrenia in people related to each other. One of these studied adult identical-twin pairs and fraternal-twin pairs in which at least one twin had been diagnosed with schizophrenia. The finding was that over 40% of the identical-twin pairs were both schizophrenic, while only 15% of the fraternal-twin pairs were both schizophrenic. Identical twins have the same genotype, whereas fraternal twins are no more similar genetically than any two non-twin siblings. This suggests that genetics plays some part in the occurrence of schizophrenia.

The full reference is: Gottesman, I. I. (1991) *Schizophrenia Genesis*, W. H. Freeman. Notice that the form of reference shows that this publication is a book, not a journal article.

Example 4: Behaviour modification in psychiatric patients

In 1968, Ayllon and Azrin reported the use of behaviour modification with patients in a psychiatric hospital. Patients were given tokens for adaptive behaviour, such as hair combing and bed making, while maladaptive behaviour such as screaming was ignored. This reversed the usual situation in the ward, in which patients were given attention when they made trouble for the staff.

This illustrates an application of the learning theory/operant conditioning perspective.

The full reference is: Ayllon, T. and Azrin, N. H. (1968) *The Token Economy: A Motivational System for Therapy and Rehabilitation,* Appleton Century Crofts, New York.

Designing your own study

Although you do not have to carry out a study of your own, there are some advantages to doing this:

+ You are likely to find the work for the report more interesting.
+ It will give you useful material to show your ability to evaluate studies.
+ Designing your own study also enables you to write about a study that links more than one perspective.

Such a study does not have to be completely original. In fact, there are advantages in designing a modified (probably simplified) version of a study you have read about.

If you decide to carry out your own study, it is important to discuss your plans with your teacher. This should help you avoid attempting a study that might be unethical or too ambitious.

Fewest ethical issues are raised in studies of fellow students or adults. You should only carry out a study involving children under the age of 16 if you have obtained informed consent from participants and their parents or head teacher, and only if the study does not involve causing distress. If you carry out a study using participants under the age of 16, a teacher should be present.

You should not carry out studies that involve applying treatment, such as medication or counselling, to participants.

You should describe your study in the 'Evidence' section of your report. Material such as raw data and copies of a questionnaire or interview schedule should be included in an appendix to your report.

Writing the report

Before you start to write your report, try to get the following ideas clear in your mind:

+ The topic you are going to write about and, in particular, what you are going to include. For example, if you are writing about psychological perspectives in eating disorders, are you going to concentrate on explanations of eating disorders or treatment, or both?
+ The perspectives that are relevant to your topic. If you cannot see the connection between your topic and at least two of the perspectives described above, then your topic is probably not suitable. If you try to link your topic with an irrelevant perspective, you risk losing marks.
+ The connection that your topic has with early years – and social care. It is easy to become sidetracked into an irrelevant topic, such as health for example, because you find Milgram's study of obedience quite interesting.

Structuring the report

The unit specification gives detailed guidance on how to structure your report and what to include in each section. You should keep a copy of this guidance to hand when you are writing the report. It is important to follow this structure and to ensure that your report contains the five sections required.

If you do not have access to a copy of the specification, you can find it on the AQA website (www.aqa.org.uk).

Achieving high marks

The assessment criteria for this unit indicate that your report should have the following features:

+ It should be complete, i.e. contain all the five sections required.
+ It should include clear, concise (not rambling or long-winded) and accurate descriptions of the perspectives relevant to your topic, with use of appropriate terminology.
+ There should be no irrelevant studies or perspectives.
+ References should be in the correct form (for guidance, see Chapter 11).
+ The chosen perspectives should be applied to the topic in a way that is logical and serves to explain the topic.
+ There should be evidence of knowledge and genuine understanding of the 'real world' of health and social care.
+ At least two studies should be described. Their implications for the topic – for example, likely benefits – and their link with one or more perspectives should be explained. This is likely to reveal how well you understand scientific psychology.
+ There should be sound evaluation of the studies and perspectives described. This should include reasoned arguments to justify your evaluations. Evaluation of perspectives involves more than simply reproducing the evaluations given in each of the sections on perspectives in this chapter. It requires an assessment of how well or how convincingly each chosen perspective applies to, or explains, your topic.

Sound evaluation is likely to avoid overstatement of the positive or negative features of studies and perspectives.

Further reading

Davison, G. C. (2003) *Abnormal Psychology*, John Wiley and Sons.
Gross, R. (2001) *Psychology: The Science of Mind and Behaviour* (4th edn), Hodder and Stoughton.
Ogden, J. (2004) *Health Psychology: A Textbook* (3rd edn), Open University Press.
Pennington, D. et al. (2003) *Advanced Psychology: Child Development, Perspectives and Methods*, Hodder and Stoughton.
Turner, L. (2003) *Advanced Psychology: Atypical Behaviour*, Hodder and Stoughton.

Websites

The British Journal of Health Psychology:
www.bps.org.uk/publications/journals/bjhp/
Nursing Times:
www.nursingtimes.net
The Resource Discovery Network:
www.rdn.ac.uk

Study skills

This chapter provides tips to maximise your performance in assessments. You will probably find it useful if you apply the same principles to subjects other than health and social care.

Units assessed by examination

The information given in the chapters of this book that cover examination-assessed units should be enough to enable you to gain high marks in the unit tests.

If you can understand and learn most or all of this information, you will have taken an important step to doing well in your examination. This step involves both understanding and revision.

Understanding

The first time you hear or read about a topic, you should not expect to understand it fully. You will get a rough impression of the topic, but you will forget some of the information and some of the facts you remember will be inaccurate. Your understanding will improve if the first information you come across is later supported. For example, if your teacher explains language development to you, as part of your work for Unit 4, your understanding is likely to increase if you then read the section relating to language development in this book. Reading the information a second time will also help your understanding.

There will be times when some aspect of a topic does not make sense to you. Perhaps you have read the section in Chapter 2 about processing attitude scores, but still cannot see how to do this. Then you should ask someone else – a fellow student or your teacher.

Another important aid to understanding is to talk about what you are learning. If a friend or parent asks you, 'What did you learn about today?', take the opportunity to try to describe and explain what you studied.

Homework is also useful. Writing answers to questions helps to develop familiarity with the material.

The Workbook designed to accompany this text includes exercises to help you understand the topics covered in the compulsory units (Units 1, 2 and 3).

Effective revision

You should understand that effective revision can make a very big difference to how well you perform in an examination. Whatever you did to prepare for your GCSEs, you can expect to succeed in examinations at AS only if you revise, and you do this effectively.

Revision materials

Revision is likely to be effective only if the materials you revise from are organised in an appropriate form. Appropriate materials include summary tables (such as those included in this book), diagrams, mnemonics and single-page topic notes.

Diagrams

Diagrams, such as those showing the anatomy of the eye or spider diagrams linking facts and ideas to a topic heading, can be quite easy to learn.

Mnemonics

Mnemonics are simple devices for learning lists. Take the first letter of each item in the list, then make up a sentence with a sequence of words starting with the same letters. The sentence should be easily memorable itself.

For example, in Unit 6 you have to learn about several different types of infection and their causal agents. The lists of infections can be shown like this:

+ **B**acteria:
    + **M**eningitis
    + **P**neumonia
    + **G**onorrhoea
+ **F**ungi:
    + **A**thlete's foot
    + **R**ingworm
    + **T**hrush
+ **V**iruses:
    + **C**ommon cold
    + **I**nfluenza
+ **P**arasites:
    + **H**ead lice
    + **S**cabies
    + **T**apeworm

Taking the first letter of all fifteen words gives the sequence:

B, M, P, G, F, A, R, T, V, C, I, P, H, S, T

Now try to make up a sentence with fifteen words, starting with those same letters. It might not be easy, but in the process of trying you are also learning. The ideal mnemonic is easy to remember because it tells a story or is funny in some way.

For the list of letters above, one mnemonic imagines two girlfriends on a holiday in South America: **B**eryl's **M**ate **P**auline **G**oes **F**or **A** **R**eally **T**all **V**enezuelan **C**alled **I**gnacio — **P**erhaps **H**e's **S**exy **T**oo.

A mnemonic like this is really useful if you then elaborate on the story. For example, you could think of a scenario where the two friends (Beryl and Pauline) unfortunately catch all the listed diseases during their holiday, for example by eating undercooked seafood, being in crowded conditions in Ignacio's flat and so on.

By jotting down the mnemonic in an examination, it should trigger your memory of the list, because you know the first letter of each word.

Single-page topic notes

While summary tables, diagrams and mnemonics are useful, they cannot be applied to all the information you need to learn. Single-page topic notes can be used for everything. The idea is to take a topic within a unit, for example *Cognitive and Language Development* from Unit 4, and summarise all the key information on one side of paper. You should not include too many words. The idea is that the topic notes should help unlock other details already stored in your memory.

The secret of successful revision

For some reason, very few students know this secret. It's very simple. The secret of successful revision is **self-testing**.

How self-testing works

+ Take a summary table, diagram, mnemonic or page of topic notes.
+ Study it carefully for a few minutes, thinking about what it means.
+ Turn the page over.
+ Take a fresh sheet of paper and try to reproduce the information you have just been reading.
+ Compare what you wrote with the original.

The first time, you will probably not remember much, so look carefully at what you did not remember (perhaps you could highlight it on the original sheet) and then try to reproduce the sheet again.

For any one unit, you might have perhaps twenty different sheets. Once you have succeeded in reliably reproducing a sheet without errors or omissions (over a period of several days), you should occasionally self-test again, to keep the information stored accurately in your memory.

The evening before the examination, your revision could take the form of self-testing on all the sheets for that unit (which might take an hour or two).

The advantage of self-testing is that, not only do you end up knowing the necessary information, but also you know that you know it. Therefore, you can go into the examination with more confidence than if you had used less effective methods of revision.

How long should you spend?

Some students make the mistake of thinking that what is important is the amount of time they spend revising. It is possible to spend many hours leafing through classroom notes or textbooks, yet learning hardly anything. What is important is not the overall time, but the effectiveness of the method.

The method suggested here — of assembling useful revision materials and self-testing — should not take very long. However, the time spent is best spread over several weeks rather than being concentrated into a few days before the examination.

Examination technique

The other important step towards doing well in your examination involves developing an effective examination technique.

Be in control

Some students adopt a fatalistic attitude to examinations. They act like helpless victims. The result is that, on reading a question, they tend to write down the first thing that comes into their heads. Sometimes this approach means they do not read the question carefully enough and, as a consequence, give the answer to a different question.

A more useful attitude is to see yourself as being in control of what happens in the examination room. You can do this by preparing effectively. Of course, this means revising effectively. However, you should also try to anticipate what the examination will be like. For example, you could look at sample papers or past papers for that unit, as well as the unit specifications.

It is important to know what to expect. For example, in Unit 1: Effective caring, you should expect to have to suggest some service provision for a particular client and to suggest an effective skill or technique for dealing with a particular situation. Then, when you look at the examination paper and it has a question asking about suitable provision for an elderly person who has become disabled, you will be able to say to yourself, 'I was expecting something like this'.

Interrogate the question

An examination question contains much information to guide you. Your examination performance will be better if you make use of it all. When you interrogate a question, you should pay attention to:

+ the key topic
+ specific instructions about the number of responses required
+ whether examples should be given
+ the number of marks available

Look at this section from an example question given in Chapter 1: Effective caring.

> Isobel is 90 years old and lives alone. She receives neither formal nor informal care. She has osteoarthritis, which makes it difficult for her to move about and handle objects. She recently scalded herself when she spilt a pan of boiling water.

(a) Suggest three different physical life-quality factors that Isobel is
    likely to lack. Illustrate each with reference to the description
    of Isobel. (6 marks)

Interrogating this question tells us the following:

+ It is mainly about **physical** life-quality factors. This means *not* psychological factors, so, for example, not social isolation.
+ Three factors are required.
+ The answers must be specifically linked to the description of Isobel – for example, by quoting from the question.
+ There are 6 marks available – 2 marks per life-quality factor.

It should now be clear that all you have to do is to name correctly a life-quality factor relevant to the description (1 mark), and make the link with the description (1 mark). This process has to be repeated for three factors.

One of the answers could be:

Adequate nutrition (1 mark). Isobel finds it difficult to move about and handle objects, so she might not be able to go shopping for food, or to cook it (1 mark).

This seems simple enough. However, a student who did not interrogate the question would be quite likely to give an answer about a psychological life-quality factor or launch into a long, rambling description of what needs to be done for Isobel – all irrelevant to the question asked.

Keep it together

Some students underperform in examinations because they are over-anxious. It is important to put an examination into perspective on the scale of frightening events. Unlike drink-driving or falling down stairs, an examination cannot hurt you.

In the event of over-anxiety it is useful to have an action plan to help you cope. When you panic, there must be a well-learned, familiar activity to help you get over it. One approach is to jot down some of the mnemonics or diagrams you have revised (even if you don't immediately see their relevance to the questions asked). This gives you time to calm down. As you relax, you will begin to understand the questions. This is an example of a distraction technique designed to reduce the attention you give to your own anxiety.

Visualisation

Visualisation can also help. Visualisation is a technique based on scientific psychology that is used by sports players and others to improve performance under pressure. Visualisation helps by preparing you for events, so that you are more likely to produce an effective response.

Visualisation before an examination could prepare you for events that might otherwise cause you to become over-anxious. When you visualise, you might think through the following plausible scenario:

In the morning the bus will probably be late, but it won't be a problem because the exam doesn't start until half past nine. The others will all be in a crowd, twittering about how they haven't done enough work. I shall stay away from them and probably walk about a bit. In the exam room, there will probably be a mix-up with us getting the wrong papers or maybe having to go to a different room. In other words, situation normal.

When I get the exam paper and open it, my mind will probably go blank. Again, situation normal. I'll scribble down my mnemonic for life-quality factors. Meanwhile, the others will already have covered about half a page. I'll read the questions carefully again and begin to interrogate them. This time I will be able to see how to answer some of them. I'll start writing and my pen will run out. Luckily, I will have remembered to bring a spare.

While this seems rather pessimistic, it does prepare you for the worst, with the advantage that the reality is likely to be better.

Writing style

An approach that some students adopt is to write as much as possible in answer to any question. They seem to believe that the more words they write, the more marks they will gain. This is not usually true. Long passages of unfocused waffle are unlikely to gain many, if any, marks. Shorter answers that actually address the question asked are likely to gain more marks. One way to ensure that you adopt this approach is to try, where possible, to start your answer in the same terms in which the question is asked.

For example, if the question asks you to 'Identify two minerals and outline the possible effects of deficiency of these minerals in the diet', you might start your answer by saying, 'One important mineral is iodine. One possible effect of an iodine deficiency is goitre...'

Starting with phrases used in the question increases the likelihood that your answer will be relevant.

Some students choose to answer questions not in continuous sentences, but in the form of tables or lists. This technique is unlikely to gain high marks because it makes it more difficult to develop a structured argument, illustrated by examples.

Elaboration

Sometimes you might notice that an apparently simple question has a lot of marks allocated to it. In cases like this, you should give plenty of factual elaboration.

For example, if the question was about dental caries (Unit 6), you might gain elaboration marks for naming the different parts of a tooth in your answer (i.e. the crown, enamel, dentine, pulp and root canal).

Even if a question has only 2 marks available, you should still try to ensure that you say two things (e.g. name a factor and give an example of it).

Describing and explaining

A useful way of elaboration when describing and explaining is to give illustrative examples. For example, if in Unit 1 you are asked to explain how ignorance can act as a barrier to accessing services, you should explain what ignorance means (not knowing about the service or its purpose) and illustrate this with an example (e.g. an elderly person has not heard about Aid-Call, and so cannot use this service).

Discussing and evaluating

When you are asked to discuss, this often requires an extended description plus explanation. Sometimes — but not always — it is also appropriate to include some evaluation.

Evaluation usually involves describing the advantages and disadvantages of something. It is important to consider both sides. One way of doing this is to make a point and then give a counter-argument. Counter-arguments often start with 'However,...'

For example, if in Unit 4 you are asked to evaluate the influence of parents on the development of language, you could make the point that, 'Parents produce examples of language from which infants can learn the meanings of words. For example, if they keep talking about the fridge, while opening and shutting it, the child will learn to associate the word 'fridge' with that buzzing white metal box in the kitchen. However, parents are not the only influence on the child's development of language...'

Units assessed by portfolio

Useful tips

Be in control

Students tend to do better in portfolio assessments if they take control of their own work, instead of the teacher having to push them at every step. To take control, you need to have a clear idea of the portfolio task right from the start. This means you must make sure that you have a copy of the specification for the unit you are studying. If you do not have a copy, you should look at the AQA website (www.aqa.org.uk), where the specification is available.

If you understand what you have to do, you will be able to make the best use of the resources available. For example, you may come across relevant ideas on television and in magazines. You will also be able to select information you need from material teachers have provided.

It is advisable to take opportunities to discuss your coursework plans and progress with your teacher. However, you should not become too dependent on your teacher to tell you what to do next. If you rely on the teacher too much, this will be taken into account when assessing your work.

You are likely to score higher marks if the work you present is clearly your own. For example, if several students from the same centre present very similar work, there is a risk that this will be seen as a shared or group task. That is why, in units in which you choose your own topic, you should try to do something different from everyone else.

Keep it together

A portfolio unit usually involves collecting quite a lot of resources, so you should have a large file to keep together all the paper material, including your notes, for any one unit.

Losing this file would be like forgetting to turn up for an examination, so it is advisable to keep backup photocopies of essential documents. Similarly, you should keep backup copies of electronic files. Wherever possible, word-process the text you intend to include in your portfolio.

Scoring high marks

Students sometimes put a lot of effort (on occasion too much effort) into coursework, without scoring very high marks. The key to scoring high marks is to make sure that what you produce is what the specification actually requires. In this respect, the most important part of the specification is the table of assessment criteria at the end of the specification for each unit. You should study this early on in your work for the unit.

Assessment criteria

The first thing to notice is that the assessment criteria are divided into four sections:
+ AO1 marks are mainly for description.
+ AO2 marks are for applying knowledge, ideas and concepts to the topic.
+ AO3 marks are for research and analysis.
+ AO4 marks are for evaluation.

There is a different maximum mark for each of these sections. In the compulsory units (2 and 3) the highest number of marks is given for AO2 (Application). In the optional units (7, 8, 9 and 10) the highest number of marks is given for AO1 (Knowledge). It is important not to skimp on the highest-scoring section.

You should find out what you have to do to obtain the marks allocated to each section of each unit.

For example, if you look at the 13–16 mark box of the AO4 mark section for Unit 2, you will see that to gain these marks, you have to:
+ evaluate your own communication skills
+ make judgements about how reliable your feedback was
+ justify the decisions you made when you planned your talk
+ express all this clearly

If you do not do all of these things — for example, if you do not say anything about your 'design decisions' — you cannot score marks in this 13–16 mark range.

Another useful tip in writing your report is to use subheadings to draw attention to sections of the report that are required by the assessment criteria. For example, you could include a section headed 'Design decisions'.

Another example relates to the assessment criteria for Unit 3. AO3 marks are available for drawing conclusions from the questionnaire data. So you should have a subheading 'Conclusions', to make sure that this is noticed by the person assessing your work.

Report guidance

Most of the unit specifications include very specific guidance on how a report should be structured. You will find it useful to stick to this guidance — although remember that, if in doubt, the assessment criteria carry the most weight.

You should not include additional sections or materials that are not required by the specification. For example, if the report guidance does not mention an appendix, you should not include one. You should not submit video- or audiotapes or other non-written material.

Try to produce slim, concise reports.

Doing research

Finding sources of information can be quite time-consuming, but remember that marks are available for this in all the portfolio units. Remember also that the information included in the chapters of this book that deal with portfolio units will not be enough to enable you to score the highest marks. This is because some AO3 marks are available for using a range of sources, i.e. more than one.

You should start collecting information from sources (books, the internet, your teacher and other people) very early on, as soon as you have grasped what the unit requires you to produce.

Some sources can only be accessed after a delay — for example, if you have requested an interlibrary loan. You must keep a record of your sources so you can refer to them in your reference section. It is very frustrating to find a good source, take some notes, and then later discover that you have lost the name of the author or title.

Avoiding plagiarism

Plagiarism means taking large sections of text from a source and presenting it, little changed, as your own. The inclusion of whole paragraphs copied from textbooks or websites and presented as your own work is likely to be regarded as cheating.

However, you may quote from such sources, provided that you state clearly the source, and give an appropriate reference. Even so, extensive quotations (say, more than a paragraph) are likely to be inappropriate. The writer you are quoting from is unlikely to have had the same aim as you, so the text is unlikely to be as appropriate as your own.

Using the internet

Search engines are useful, but often produce material that is American, and possibly not relevant to the UK. The Google homepage has an option you can select that will restrict your search to UK sites. This would save trouble if you were trying to look up services provided in your local town, and then discovered you had spent half an hour reading about a town with the same name in Oklahoma.

The Resource Discovery Notebook (**www.rdn.ac.uk**) is useful for finding the titles and contents of articles in journals. It will also direct you to sites that have been approved by academics and which are, therefore, less likely to have inaccurate information than some other sites.

Writing reference sections

Books and journals

The recommended way to write references for published sources is as follows:

For a book, the order of information is:

+ name and initials of the author or authors
+ the year of the publication (in brackets)
+ the title of the book (in italics)
+ the publisher

An example is: Bowlby, J. (1975) *Attachment and Loss, Volume 1: Attachment,* Pelican.

The order is: name(s), initials, year, title, publisher.

For a journal or magazine article, the order is similar:

+ the name and initials of the author(s)
+ the date (in brackets)
+ the title of the article
+ title of the publication (in italics)
+ the issue number (or volume number)
+ the numbers of the pages on which the article appears

An example is: Baron-Cohen, S., Leslie, A. M. and Frith, U. (1985) 'Does the autistic child have a theory of mind?' *Cognition,* Vol. 21, pp. 37–46.

References are usually presented in alphabetical order of the authors' surnames. If there are several joint authors, it is the first surname that counts. So of the two references above, Baron-Cohen should come before Bowlby.

Books and journal/magazine articles can be listed together.

Other examples of appropriate presentation of references can be found at the back of psychology textbooks (before the Index).

Websites

Websites should be referenced separately from books and journals. The recommended way is to give the title of the organisation whose website it is, the web address and the date and time at which you accessed this site. Website addresses should be presented in alphabetical order of the start of the first part of the address, following www. For example:

Nursing Times:

www.nursingtimes.net 20/01/06, 1.45 p.m.

SureStart:

www.surestart.gov.uk 17/10/05, 9.17 a.m.

index